Principles of Forensic
Mental Health Assessment

Perspectives in
Law & Psychology

Sponsored by the American Psychology-Law Society / Division 41 of the
American Psychological Association

Series Editor: RONALD ROESCH, *Simon Fraser University*
Burnaby, British Columbia, Canada

Volume 1   THE CRIMINAL JUSTICE SYSTEM
             Edited by Bruce Dennis Sales

Volume 2   THE TRIAL PROCESS
             Edited by Bruce Dennis Sales

Volume 3   JUVENILES' WAIVER OF RIGHTS
             Legal and Psychological Complications
             Thomas Grisso

Volume 4   MENTAL HEALTH LAW
             Major Issues
             David B. Wexler

Volume 5   HANDBOOK OF SCALES FOR RESEARCH IN CRIME AND
             DELINQUENCY
             Stanley L. Brodsky and H. O'Neal Smitherman

Volume 6   MENTALLY DISORDERED OFFENDERS
             Perspectives from Law and Social Science
             Edited by John Monahan and Henry J. Steadman

Volume 7   EVALUATING COMPETENCIES
             Forensic Assessments and Instruments
             Thomas Grisso

Volume 8   INSANITY ON TRIAL
             Norman J. Finkel

Volume 9   AFTER THE CRIME
             Victim Decision Making
             Martin S. Greenberg and R. Barry Ruback

Volume 10   PSYCHOLOGY AND LAW
             The State of the Discipline
             Edited by Ronald Roesch, Stephen D. Hart, and James R. P. Ogloff

Volume 11   JUDICIAL DECISION MAKING
             Is Psychology Relevant?
             Lawrence S. Wrightsman

Volume 12   PRINCIPLES OF FORENSIC MENTAL HEALTH ASSESSMENT
             Kirk Heilbrun

Principles of Forensic Mental Health Assessment

Kirk Heilbrun

MCP Hahnemann University
Philadelphia, Pennsylvania
and
Villanova University
Philadelphia, Pennsylvania

KLUWER ACADEMIC / PLENUM PUBLISHERS
NEW YORK, BOSTON, DORDRECHT, LONDON, MOSCOW

Library of Congress Cataloging-in-Publication Data

Heilbrun, Kirk.
    Principles of forensic mental health assessment/Kirk Heilbrun.
        p.   ; cm.—(Perspectives in law & psychology; v. 12)
    Includes bibliographical references and index.
    ISBN 0-306-46538-8
        1. Psychology, Forensic.   2. Mental illness—Diagnosis.   3. Evidence, Expect.   I. Title.   II.
Series.

    RA1148 .H45 2001
    614'.1—dc21

                                                                    00-067432

ISBN 0-306-46538-8

©2001 Kluwer Academic / Plenum Publishers, New York
233 Spring Street, New York, N.Y. 10013

http://www.wkap.nl/

10 9 8 7 6 5 4 3 2 1

A C.I.P. record for this book is available from the Library of Congress

To Patty and Anna

Preface

Most of the literature in forensic mental health assessment is organized around the particular legal issue that is the focus of a given assessment, tool, or research study. This book starts with a different assumption: There are broad principles of forensic assessment that are applicable across different legal issues. If such principles exist, they should be derived from and supported by sources of authority in ethics, law, science, and professional practice. This is what I seek to do in this book, with each of the 29 broad principles of forensic mental health assessment described and analyzed from the perspective of these sources of authority.

There are a number of individuals who have contributed in various ways to making this a better book. It seems best to begin with a general acknowledgment: Those interested in forensic mental health assessment, particularly my colleagues from the American Psychology–Law Society and the American Board of Forensic Psychology, have been an extraordinarily helpful and congenial group. I have learned a great deal from them over the years and they challenged me to undertake the daunting task of trying to capture the broad views of the field in this book.

I grew up in a home in which books, ideas, and achievement were valued and interspersed with love and humor. Thanks to my parents, Alfred and Marian Heilbrun, for providing such a home for my sisters, brother, and me. Special thanks to my wife Patty, and our daughter Anna; this book is dedicated to you.

I first began thinking about principles of forensic mental health assessment during my postdoctoral fellowship year under Ned Megargee. He taught me valuable organizing skills that year and showed me how to apply the highest standards to research and scholarship in criminal justice. My "inpatient forensic" years were mainly spent at the Forensic Service at Florida State Hospital in Chattahoochee, where Stewart Parsons and Sam Cunningham allowed me to learn so much, and have so much fun, that I am surprised I ever left. I am grateful to both of you.

At one time, there was discussion about making this a book with three authors. Although I did not eventually collaborate with Stan Brodsky and Norm Poythress in writing this volume, it is hard to imagine how two colleagues could have been more helpful in shaping many of the ideas that went into describing principles of forensic mental health assessment. Thanks to you both.

Work on the book began in earnest after our move to Virginia. John Monahan, Richard Bonnie, Gary Hawk, Janet Warren, Larry Fitch, Randy Thomas, and Russ Petrella were among those who contributed to making those years incredibly stimulating for me. Each contributed in valuable ways to an environment in which forensic mental health assessment was accorded the highest standards possible. In a similar way, a number of my colleagues from around the United States and Canada have been particularly helpful with concepts, standards, analysis, and providing good models as scientist-practitioners. Steve Golding, Randy Otto, Joel Dvoskin, Ira Packer, Randy Borum, Jim Ogloff, Steve Hart, Dick Rogers, and Stuart Greenberg particularly come to mind; thanks to each of you. In addition to helping in similar ways, Alan Goldstein has for years directed a superb continuing education program for the American Academy of Forensic Psychology. The workshops I have presented for AAFP over the years have forced me to organize and communicate many of these ideas in a (hopefully) more coherent way, and I appreciate the chance to do so.

My association with the Law–Psychology program at MCP Hahnemann University and Villanova School of Law, directed by Don Bersoff, has provided an invaluable opportunity to improve the conceptual and legal components of this book. Don has been a good friend and colleague during the time I have spent as codirector of the program. Several law–psychology students (David DeMatteo, Geff Marczyk, Lori Peters, and Kim Picarello) provided tireless research assistance, for which I am very grateful. Other legal and scholarly help was provided by the works of Chris Slobogin, John Petrila, and Michael Perlin. In addition, Perlin graciously agreed to review the manuscript while in town to speak at Villanova (and did so in typically Perlin-esque fashion, giving an amazingly detailed review and subsequent suggestions that took six months to implement). Ron Roesch reviewed the manuscript at a time when it needed a push; as always, Ron provided superb help in his low-key, extraordinarily effective way.

The most resounding "thank you" goes to Tom Grisso. He served as the editor for this book long after his tenure as editor for the AP-LS book series ended, and for that I am very grateful. I am even more grateful for his time, energy, substantive contributions, and insistence on adherence to the highest possible standards. His contributions to this book have been enormous. Thanks, Tom.

Contents

I. INTRODUCTION

CHAPTER 1. DEVELOPING PRINCIPLES OF FORENSIC MENTAL
HEALTH ASSESSMENT

Forensic versus Therapeutic Assessment   9
A Structure for Organizing Principles of FMHA   14
Deriving and Analyzing Principles   16

II. PREPARATION

CHAPTER 2. FIRST CONTACTS

Identify Relevant Forensic Issues   21
Accept Referrals Only within Area of Expertise   26
Decline Referral When Evaluator Impartiality Is Unlikely   36
Clarify Role with Attorney   46
Clarify Financial Arrangements   51
Obtain Appropriate Authorization   58

CHAPTER 3. DEFINING THE EVALUATOR'S ROLE

Avoid Dual-Role Relationships of Therapist and Forensic
     Evaluator   65
Determine the Role to Be Played within Forensic Assessment if
     the Referral Is Accepted   73

CHAPTER 4. USING A MODEL

Select and Employ a Model to Guide Data Gathering,
     Interpretation, and Communication   84

III. DATA COLLECTION

CHAPTER 5. SELECTION

Use Multiple Sources of Information for Each Area Being
Assessed 99
Use Relevance and Reliability (Validity) as Guides for Seeking
Information and Selecting Data Sources 107
Obtain Relevant Historical Information 115
Assess Relevant Clinical Characteristics in Reliable and Valid
Ways 121
Assess Legally Relevant Behavior 129

CHAPTER 6. ADMINISTRATION

Ensure that Conditions for Evaluation Are Quiet, Private, and
Distraction-Free 136
Provide Appropriate Notification of Purpose and/or Obtain
Appropriate Authorization before Beginning 141
Determine Whether the Individual Understands the Purpose of
the Evaluation and Associated Limits on Confidentiality 153

IV. DATA INTERPRETATION

CHAPTER 7. ASSESSING RESPONSE STYLE

Use Third-Party Information in Assessing Response Style 167
Use Testing When Indicated in Assessing Response Style 176

CHAPTER 8. INCORPORATING SCIENTIFIC REASONING AND DATA

Use Case-Specific (Idiographic) Evidence in Assessing Causal
Connection between Clinical Condition and Functional
Abilities 190
Use Nomothetic Evidence in Assessing Causal Connection
between Clinical Condition and Functional Abilities 196
Use Scientific Reasoning in Assessing Causal Connection
between Clinical Condition and Functional Abilities 206

CHAPTER 9. MAKING ASSERTIONS AND CLARIFYING LIMITS

Do Not Answer the Ultimate Legal Question Directly 213
Describe Findings and Limits so that They Need Change Little
under Cross Examination 226

V. COMMUNICATION

CHAPTER 10. COMMUNICATING CLEARLY

Attribute Information to Sources 241
Use Plain Language; Avoid Technical Jargon 246
Write Report in Sections, According to Model and Procedures 249

CHAPTER 11. TESTIFYING EFFECTIVELY

Base Testimony on Results of Properly Performed FMHA 257
Testify in an Effective Manner 267

VI. APPLYING THE PRINCIPLES
OF FORENSIC MENTAL HEALTH ASSESSMENT

CHAPTER 12. IMPLICATIONS FOR RESEARCH, TRAINING, PRACTICE, AND POLICY

Implications for Research 286
Implications for Training 299
Implications for Practice 301
Implications for Policy 305

REFERENCES 309

CASES 332

INDEX 335

I

Introduction

1

Developing Principles of Forensic Mental Health Assessment

The past 15 years have witnessed a tremendous change in forensic mental health assessment (FMHA). For present purposes, this kind of assessment will be defined as evaluation that is performed by mental health professionals as part of the legal decision-making process, for the purpose of assisting the decision-maker or helping one of the litigants in using relevant clinical and scientific data. Such legal questions in the criminal area include sanity at the time of the offense, sentencing, and competencies to confess, plead guilty, refuse an insanity defense, waive the right to counsel, testify, stand trial, be sentenced, and be executed, and juvenile transfer. Civil legal questions include civil commitment, guardianship, competencies to consent to treatment and research, testamentary capacity, fitness to work, personal injury under both workers' compensation and tort laws, child abuse and neglect, and child custody.

The professions most commonly involved in FMHA are psychiatry, psychology, and social work. Some of the procedures employed by each of these disciplines are most characteristic of the particular profession involved; when psychiatrists (e.g., Appelbaum & Gutheil, 1991) write about the process of forensic evaluation, they differ in some respects from psychologists (Grisso, 1986a, 1998a; Melton, Petrila, Poythress, & Slobogin, 1997; Shapiro, 1991).

The growth and development of FMHA during the last 20 years within psychology has been part of the broader evolution of the specialty area of law and psychology. This area has been represented primarily by the American Psychology–Law Society/Division 41 of the American Psychological Association. It includes both research and applied compo-

3

nents, and encompasses areas of psychology that include clinical, counseling, neuropsychology, and school, as well as social, developmental, community, cognitive, and human experimental (see Table 1.1). The area of "forensic psychology," defined narrowly, would encompass the research and applied components of clinical, counseling, neuropsychology, and school psychology as they relate to legal decision-making and other aspects of litigation. When defined more broadly, "forensic psychology" would also encompass the areas of social, developmental, community, cognitive, and human experimental psychology in their applications to legal proceedings.[1]

One way to conceptualize forensic psychology is to describe the overall domain of activities and interests that are pursued by psychologists in legal contexts, which might be called "Law and Psychology." Within that larger domain, one can then identify subareas within which the professions of psychology and of law may define "forensic psychology" for specific purposes. As seen in Table 1.1, the overall domain encompasses the areas of "clinical" (including clinical, counseling, and school psychology, and neuropsychology), "experimental" (social, developmental, cognitive, and human experimental psychology), and legal (law, relevant methodological and substantive areas of behavioral and medical sciences). Within this overall domain, individuals may be involved in activities identified in different cells in the table. Regardless of the breadth of any definition of "forensic psychology," however, the value of its contributions will depend on work that is done in each of the six Table 1.1 areas. For example,

---

[1]There is currently a vigorous debate within the field of law and psychology concerning how "forensic psychology" should be defined. One possible definition is broad, encompassing many specialty areas within psychology. Such a broad definition of forensic psychology is consistent with that provided in the *Specialty Guidelines for Forensic Psychologists* ("professional practice by psychologists, within any subdiscipline of psychology (e.g., clinical, developmental, social, experimental) when they are engaged regularly as experts and represent themselves as such, in an activity primarily intended to provide professional psychological expertise to the judicial system," Committee on Ethical Guidelines for Forensic Psychologists, 1991), that offered by the American Board of Forensic Psychology in the descriptive brochure on the Diplomate process ("the application of the science and profession of psychology to questions and issues relating to law and the legal system), or that given elsewhere in the literature (e.g., as "both (1) the research endeavor that examines aspects of human behavior directly related to the legal process ... and (2) the professional practice of psychology within, or in consultation with, a legal system that embraces both civil and criminal law," Bartol & Bartol, 1987, p. 3). A narrow definition, encompassing the areas of clinical, counseling, neuropsychology, and school psychology, was endorsed in 1998 by the Executive Committee of the American Psychology–Law Society/Division 41 of APA, for the purpose of pursuing specialty recognition for forensic psychology from the American Psychological Association. The "broad versus narrow" definitional question has not yet been resolved within the field (see, e.g., Brigham, 1999).

TABLE 1.1. Law and Psychology, Forensic Psychology, and Definitions

Law and psychology interest areas (with associated training)		
Clinical (clinical, counseling, school psychology)	Experimental (social, developmental, cognitive, human experimental psychology)	Legal (law, some training in behavioral science or medicine)
Research scholarship		
1. Assessment tools 2. Intervention effectiveness 3. Epidemiology of relevant behavior (e.g., violence, sexual offending) and disorders	1. Memory 2. Perception 3. Child development 4. Group decision-making	1. Mental health law 2. Other law relevant to health and science 3. Legal movements (law and social science, therapeutic jurisprudence, psychological jurisprudence)
1	3	5
Applied		
1. Forensic assessment 2. Treatment in legal context 3. Integration of science (idiographic, nomothetic, reasoning) into practice	1. Consultation on jury selection 2. Consultation on litigation strategy 3. Consultation on "state of science" 4. Expert testimony on "state of science"	1. Policy and legislative consultation 2. Model law development
2	4	6

although courts may be concerned primarily with applied questions (see cells 2 and 4), such questions cannot be answered as well by forensic psychologists without incorporating the scientific work described in cells 1 and 3, respectively.

The ongoing debate within psychology (see Brigham, 1999; footnote 1, this chapter) concerning whether "forensic psychology" should be defined narrowly (cells 1 and 2) or broadly (cells 1–4, or even 1–6) may be understood in the context of the implications for defining a specialization with the American Psychological Association, and the possible implications for training and eventual accreditation of training programs. There is little substantive disagreement that the scientific contributions of experimental psychology (cell 3) can usefully inform the legal applications of clinical psychology (cell 2). Although this book will focus primarily on research in clinical forensic psychology (cell 1), relevant legal scholarship and law (cell 5), and their respective applications (cells 2 and 6, respectively), readers should be aware that the contributions of experimental psychology to law are very important within the broader domain of law and psychology, and are described in detail elsewhere (Horowitz, Willging, & Bordens, 1998; Roesch, Hart, & Ogloff, 1999).

Within the field of psychiatry, the question of how to define "forensic psychiatry" appears to have been resolved more clearly. In the *Ethical Guidelines for the Practice of Forensic Psychiatry*, the following definition is provided: "Forensic psychiatry is a subspecialty of psychiatry in which scientific and clinical expertise is applied to legal issues in legal contexts embracing civil, criminal, correctional or legislative matters" (American Academy of Psychiatry and the Law [AAPL], 1995).

The process of FMHA is not easily divided according to the type of mental health profession involved, however. More typically, "the nature of the legal question" has served as the unifying theme and the focus of most of the literature in forensic assessment. Entire books have been devoted to a single legal question (the ultimate decision that a court makes in a given case), such as competence to stand trial (Grisso, 1988; Roesch & Golding, 1980), criminal responsibility (Rogers, 1986), competence to consent to treatment (Grisso & Appelbaum, 1998a), and child custody (Ackerman & Kane, 1998). Other books have been organized around legal questions as well, but feature separate sections on different legal questions (e.g., Greenberg & Brodsky, in press; Grisso, 1986a, 1998a; Melton et al., 1997; Shapiro, 1991; Weiner & Hess, 1987) or particular forensic issues (constructs and functional demands that are relevant to the legal question) such as response style (the nature and accuracy of the information provided by individuals being evaluated regarding their own thoughts, feelings, and behavior; see McCann, 1998; Rogers, 1997) or violence risk (Monahan & Steadman, 1994). These works begin with the legal question or forensic issue, and then identify relevant research, law, and procedures. At times a set of guidelines (e.g., Greenberg & Brodsky, in press) or a model (e.g., Grisso, 1986a) is included in the analysis.

The goals of this book are somewhat different. I will identify a core set of principles relevant to FMHA that transcends legal questions, forensic issues, and discipline. The term *principle* will be used somewhat differently than its primary definition—"fundamental truth or law"—would imply. In this book, *principle* will refer to "the essence of a body or its constituent parts," as well as the "theoretical part of a science" (Black, 1983). The process of identifying and describing "principles" will begin with the "constituent parts" of FMHA, and ultimately yield specific, procedural guidelines for forensic clinicians.

Why does the field need such principles? Principles are valuable for (1) training, (2) to assist research and theory, and potentially (3) to improve the establishment of policy and the quality of practice of FMHA. Each of these reasons will be discussed briefly.

Concerning the first of these objectives, the training of mental health professionals in the understanding and practice of FMHA is not guided by a core model. Rather, training appears to be presented according to discipline, substantive area within mental health (e.g., age of population, severity of disorder), and by legal issue (see the special issue on training, *Behavioral Sciences & the Law*, Vol. 8, 1990). The identification of basic principles common to all forms of FMHA is an important first step in the development of a training model for mental health professionals. Such a model would provide trainees with a generalizable approach to FMHA and allow specific proficiencies (i.e., with certain populations and particular legal issues) to be developed in accordance with the trainee's goals and skills. However, the trainee would not be asked to evaluate a legal issue without general training in FMHA procedures. The trainee would not be forced to generalize from limited experience with one forensic issue to procedures associated with another.[2]

Second, the identification of core principles of FMHA should have a favorable impact on research in forensic assessment. In some areas, the existing empirical support for an identified principle is reasonably good. In others, however, the research support is weak or inconsistent; often such research simply has not yet been done. There will be other criteria used in identifying principles—legal, ethical, and standard of practice— but the determination that research remains to be done in a given area hopefully will stimulate investigators to pursue these issues.

This process may have implications for theory-building in FMHA as well. Some of the identified principles, when tested empirically, may become further established as components of a larger theory, while others may be rejected for lack of empirical support. Still other principles may already have the necessary empirical support to be considered established

[2]I am aware of no data demonstrating that trainees are performing evaluations for which they are not properly supervised. Such data would be difficult to obtain and potentially sensitive, given their possible implication of a violation of training policies and ethical standards. However, my observation has been that the demand for FMHA services in the United States apparently far exceeds the supply of highly trained forensic specialists. Consequently, many FMHA services are delivered by otherwise qualified mental health professionals with limited forensic training and experience. It is for these individuals that such training could be most beneficial.

components of a relevant theory. It is beyond the scope of this book to develop a larger theory of FMHA, however. The field has not yet developed sufficiently. Rather, a core set of principles may be considered one step in the direction of larger theory-building.

Finally, principles are relevant to policy. Whether it is the shaping or interpretation of legislation or administrative code relevant to performing and using forensic assessments, or the development and implementation of court or agency policy intended to increase the consistency and quality of FMHA, the availability of a core set of principles to inform the application and quality improvement of forensic assessment may be helpful.

The description of these principles can also have implications for the practice of FMHA. Criticisms of the practice of forensic assessment, summarized by Grisso (1986a), include (1) *ignorance and irrelevance* (the failure to focus the assessment on relevant legal standards), (2) *intrusion* (going beyond the scope of the evaluation and into the domain of the legal decision-maker), and (3) *insufficiency and incredibility* (the failure to provide adequate, credible information consistent with the conclusions drawn). A general set of principles, applicable to all forensic evaluations, would provide guidance to practitioners in avoiding such problems. Further, the widespread acceptance of such general principles would undoubtedly increase the uniformity of FMHA. Fewer deficits and greater uniformity might in turn improve the satisfaction of FMHA consumers, such as attorneys, judges, and public sector agencies.

How will such principles change as the field of FMHA develops? In certain areas, the principles may be sufficiently established and generalizable that they will change little as the field matures. Other principles described in this book are neither consistently supported nor firmly established. Further theory development, empirical research, and developments in case law and forensic practice may refine them significantly. It is important to distinguish between principles accordingly. Thus, principles will be classified as either *established* (largely supported by research, accepted in practice, and consistent with ethical and legal standards) or *emerging* (supported in some areas, but with mixed or absent evidence from others, or supported by some evidence but with continuing disagreement among professionals regarding their application). Established principles of FMHA will probably be those that will change little, while emerging principles may appear considerably different in another decade.

Before discussing such principles, it is necessary to review the differences between forensic assessments and other clinical assessments, and the content areas in which the principles will be based. There are important differences between FMHA and evaluation that is performed for "therapeutic" purposes such as diagnosis, behavioral description, and treatment-planning. These types of evaluation will be termed *forensic* and *therapeutic*, respectively. Existing principles for *therapeutic* assessment are not adequate to describe the more specialized activity of *forensic* assessment. The following review of differences between the two will clarify why.

FORENSIC VERSUS THERAPEUTIC ASSESSMENT

A comparison of forensic versus therapeutic evaluation is presented in Table 1.2. A total of 10 dimensions are described: (1) purpose, (2) examiner–examinee relationship, (3) notification of purpose, (4) who is being served, (5) the nature of the standard being considered, (6) data sources, (7) the response style of the examinee, (8) clarification of reasoning and the limits of knowledge, (9) the role of the written report, and (10) the role of testimony.

The primary purpose of the forensic evaluation is to assist a legal

TABLE 1.2. DIFFERENCES BETWEEN TREATMENT AND FORENSIC ROLES FOR MENTAL HEALTH PROFESSIONALS

	Therapeutic	Forensic
Purpose	Diagnose and treat symptoms of illness	Assist decision-maker or attorney
Examiner–examinee relationship	Helping role	Objective or quasi-objective stance
Notification of purpose	Implicit assumptions about purpose shared by doctor and patient Formal, explicit notification typically not done	Assumptions about purpose not necessarily shared Formal and explicit notification
Who is being served	Individual patient	Variable; may be court, attorney, and client
Nature of standard being considered	Medical, psychiatric, psychological	Medical, psychiatric, psychological, and legal
Data sources	Self-report Psychological testing Behavioral assessment Medical procedures	Self-report Psychological testing Behavioral assessment Medical procedures Observation of others
Response style of examine	Assumed to be reliable	Not assumed to be reliable
Clarification of reasoning and limits of knowledge	Optional	Very important
Written report	Brief, conclusory statement	Lengthy and detailed Documents findings, reasonings, and conclusions
Court testimony	Not expected	Expected

decision-maker in addressing a given legal issue. The forensic evaluation should contribute to this decision-making process by helping to determine whether, and to what extent, the individual being evaluated is (or was) able to know, think, feel, or act in a certain fashion. These capacities underlie the fitness to satisfy the demands of a given legal role, such as making a will (testamentary capacity), functioning as a criminal defendant (competence to stand trial) or hospitalized patient (competence to consent to treatment), or meeting criteria prescribed by law to satisfy a given standard (e.g., criminal responsibility, fitness to parent). In contrast, a therapeutic evaluation is performed for reasons traditionally associated with the role of the mental health professional: a need to describe the symptoms, characteristics, and behavior relevant to mental health functioning. That description is then used in planning a treatment intervention, with the goal of improving or ameliorating the difficulty.

Our society holds certain expectations about the relationship between doctor (including psychiatrists and psychologists) and patient. One of the most basic of these assumptions is that of the "helping role" of the therapist—that the "helper" will act in the best interest of the individual seeking help. Because individuals in the "patient" role are typically aware of these expectations, at least to some extent, there is little need for formal clarification. In contrast, there is a considerably different set of assumptions underlying forensic evaluation. Rather than assuming a helping role, the forensic clinician performing FMHA operates from an objective or quasi-objective stance, neither accepting nor rejecting the accuracy of information that is provided until it can be checked against information from other sources. It is important to begin a forensic evaluation by notifying the individual being evaluated about the specific purpose(s) of the evaluation. A forensic evaluation will certainly differ from a therapeutic evaluation in purpose, and different kinds of forensic evaluations will also differ from one another.

A therapeutic evaluation is performed to serve an individual, couple, or family in the role of "identified client." In contrast, there may be multiple "clients" in a forensic evaluation (Monahan, 1980). The "primary client" is usually the legal decision-maker when the evaluation is court-ordered, and the forensic clinician is striving to help the court make a better-informed decision by providing relevant, accurate information. Alternatively, the "primary client" may be the attorney and the litigant, when the forensic clinician is performing an evaluation at the request of the individual in the context of litigation. However, such assistance still differs from treatment in one important respect, namely, the goal is to provide accurate information for use in litigation, not to enhance the individual's mental health functioning.

The nature of the standard used in the evaluation differs between therapeutic and forensic evaluation. In therapeutic evaluation, three kinds of standards have been widely used: (1) diagnostic (using the current version of the *Diagnostic and Statistical Manual* of the American Psychiatric Association), (2) behavioral, and (3) psychodynamic. These standards serve organizing, condensing, and orienting functions. They help to identify relevant areas for investigation, reduce the obtained information into a shorthand that is readily communicated to other mental health professionals, and translate the findings into implications for action. In contrast, a forensic evaluation must address both a medical or mental health standard *and* a legal standard. The accurate identification of the appropriate legal standard is crucial in forensic evaluation, because the intersection of the two standards—for example, the description of how the ability to perform tasks relevant for the legal standard is impaired by mental disorder—is one of the most important areas addressed in the evaluation.

The sources of information used can vary between therapeutic and forensic evaluation. Standard data sources for therapeutic evaluation include self-report, medical procedures, psychological testing, and behavioral assessment. These sources often are used in forensic assessment as well. In the forensic context, however, it is important to use additional information, such as relevant documents (e.g., arrest history, arrest report, prior evaluations, medical records, and records of job, school, and military performance) and the observations of others, for two reasons. First, the usual sources of information for therapeutic evaluation will provide limited data about the individual's behavior on legally relevant dimensions. More specifically, such information will usually not pertain directly to the functional components (what an individual must be able to do, say, think, decide, and the like) of a specific legal standard, because it has not been collected with those particular areas in mind. Second, since self-report cannot be assumed to be accurate, these additional sources of information are used to "cross-check" the consistency of self-report with other observations.

Response style refers to the nature and accuracy of the information provided by individuals being evaluated regarding their own thoughts, feelings, and behavior (see Rogers, 1984, 1997). Clinicians performing a therapeutic evaluation are aware that intrapersonal (feelings evoked by sensitive topics) and interpersonal (the reactions involved in discussing these topics with another person) influences may interfere with the accuracy of clients' self-report. However, there is no *consistent* expectation by clinicians conducting therapeutic evaluation that the individuals being evaluated will have an incentive to exaggerate or minimize the extent of certain symptoms or experiences.[3] In a forensic evaluation, in contrast, there is a much more *consistent* expectation, as the individual being evaluated stands to gain (or lose) from the outcome of the case. Understandably, that individual might be more likely to respond to the *situationally based* incentive to present herself in an advantageous light, in the same way that people would be comparably motivated under a variety of other circumstances (e.g., when applying for a job). It is the *consistent* presence of this situationally based incentive, created by the circumstances of litigation, that distinguishes forensic from therapeutic evaluation in the importance of response style.

The process of clarifying reasoning and the limits on knowledge differs sharply between therapeutic and forensic evaluation. A therapeutic evaluator typically holds assumptions, uses methods, and draws conclusions without the expectation that they will be challenged.[4] Therapeutic evaluation is performed within a collaborative professional model that carries the implicit reliance on the professional knowledge and skill of the evaluator. In contrast, a forensic evaluation is performed in the context of an adversarial legal system. If findings are used in a given case, it is presumably because they are expected to be helpful to the party presenting them. They are subject to challenge within the rules of evidence by opposing counsel. Such challenges may include direct and indirect attempts to undermine the evaluator's credibility, and may also include the presentation of testimony by a mental health expert who has reached different conclusions on the same legally relevant questions.

There is no clear, consistent expectation about the nature of the writ-

---

[3]There are a number of clinical influences that may result in distorted self-report by patients. These include, for instance, exaggerating symptoms as a "cry for help" or the wish to assume the patient role, or denying unusual thoughts or feelings in the exercise of psychological defenses. However, these are largely *internal* motivations rather than situationally generated incentives. It is true, of course, that there are certain kinds of "therapeutic evaluation" cases which may involve a patient's *externally* induced motivation to exaggerate or minimize symptoms of psychopathology. Issues related to actual or perceived coercion into treatment, third-party reimbursement, the social implications of seeking mental health treatment, the avoidance of military service, or the maintaining of V.A. or insurance benefits may arise. Some apparent exceptions, however, may occur in evaluations that are actually forensic rather than therapeutic. For example, when a mental health professional evaluates a patient to determine whether she continues to require mental health disability benefits, this particular evaluation more closely resembles the forensic than the therapeutic evaluation process described in this chapter.

[4]In this era of managed care, clinicians may perceive challenges to both evaluations and interventions from third-party payers. When this is considered, therapeutic evaluation is less distinct from forensic evaluation on the "expectation of challenge" dimension than was once the case.

ten report needed to document a therapeutic evaluation. Such evaluation may be recorded in brief fashion, such as a file note, chart note, or letter to the referring source. A more elaborate report may be written under some circumstances, but often is not needed. In contrast, the documentation requirement for a forensic evaluation is much more detailed; a lengthy report is usually needed, describing the findings, reasoning, and conclusions. Such a report is useful for describing the evaluation's procedures, some of which are selected specifically for the legal issue in question. However, extensive documentation is important for other reasons as well. Since the evaluation is being performed as part of legal proceedings, it will serve as evidence relevant to the arguments prepared by both sides, and to the court as decision-maker. The preparation of a detailed report facilitates the use of the forensic evaluation as evidence.[5]

Finally, clinicians performing a therapeutic evaluation need not expect that the results will become a part of litigation, or that they will subsequently testify in legal proceedings based on this evaluation. Under rare circumstances, a given patient might become involved in legal proceedings, and the therapeutic evaluation made part of the legal record. Even under such circumstances, however, the therapeutic evaluation should not be considered a forensic evaluation, and the evaluating clinician should not testify as an expert. In contrast, the clinician doing a forensic evaluation should always anticipate that testimony in a deposition, hearing, or trial will be associated with the evaluation. Not all forensic evaluations result in the clinician being called to testify, of course. However, the evaluation should be performed so that *if* testimony is needed, it will be of high quality and follow logically from the substance of the evaluation.

In summary, the process of forensic assessment differs in important

---

[5]Under some circumstances, the forensic evaluator might not prepare a report. For example, if the attorney retaining the clinician's services wanted to discuss the results of the evaluation before having them written (to prevent the possibility of unfavorable results being obtained through discovery by opposing counsel), then the writing of a report would be delayed. However, any time the results of the valuation are presented in testimony, they should be documented in a detailed written report. For reasons to be discussed at length later, this recommendation appears sound. Nonetheless, there is a school of thought among some attorneys and forensic clinicians that the report should not document all of the results obtained and reasoning used in drawing conclusions. Part of this practice is apparently strategic, to avoid providing the opposing attorney with material to use in preparation for cross-examining the forensic clinician. This approach can have significant strategic disadvantages, however, if the notes and other materials used in the evaluation are obtained by the opposing attorney and incorporated into cross-examination. In such instances, the forensic clinician can appear to have deemphasized important data in reaching conclusions, and may appear less credible as a result.

ways from that of therapeutic assessment. Accordingly, it follows that any set of general principles applicable to therapeutic assessment will be insufficient at best, and misleading at worst, when applied to FMHA.

A STRUCTURE FOR ORGANIZING PRINCIPLES OF FMHA

This section describes a structure within which the principles of FMHA can be derived and organized, and which will be used throughout subsequent chapters. The structure contains four broad areas, presented in an order that corresponds to the sequence within the evaluation process: (1) preparation, (2) data collection, (3) data interpretation, and (4) communication. Within each of these broader areas, subareas will be identified that involve discrete steps in the forensic evaluation process. An outline of the steps to be taken in each of these areas is presented in Table 1.3.

PREPARATION

The major question within the preparation task is the focus of the evaluation. What are the legal issues to be decided by the court? This question has a number of implications for the evaluation, because the legal issues will be used to identify the relevant functional abilities to be evaluated.

A related question at the preparation stage involves the definition of the evaluator's role. Determining which of these roles will be played in

TABLE 1.3. OUTLINE OF STRUCTURE
FOR ORGANIZING PRINCIPLES
OF FORENSIC MENTAL HEALTH ASSESSMENT

Preparation
  • First contacts (Chapter 2)
  • Defining the evaluator's role (Chapter 3)
  • Using a model (Chapter 4)
Data collection
  • Selection (Chapter 5)
  • Administration (Chapter 6)
Data interpretation
  • Assessing response style (Chapter 7)
  • Incorporating scientific reasoning and data (Chapter 8)
  • Making assertions and clarifying limits (Chapter 9)
Communication
  • Communicating clearly (Chapter 10)
  • Testifying effectively (Chapter 11)

the immediate case will have important implications for how the overall FMHA task is defined and addressed. Accordingly, this question will be included in the structure used to develop and describe principles of FMHA.

DATA COLLECTION

The first step in the data collection task is conceptual, involving the selection of a model to guide the presentation of information and clarify the reasoning used by the evaluator. There are two general models, applicable to FMHA, that have been described in the literature: Morse's (1978a) and Grisso's (1986a). The strengths and weaknesses of each will be discussed.

The next data collection step involves the selection of relevant sources of data, and the administration of the necessary procedures. Considerable differences will be apparent between therapeutic and forensic assessment at this point; the guiding principles for data source selection involve relevance to the legal issue and its associated constructs, as well as validity (often termed *reliability* by courts; see, e.g., *Daubert v. Merrell Dow Pharmaceuticals, Inc.*, 1993).

DATA INTERPRETATION

The data interpretation task begins with consideration of response style. Before meaningful conclusions can be drawn about relevant clinical and behavioral characteristics, an evaluator must weigh the contributions of self-report of various kinds, including testing (if administered). To the extent that the individual being evaluated responds inaccurately, then self-report and testing data must be deemphasized and the role of collateral information expanded.

Both scientific reasoning and empirical data should play a role in interpretation. The use of such empirical data depends on several considerations. Are there studies relevant to the clinical and legal issues raised by a given case? What is their scientific quality, and to what extent are they generalizable to cases like the one at hand? What is the pattern of results from these studies, and their implications for the present case? Likewise, the process of scientific reasoning can serve as a model for the reasoning used in FMHA.

COMMUNICATION

The final task in forensic assessment is communication. This may include written communication (in the form of a report), informal oral communication (in feedback to attorneys or decision-makers), and formal oral communication (testimony in a deposition, hearing, or trial). Since written and oral communication differ in important ways, they will be discussed separately. Effective communication requires more attention in forensic work than in general clinical practice, because forensic examiners must write for readers who are not mental health professionals. Thus, they must avoid technical terms whenever possible (Melton et al., 1997), while providing detailed documentation of the evaluation process, including the sources of information, observations and results, conclusions, and reasoning process. Important principles for report writing will be addressed in this section of the book.

Effective expert testimony in legal proceedings has both a substantive and a procedural component. The substantive aspect relates directly to the forensic evaluation and the report; when these have been done properly, the expert witness can present them in testimony that describes (in much the same way the report has done) what has been performed. However, expert testimony in an adversarial context is never so straightforward as having the expert simply describe the evaluation. The expert will need to present this information effectively and convincingly while being challenged. This is the procedural dimension, involving the use of style and presentation techniques to enhance effectiveness and credibility in communication. Indeed, this is the aspect of expert testimony that receives particular attention in highly publicized cases. Both substantive and procedural aspects of expert testimony will be discussed in this book.

Four broad tasks have just been described: preparation, data collection, data interpretation, and communication. Taken together, these four tasks will provide the organizing structure within which principles of FMHA will be described.

DERIVING AND ANALYZING PRINCIPLES

Having identified a structure that will assist in examining principles of FMHA, and having organized it sequentially, it is necessary to describe how the principles in this book were derived. I have used several sources of authority when considering principles for FMHA: (1) the legal and behavioral science literatures, (2) consultation from authorities in the field of forensic assessment, and (3) my own experience with FMHA. When a prospective principle is identified, it will be evaluated by addressing each of four questions: Is the principle consistent with ethical guidelines? Is the principle consistent with law? Does the principle have scientific support? To what extent is the principle recognized by authorities as important for practice, and practiced by forensic clinicians? Based on the answers to these questions, each principle will be classified as either *established* or *emerging*.

Concerning the third of these, support from the behavioral science literature was assessed by reviewing the major data bases (PSYCHLIT and MEDLINE) for works published between 1979 and 1999. Additional articles, chapters, and books published prior to 1979 that are particularly important have been included as well. Journal articles from psychiatry, psychology, and social work have been applied to evaluating each principle, as have studies and reviews published in interdisciplinary journals in criminal and civil law.

The first subsection for evaluating each principle will focus on *ethical standards*. The ethical standards for psychology (*The Ethical Principles of Psychologists and Code of Conduct*, American Psychological Association, 1992) will be considered, along with the most applicable forensic psychology ethical guidelines (*The Specialty Guidelines for Forensic Psychologists*, Committee on Ethical Guidelines for Forensic Psychologists, 1991). Also, the ethical standards for psychiatry (*The Principles of Medical Ethics with Annotations Especially Applicable to Psychiatry*, American Psychiatric Association, 1998) and forensic psychiatry (*The Ethical Guidelines for the Practice of Forensic Psychiatry*, American Academy of Psychiatry and the Law, 1995) will be considered for their relevance to each principle.

The second evaluative criterion is *law*. Relevant case law, identified primarily at the level of the U.S. Supreme Court and federal appellate courts, has been identified using LEXIS and WESTLAW. Although relevant statutory and administrative law may differ considerably between states, there will be no attempt to review legal standards as they exist in each of the 50 U.S. states. However, relevant statutes and administrative code at the federal level will be examined. Works such as the *Criminal Justice Mental Health Standards* (American Bar Association, 1989), describing "model" mental health law, will also be considered; taken together, these sources of legal authority will be used to evaluate and illuminate the respective principle.[6]

The third evaluative criterion is *scientific support*. Examining the exist-

---

[6]Although there are clearly relationships between science, ethics, law, and practice standards, one might question the functional difference between ethics and law. The two are conceptually distinct (see, e.g., Bersoff, 1995), but are ethical standards incorporated into judicial decision-making on issues of concern to both areas? Some case law is consistent with court's use of ethical principles to help frame the specific limits of a legal duty (*Brandt v. Medical Defense Association*, 1993), and the use of ethical standards as one justification for a legal decision when they are consistent with public policy (*Wood v. Upjohn Company*, 1984). However, other courts have held that ethical principles are independent of state supervision (*Arizona State Board of Medical Examiners v. Clark*, 1965; *Nash v. Wennar*, 1986), that an ethical duty may be distinguished from a legal duty (*Thompson v. Sun City Community Hospital, Inc.*, 1984; *Hiser v. Randolph*, 1980), and that a breach of ethical standards may establish grounds for professional discipline, but not a civil cause of action (*Noble v. Sartori*, 1989). There seems to be sufficient justification for treating ethics and law as distinct sources of authority, both on conceptual and empirical grounds.

ing behavioral science literature and focusing primarily on well-designed empirical studies will provide information about the research base of each principle that is identified. Good empirical studies will not exist for some principles, so there will be discussion of the empirical work that has been done and analysis about the meaning and generalizability of such work. In some instances, relevant theoretical work will be considered as well.

In addition to using the *outcome* of scientific research as it applies to these principles, the *process* of science will provide an important contribution to FMHA as it is described in this book. There are noteworthy similarities between science and forensic assessment in the development of hypotheses, the operationalization of variables, the testing of hypotheses, and the interpretation of results. This will be discussed in detail in later chapters.

The fourth evaluative criterion might be described as *standard of practice*. This will focus on the extent to which the principle is recognized by authorities as important for FMHA practice. When possible, this area will also include the extent to which the principle is practiced by forensic clinicians, although the literature describing the normative aspects of forensic practice is rarely sufficiently developed to address this second question effectively. Using these two questions as guides to analyzing each principle requires the incorporation of information from professional publications, CE training, available base rates, and my own experience in conducting, supervising, teaching, and testifying about forensic assessment, and observing the assessments performed by others.

The overall process of FMHA has a number of discrete steps and an associated set of underlying principles. In these respects, FMHA might be compared to building a house. Beginning with the decision to build, the process then encompasses drawing up plans, excavating, building the foundation, framing the structure, building the walls, incorporating the systems, trimming the details, and checking for functions before it is completed. The successful completion of later steps depends on how well earlier tasks have been performed. In Chapter 2, we begin the process of identifying principles of FMHA with the earliest tasks—figuratively, the "planning" and "foundation" of the evaluation process.

II

Preparation

2

First Contacts

This chapter will describe and analyze principles encompassed within the first part of the structure. These principles will refer to the earliest steps taken in the FMHA process. Some questions of definition must be clarified, however, early in this discussion. There are a number of terms or phrases that have been used to describe various aspects of the legal decision to be made. *Forensic issue, clinical-legal issue, legal question, defining criteria,* and *issue being litigated* are common examples. For present purposes, I will use *forensic issue* to refer to the questions addressed by FMHA within the context of the larger legal question that the court must ultimately decide. The forensic issues and larger legal questions are not synonymous. In some instances, the forensic issue and larger legal question are relatively similar. For example, for competence to stand trial, FMHA describes the defendant's abilities to participate in a trial, and the legal standard itself focuses primarily on those abilities. At other times, however, the forensic issues constitute only a part of the overall legal question. For example, in juvenile transfer, the forensic issues addressed in FMHA include risk assessment and treatment needs/amenability, but the legal standard may depend on additional criteria that FMHA is not asked to address, such as the seriousness of the alleged offense and whether it appears to have been premeditated (Heilbrun, Leheny, Thomas, & Huneycutt, 1997). The relationship between forensic issues and the larger legal question will be discussed in detail in the principle on answering the "ultimate legal question."

IDENTIFY RELEVANT FORENSIC ISSUES

Forensic issues are the capacities, skills, and functional abilities that are relevant to the broader legal question that a court must decide in a

21

given case. Since forensic evaluations are performed because there are larger legal issues to be decided, an important first step is to identify the forensic issues contained in these legal questions that have triggered the need for the evaluation. This can be straightforward when it involves a well-recognized legal question (e.g., competence to stand trial) in which the included forensic issues are clear. At other times, however, the mental health professional may be asked to perform an evaluation involving a forensic issue that is vaguely or inappropriately stated, or a larger legal question that is poorly defined by statute or case law. In such cases, further clarification of the legal questions, and the included forensic issues, is needed. Such information may be obtained from consultation with the referring attorney, a search of relevant statutes, case law, or administrative code, and an examination of the relevant behavioral sciences literature.

In other cases, the forensic clinician may be asked to address a forensic issue that is relevant to only a part of the larger legal question. For example, in a case involving an insanity defense, a psychologist might be asked to perform testing to help clarify the issues of response style and presence of a mental disorder, but not to provide information relevant to the defendant's thoughts and feelings around the time of the offense. In another example—a malpractice case—the ultimate legal decision might involve the application of a therapist's duty to protect others from a patient's future violent acts. A clinician familiar with the clinical and re-search literature on risk assessment might be asked to determine whether the therapist's evaluation of her patient's potential for violence toward others was consistent with the literature and standard of practice at the time she evaluated this patient.

In cases like these, even a good awareness of the legal question being addressed may offer insufficient guidance to the forensic clinician. Clari-fication of the forensic issues to be evaluated *in the context of the legal question* may come, in part, through the legal and behavioral science literatures, but may also need to be refined through discussion with the referring attorney. Such discussion should aim to modify attorneys' re-quests to address forensic issues in ways that are not meaningful or realistic.

ETHICS

None of the sources describing ethics for forensic assessments directly addresses the need to identify relevant forensic issues. However, the *Specialty Guidelines for Forensic Psychologists* describes the importance of the forensic clinician having "a fundamental and reasonable level of knowl-edge and understanding of the legal ... standards that govern their participation as experts in legal proceedings" (Committee on Ethical Guidelines for Forensic Psychologists, 1991, p. 658). Also, the *Specialty Guidelines* indicates that forensic psychologists "have an obligation to ensure that prospective clients are informed of ... the purposes of any evaluation" (p. 659), which presumably would include a notification of the forensic issue(s) being evaluated.

LAW

The importance of specifying the particular forensic issue is consistent with the evidentiary principle of relevance; under the *Federal Rules of Evidence*, evidence is relevant if it has "any tendency to make the existence of any fact that is of consequence to the determination of the action more probable or less probable than it would be without the evidence" (F.R.E. 401). Several cases appear supportive. In *United States v. Green* (1977), the Sixth Circuit Court of Appeals held that the trial court's admission of expert testimony concerning the bizarre physiological effects of a certain drug on the body was held to be an abuse of discretion, since the expert testimony was irrelevant to the charge of manufacturing the drug. As part of this ruling, the Court adopted four criteria for review of trial court decisions involving expert testimony: (1) qualified expert, (2) proper subject, (3) conformity to a generally accepted explanatory theory, and (4) probative value compared with prejudicial effect. The "proper subject," in particular, was used by the Sixth Circuit subsequently to rule that expert evidence had been properly excluded by the trial court on the basis of relevance (*United States v. Smith*, 1984). In both of these cases, the nature of the expert testimony centered around eyewitness identification. Other cases from the Third Circuit (*United States v. Downing*, 1985) and the Ninth Circuit (*United States v. Brewer*, 1986) have also supported the exclusion of expert testimony regarding eyewitness identification on the basis of relevance, as has the U.S. Air Force Court of Military Review (*United States v. Garcia*, 1994).

A priori specification of the forensic issue in FMHA is also consistent with case law and statutes describing particular legal tests. For example, in *Dusky v. United States* (1960), the U.S. Supreme Court, addressing the issue of competence to stand trial, rejected a vague standard with several clinical components (oriented to time and place, and having some recollection of events) in favor of a more specific standard with functional legal elements (sufficient present ability to consult with his lawyer with a reasonable degree of rational understanding, and rational as well as factual understanding of the proceedings against him).

A specific example of how a court can weigh an opinion on a forensic issue that was not specifically the focus of the evaluation may be seen in the U.S. District Court's refusal, in *U.S. v. Mason* (1996), to grant a new trial to a defendant based on the possibility that he may have been incompetent to stand trial at the time of his trial 39 months previously. The speculation that the defendant may not have been competent for trial was made by a mental health professional who evaluated the defendant for another purpose. However, the court weighed more heavily the opinion of the consulting psychologist who had been ordered to provide an evaluation (retrospectively) of the *defendant's* trial competence (*U.S. v. Mason*, 1996).

EMPIRICAL

Limited research has directly addressed the impact of specifying the forensic issue on the quality of the evaluation. McGarry (1965) observed over 30 years ago that none of 106 reports reviewed addressed the issue of the defendant's competence to stand trial, even though that was one reason for the evaluations being conducted. The problem with these results, and those of research conducted since that time on the normative aspects of FMHA, is that they refer to addressing the legal question (the so-called ultimate legal issue) rather than the relevant forensic issues, and also do not provide a basis for gauging the *impact* of such deficits.

However, two studies have addressed the preferences of judges for the various forensic issues that might be considered as part of a legal decision. In one (Poythress, 1981) involving a survey of 30 Michigan circuit court judges, the judges were asked to rate as essential, desirable, or undesirable a total of eight aspects of FMHA results communicated in testimony. Three such aspects—statistical/actuarial data on the relationship between clinical and legally relevant behavior, theoretical accounts or explanations for legally relevant behavior, and weighing different motives or explanations for legally relevant behavior—are somewhat relevant to this principle (information concerning legally relevant behavior is harder to provide without specifying the nature of such legally relevant behavior). Judges rated the second and third aspects as desirable, while the first was considered either unnecessary, uninformative, or undesirable.

In the second study (Lowery, 1981), a total of 57 judges in Kentucky (representing a 68% response rate) responded to a survey on the importance of various forensic issues in child custody litigation. Results of this survey revealed that 18 of the total 20 items were rated by judges at the midpoint or higher of a scale ranging from "of little importance" to "highly important." The elements rated as most important were mental stability of each parent, each parent's sense of responsibility to the child, the biological relationship to the child, and each parent's moral character.

Additional information is available on the desirability of identifying the relevant forensic issues (Borum & Grisso, 1996). In a national survey of forensic psychologists and forensic psychiatrists on the legal questions of trial competence ($N = 102$ respondents) and criminal responsibility ($N = 96$ respondents), over 90% of those surveyed described it as "essential" to identify the basic purpose of performing the evaluation (identifying at least the legal question) for both competence to stand trial and criminal responsibility.

The longstanding acceptance of this principle among forensic specialists and researchers is probably one reason for the very limited research. Although researchers and scholars use legal question to define sample groups (for example, defendants who are Incompetent to Stand Trial or Not Guilty by Reason of Insanity; see, e.g., Monahan & Steadman, 1983; Roesch & Golding, 1980; Rogers, 1986; Shapiro, 1991; Steadman et al., 1993; Weiner & Hess, 1987), there has apparently been no research on the impact of failing to specify the legal question or related forensic issues on the quality of the FMHA. Perhaps this can be understood by noting that any FMHA that did not specify the legal question and relevant forensic issues would resemble a therapeutic evaluation far more than a forensic evaluation (see Chapter 1), and research attention is not needed to make this clearer.

STANDARD OF PRACTICE

In most practice-relevant books, the topics are divided according to the legal question being evaluated, with related forensic issues discussed within this larger context (e.g., Grisso, 1988, 1998a; Melton et al., 1997; Rogers, 1986; Shapiro, 1991; Weiner & Hess, 1987). Most of these authors explicitly indicate that the forensic examiner should begin by identifying the relevant forensic issues. Judging as well from the internal logic of these works, the identification of the relevant legal question, with included forensic issues, is an essential early step in FMHA. Forensic training conducted at the state level stresses the importance of considering different kinds of evaluations according to legal question and related forensic issues (Florida Mental Health Institute, 1989; Institute of Law, Psychiatry, and Public Policy, 1995). Instruments that have been developed for use in one kind of evaluation, such as the Interdisciplinary Fitness Interview-Revised (Golding, 1993) or the MacArthur Competence Assessment Tool–Criminal Adjudication (Polythress, Monahan, Bonnie, & Hodge, 1999) for evaluating competence to stand trial, are not interchangeable with other legal questions.

While the importance of identifying relevant forensic issues may seem obvious, the failure to do so can immediately create problems for FMHA. Naive clinicians may believe that a good "clinical" evaluation will serve in forensic cases; others may fail to distinguish properly between different forensic issues. As Grisso (1986a) pointed out, insufficiency and irrelevance have been common criticisms of forensic assessments.

DISCUSSION

The identification of the relevant legal question and the associated forensic issues is a very basic part of FMHA. Every authoritative text on forensic assessment cited emphasizes that the legally relevant question must be identified in order to guide the assessment. A major complaint regarding FMHA cited by Grisso (1986a) is "irrelevance"—performing clinical evaluation without reference to legally relevant abilities. Relevance is an importance criterion in the law of evidence. For ethical standards, there is more of an implicit assumption that the forensic issue will be identified and properly addressed than an explicit discussion of the need to do this. In empirical research, however, investigators often use legal status (determined by the legal question the court has addressed, or will address, such as competence to stand trial or competence to consent to treatment) as a variable. Thus, this principle will be classified as *established*.

ACCEPT REFERRALS ONLY WITHIN AREA OF EXPERTISE

This principle states that forensic clinicians must have sufficient expertise in a forensic area to perform an FMHA in that area. Whether a forensic clinician's expertise is sufficient to permit her to ethically accept a referral for an evaluation in a given case will depend on considerations such as the clinician's training and experience with specific populations, with the clinical issues associated with the person(s) to be evaluated, and with the application of clinical expertise in a forensic context. Separate from the ethical imperative, courts apply legal criteria to determine whether a clinician will be qualified as an expert. In this section, I will consider various sources of authority for this principle, address the issues of ethically driven versus legally granted expertise, and discuss how such factors might apply in various cases.

ETHICS

The APA's *Ethical Principles* (1992) addresses the issue of professional competence as follows:

Psychologists strive to maintain high standards of competence in their work. They recognize the boundaries of their particular competencies and the limitations of their expertise. They provide only those services and use only those techniques for which they are qualified by education, training, or experience. Psychologists are cognizant of the fact that the competencies required in serving, teaching, and/or studying groups of people vary with the distinctive characteristics of those groups. In those areas in which recognized professional standards do not yet exist, psychologists exercise careful judgment and take appropriate precautions to protect the welfare of those with whom they work. They maintain knowledge of relevant scientific and professional information related to the services they render, and they recognize the need for ongoing education. Psychologists make appropriate use of scientific, professional, technical, and administrative resources. (p. 1599)

The *Specialty Guidelines* (1991) elaborates on the issue of competence for forensic practice, noting that services are provided "only in areas of psychology in which [forensic psychologists] have specialized knowledge, skill, experience, and education" (p. 658). Further, there is

an obligation to present to the court, regarding the specific matters to which they will testify, the boundaries of their competence, the factual bases (knowledge, skill, experience, training, and education) for their qualifications as an expert, and the relevance of those factual bases to their qualification as an expert on the specific matters at issue. (p. 658)

There is also a responsibility for

a fundamental and reasonable level of knowledge and understanding of the legal and professional standards that govern their participation as experts in legal proceedings. (p. 658)

Finally, it is noted that

Forensic psychologists recognize that their own personal values, moral beliefs, or personal and professional relationships with parties to a legal proceeding may interfere with their ability to practice competently. Under such circumstances, forensic psychologists are obligated to decline participation or to limit their assistance in a manner consistent with professional obligation. (p. 658).

The *Principles of Medical Ethics with Annotations Especially Applicable to Psychiatry* (American Psychiatric Association, 1998) also discusses the issue of competence and expertise, albeit less directly. In Section 2 ("A physician shall deal honestly with patients and colleagues, and strive to expose those physicians deficient in character or competence, or who engage in fraud or deception"), it is noted that a "psychiatrist who regularly practices outside his/her area of professional competence should be considered unethical" (p. 3).

Finally, the *Ethical Guidelines for the Practice of Forensic Psychiatry* (AAPL, 1995) addresses the issue of competence by indicating that "[e]xpertise in the practice of forensic psychiatry is claimed only in areas of actual knowledge and skills, training and experience" (p. 4). Further commentary yields this elaboration:

> As regards expert opinions, reports and testimony, the expert's qualifications should be presented accurately and precisely. As a correlate of the principle that expertise may be appropriately claimed only in areas of actual knowledge, skill, training and experience, there are areas of special expertise, such as the evaluation of children or persons of foreign cultures, or prisoners, that may require special training and expertise. (p. 4).

Clearly, each of these four sets of ethical standards recognizes the importance of competence in a particular area as a prerequisite for practice in that area. The boundaries of competence are defined by knowledge, skill, experience, and education/training.[1] Interestingly, however, the concept of professional "competence" is not described in detailed fashion (particularly considering how widely accepted the dictum of "practice within one's area of competence" seems to be). One way to explore the boundaries of this principle is to inquire about exceptions: Does it apply consistently, or is occasional practice outside the bounds of one's competence acceptable?

Two of the sources of ethics authority being used in this book—the APA's *Ethical Principles* and the AAPL's *Ethical Guidelines for the Practice of Forensic Psychiatry*—provide no exceptions to their description of the need for competence in the area of practice. Both define competence in a similar manner, emphasizing training and experience; the *Ethical Principles* includes "education" among the criteria to be considered for competence, while the *Ethical Guidelines* considers "knowledge" and "skills." The other two sources of ethics authority—the *Specialty Guidelines for Forensic Psychologists* and the *Principles of Medical Ethics with Annotations*—do provide a "regular practice" modifier to the stipulation that competence is necessary for practice in an area. More specifically, the *Specialty Guidelines* note that they apply to individuals who "*regularly* [italics added] engage in the practice of forensic psychology" involving "... acting, *with definable foreknowledge* [italics added], as a psychological expert on explicitly psycho-

---

[1]Formal forensic training for psychiatrists and psychologists, while not universally available, has nevertheless expanded significantly in the last decade. There are currently 38 forensic psychiatry fellowships (postresidency) in the United States and Canada, and some exposure to forensic evaluation is now a requirement for psychiatry residency training in the United States. Forensic training opportunities within psychology are available at the predoctoral and internship levels (Vant Zelfde & Otto, 1997). In addition, postdoctoral forensic psychology training is available at 11 sites in the United States (Bersoff et al., 1997). For a detailed discussion of forensic training at all levels, see the entire issue of *Behavioral Sciences & the Law*, Vol. 8, 1990.

legal issues, in direct assistance to courts, parties to legal proceedings, correctional and forensic mental health facilities, and administrative, judicial, and legislative agencies acting in an adjudicative capacity" (p. 657). The *Principles of Medical Ethics with Annotations* simply notes that regular practice outside one's area of competence is unethical. Thus, there is no consistent guidance on this question from these sources of ethics authority. There is a "regular practice" exception from the most applicable ethical principles to psychiatry generally, but no such exception from the APA's *Ethical Principles*, which applies to psychologists. There is agreement between all of these sources, however, that those who are regularly involved in practice in a given area should be competent to do so.

LAW

Under the *Federal Rules of Evidence*, Rule 702 (1987), the definition of an expert is much briefer. Such an individual may be prepared to offer evidence in scientific matters, or those pertaining to technical or other areas of specialized knowledge. Further, the prospective expert must have acquired special knowledge, skill, experience, training, or education that would allow that individual to assist the court in the resolution of disputed questions of fact.

The question of whether the courts will use general expertise in an area (e.g., a doctorate in psychology or a medical degree plus a residency in psychiatry), or will go beyond that to require more specialized expertise, particularly in cases with very specific issues before the court, is likely to be addressed with increasing frequency during the coming years as the mental health professions move toward greater specialization. In one recent case concerning repressed memory, for example, the court determined that testimony on issues such as posttraumatic stress disorder and repressed memory would require specialization in these areas, going beyond general training in clinical psychology (*Isely v. Capuchin Province*, 1995).

Mental health expertise in the forensic context has been described in three ideal steps: (1) expertise beyond ordinary knowledge and understanding, which will assist the trier of fact in understanding evidence or determining a fact, (2) the expert is qualified by virtue of knowledge, skill, experience, training, or education, and (3) the basis for the expert's opinion is reliable, and more probative than "prejudicial, confusing, misleading, or redundant with other evidence" (Golding, 1990, p. 284). This is essentially the law's definition of expertise, which may have been expanded beyond "general acceptance" (at least in terms of the nature of the evidence considered) by the U.S. Supreme Court's decision in *Daubert v. Merrell Dow*

Pharmaceuticals (1993) to include the following criteria: (1) the proposition to which the evidence pertains is testable, (2) it has been tested, (3) the technique used to test it has a known error rate, (4) there are accepted standards for operation of the technique, and (5) the evidence has been subjected to peer review and publication (Giannelli & Imwinkelried, 1993). While it is not yet clear whether and to what extent *Daubert* will apply to FMHA, it can be demonstrated that a few rulings (11 cases of the 276 citing *Daubert* between 1993 and March 1996) have applied *Daubert* criteria to psychological testing, diagnosis, specialized techniques, and "profiling" (Heilbrun, 1996).

STANDARD OF PRACTICE

The question of when a forensic clinician is sufficiently "expert" to perform a forensic assessment is addressed in the ABA's *Criminal Justice Mental Health Standards* (1989), which has delineated four possible roles for mental health professionals in the criminal process: (1) evaluator, (2) scientist, (3) consultant, and (4) treatment agent. For the role of evaluator, the *Standards* addresses "expertise" under two related circumstances: qualifications for court-appointed evaluations and qualifications for testifying about a person's mental condition.[2] The *Standards* also addresses the issue of establishing minimum professional education and clinical training requirements for evaluators and expert witnesses, with recommendations for implementing these requirements.

Under Standard 7-3.10, no professional should be appointed by the court to evaluate a person's mental condition unless their qualifications include

---

[2]A brief clarification regarding the meanings of "expertise" and "qualification" is necessary. In the previous section, the emphasis was on competence rather than expertise. In some respects, competence and expertise are overlapping constructs; both emphasize the importance of knowledge, skill, training, and experience. The most important difference between the two concerns the source of the judgment, however. Courts have broad latitude in determining who may be considered an expert for legal purposes, with part of this discretion influenced by whether the testimony would be likely to assist the trier of fact in understanding evidence or determining facts in issue. Legal competence (reflecting the presence of characteristics and absence of disabilities making a witness qualified to testify) is part of the expertise determination, although broadly applicable to all potential witnesses, not just experts. Professional competence, in contrast, is applied by a profession (via ethical standards) to the individuals in that profession, and is more affected by broad professional consensus than the circumstances of an individual case. "Qualification" has two important meanings in the legal sense: (1) attributes of an individual relevant to legal expertise and (2) the process necessary to prepare an individual to exercise the function of performing as an expert.

   (a) sufficient professional education and sufficient clinical training and experi-
      ence to establish the clinical knowledge required for the specific type(s) of
      evaluation(s) being conducted; and
   (b) sufficient forensic knowledge, gained through specialized training or an
      acceptable substitute therefor, necessary for understanding the relevant
      legal matter(s) and for satisfying the specific purpose(s) for which the
      evaluation is being ordered. (p. 130)

Testimony as an evaluating expert, under Standard 7-3.11, would
require that the witness have

   (i) sufficient professional education and sufficient clinical training and expe-
      rience to establish the clinical knowledge required to formulate an expert
      opinion; and
  (ii) has either:
     (a) acquired sufficient knowledge, through forensic training or an accept-
        able substitute therefor, relevant to conducting the specific type(s) of
        mental evaluation actually conducted in the case, and relevant to the
        substantive law concerning the specific matter(s) on which expert
        opinion is to be proffered; or
     (b) has had a professional therapeutic or habilitative relationship with the
        person whose mental condition is in question; and
 (iii) has performed an adequate evaluation, including a personal interview
      with the individual whose mental condition is in question, relevant to the
      legal and clinical matter(s) upon which the witness is being called to
      testify. (p. 132)

If the criteria for expertise described in these *Standards* refer only to
testimony about clinical status relevant to the legal question, then this
would not qualify as a forensic assessment as this has been described in
this book. There is the potential for confusion among legal professionals
regarding such a clinical role in legal proceedings, as contrasted with a
forensic role, that should be noted. However, if the *Standards* refer to a
therapeutic or habilitative relationship as a basis for testimony in a forensic
role, then they appear misguided on this point. For reasons discussed in
detail in Chapter 1, it seems inappropriate to describe a professional therapeutic or habilitative relationship as an adequate basis for forensic expertise, or to suggest that a forensic and a therapeutic relationship should not
only coexist within the same case, but also have the therapeutically acquired knowledge actually strengthen the forensic expertise. Forensic and
therapeutic evaluations differ on a number of relevant dimensions (see
Chapter 1), including six that are particularly important to the relevance
and accuracy of testimony in legal proceedings. These six dimensions are
(1) nature of the standard being considered, (2) sources of data used to present facts and reach opinions, (3) response style of the patient, (4) clarification of reasoning and limits on knowledge, (5) nature of the written report,
and (6) *a priori* expectation of court testimony. These differences are such

that a therapeutic/habilitative relationship should not be considered an adequate substitute for a forensic evaluative relationship in its potential for yielding information that is both *relevant* to the legal question and as *reliable* as possible.[3]

Regarding minimum professional educational and clinical training requirements for evaluators and expert witnesses, the *Standards* notes that the necessary and desirable education and training requirements differ according to the subject matter of the evaluation and the specific legal issue. For instance, evaluations concerning a person's present mental competence would require a psychiatrist, a doctoral-level psychologist (clinical, counseling, or school), a master's-level clinical social worker, or a master's-level psychiatric nurse. For an evaluation concerning a person's mental condition at the time of an alleged offense, or a person's future mental condition or behavior when these issues arise as part of a sentencing proceeding or special commitment proceeding, the *Standards* indicates that the evaluator should be a psychiatrist or doctoral-level psychologist (clinical or counseling).

The following discussion proposes a two-step process in evaluating the question of expertise in the context of forensic assessment (originally suggested by Heilbrun, 1995). The first step is determining whether the clinician has *substantive expertise* with a given population; the second involves whether this expertise has been *applied in forensic contexts*.

Concerning the first step, substantive expertise involves formal training and experience (both supervised and independent) with a given population. For example, for a mental health professional to conclude that she has sufficient substantive expertise to perform child custody evaluations, her substantive training should include graduate, internship, or postgraduate work in child and family areas. There should also be supervised clinical experience with children and families, particularly in the assessment area, and provision of such services on an independent (postlicensure) basis. The extent of the "specialization"—the percentage of work devoted to a specific population—could obviously vary, but I suggested that a minimum of 25% of the clinical work that is done postlicensure be in the particular area of specialization.[4] If this level of experience has not been

---

[3]Relevance and reliability are distinct from the professional ethical problems that may arise from serving as both a treating therapist and a forensic evaluator in the same case. This is discussed further in the principles on dual relationships in Chapter 3.

[4]This is not to suggest that an individual would need to spend 25% of his or her time doing clinical work in the specialization area. Rather, it means that for the clinical work that *is* done, at least 25% of it should be in this particular area. Professionals who engage in a variety of activities, including research, teaching, consultation, and training, as well as clinical and forensic work, may be quite appropriate as specialists under this definition.

acquired through formal predoctoral or postdoctoral/residence training, then an individual seeking to respecialize (or add an area of specialization) would have several options. He could contract with a specialist in that area, arranging to receive supervision in exchange for payment and possibly the opportunity for clinical-forensic experience. He could also seek a more formal period of postdoctoral training in an accredited facility providing supervised experience with such a population.

While licensure through the appropriate state board in the clinician's discipline is essential, there are additional reflections of professional standing (e.g., the National Register of Health Service Providers in Psychology) and competence (e.g., certification through the American Board of Professional Psychology or the American Board of Psychiatry and Neurology). In addition, it is useful to consider whether the mental health professional's expertise has been reflected in related professional activities— research, scholarly or professional articles, conference presentations, teaching, training of graduate students or mental health professionals, and university appointments. Taken together, the nature of the clinician's training, the degree of specialization with a given population, licensure and other certification, and related professional activities can provide the information necessary to assess whether the clinician has *substantive* expertise with a given population.

There should be a second step in assessing expertise in the forensic context, however, also important but frequently overlooked. What kind of specialization,[5] formal training,[6] supervised experience, advanced certification, and related professional activities can be demonstrated in *forensic* applications? To what extent has the clinician applied substantive expertise with a particular population to issues arising in the course of litigation? How often has the clinician applied substantive expertise (e.g., with children and families) to a legal issue relevant to that expertise (e.g., the assessment of child custody)?

---

[5]The term *specialization* is used without the specific connotation that it may have as a result of an ongoing initiative sponsored by the APA, where the Committee for the Recognition of Specialties and Proficiencies in Professional Psychology (CRSPPP) will make recommendations to designate a "specialty" (requiring advanced knowledge acquired through organized education and training) or a "proficiency" (a circumscribed activity in the practice of general psychology or any of its specialties, competence for which may be obtained through continuing education) (APA, 1995).

[6]Formal training in forensic psychiatry and psychology was largely unavailable before 1975. Currently, there are 46 forensic psychiatry fellowship (postresidency) programs in the United States and Canada (AAPL, Association of Directors of Forensic Psychiatry Fellowships, 2000), and 11 forensic psychology postdoctoral fellowships (Bersoff et al., 1997). Nonetheless, the supply of fellowship training opportunities still appears insufficient to meet the demand for forensic specialization.

In a 1995 national conference on training in various areas of law and psychology (Bersoff et al., 1997), three levels of clinical forensic specialization were designated. The first of these is the "legally informed" clinician:

> Beyond general clinical training, all professional psychologists would receive basic education in law as it applies to professional practice, including information about confidentiality and privileged communications, and appropriate procedures for responding to subpoenas for clinical records and personal notes. Some of this forensic content can be introduced in many, if not all, required clinical courses, especially those on assessment, intervention, and ethics. Ethics courses would include discussion not only of the APA's ethical code of conduct (APA, 1992) and other policy documents but of the *Specialty Guidelines for Forensic Psychologists* (Committee on Ethical Guidelines for Forensic Psychologists, 1991) as well.
>
> Dissemination of other important didactic content would require the periodic offering of an overview course in mental health law. Such a course would provide a basic understanding of the theoretical and practical differences between law and psychology, fundamental knowledge of how the civil and criminal justice systems operate, a primer on how to find and read the law, and advanced consideration of ethical issues that are unique to forensic practice. (pp. 1305–1306)

An intermediate degree of specialization was described as *proficiency* in forensic psychology:

> Psychologists attaining this mid-level expertise may be trained through general professional programs, with an emphasis on forensics; training programs offering a "concentration" in forensic psychology; or, for already trained clinicians, through extensive continuing education or postdoctoral programs.... Beyond course work that would focus on didactics, students concentrating on forensics would receive practical training in court clinics, forensic hospitals, juvenile facilities, public defenders' offices, or workers' compensation clinics. There would be greater exposure, compared with entry-level students, to legal concepts and to training in testifying as an expert witness, consulting with legal counsel, and performing forensic evaluations related to their clinical specialties. Students in this concentration would most likely do their dissertation research on forensic topics. (p. 1306)

The third, and highest, level of specialization in forensic psychology was described as *specialized*:

> Those professional psychologists wishing to attain the highest level of training would almost assuredly be educated in programs dedicated to producing forensic psychologists. These programs would have an integrated, carefully developed sequence of training with an identifiable, experienced forensic faculty with recognized credentials. Beyond intensive and in-depth understanding of case law and extensive training in forensic skills, the forensic specialist would work with a variety of populations (e.g., children, victims of sex offenders, sex offenders and other criminal defendants, elderly adults, and those for whom civil commitment is sought). (p. 1306)

These identified levels may serve increasingly as relevant expertise markers for practitioners of FMHA. However, it may not be sufficient to determine whether an individual has forensic training and experience in a broad sense; there may be interest as well in determining whether the clinician has training and experience in a very specific kind of evaluation. There are some kinds of forensic assessment (e.g., capital sentencing, child sexual abuse) that may be sufficiently specialized so that even experience in related kinds of FMHA may not be enough to allow the clinician to perform them without additional preparation. Such preparation could include a review of relevant literature and law, direct supervision from a clinician experienced with that issue for at least three to six evaluations, and ongoing consultation from an experienced forensic clinician as questions arise on such evaluations over the course of a year. Depending on the levels of knowledge, skill, training, and experience on the part of the supervised clinician in related areas, it could take longer to accomplish this transition—but it seems unlikely that it could be done in a shorter period of time.

DISCUSSION

There is clear agreement within the ethical standards of psychology and psychiatry about the importance of providing services only within areas of competence. A number of sources of legal authority provide definitions of expertise in the forensic context, underscoring the importance of education, training, and experience in the practice of FMHA. The limited available empirical evidence suggests that competence in FMHA is more strongly related to specific experience and training than it is to disciplinary differences, but there are no empirical studies comparing the work of clinicians of varying levels of expertise. Finally, the available literature in the area of standard of practice strongly supports the principle of providing services only in areas of competence, with more recent literature offering a better delineation of levels of competence in both substantive areas and forensic applications. Hence, this principle will be classified as *established*.

It is very likely that this principle will be sorely tested, however, in the coming decade. In the face of pressure exerted by changing patterns of third-party reimbursement for mental health services on more traditional forms of practice in psychology and psychiatry, there is a movement toward "expanding existing markets" to compensate for the loss of opportunities involving fee-for-service activities. This could be a source of significant concern. When clinicians are not appropriately trained and experienced in forensic areas, they may continue to make the kinds of errors in

FMHA that have become a recognized part of the forensic assessment literature (see, e.g., Faust & Ziskin, 1991; Grisso, 1986a; Melton et al., 1997), and played a large part in convincing some in the legal community (e.g., Bazelon, 1974, 1978) that FMHA seemed to promise far more than it could deliver.

Nonetheless, it also appears that the legal system is underserved relative to the number of available forensic specialists, or even mental health professionals proficient in FMHA. The challenge during the next decade will be to continue to expand specialized forensic training opportunities, which seem to have increased significantly during the last decade, so they are even better integrated with graduate programs and internships in psychology,[7] and residency training in psychiatry. If this can be done, then future practitioners of FMHA can be better prepared for competent practice in this area. It should also be observed that the proposal of varying levels of competence in this area (such as the "specialty/proficiency" distinction in psychology) may help to meet the needs of the legal system while allowing courts and attorneys a more straightforward way of identifying expertise. Finally, research is needed on the relation between potential "markers" of competence, such as training, experience, licensure, and board-certification, and quality of performance on FMHA tasks.

DECLINE REFERRAL WHEN EVALUATOR IMPARTIALITY IS UNLIKELY

The absence of *a priori* bias on the part of the examiner is important in most FMHA cases, but not all. This principle addresses the nature of impartiality and describes the importance of declining to perform forensic assessment in those instances in which impartiality is important, while describing the exceptional cases in which it is not. "Impartiality" is defined as the evaluator's freedom from significant interference from factors that

---

[7]For a current listing of training opportunities in clinical forensic psychology, see Vant Zelfde and Otto (1997). They cited surveys performed following the National Invitational Conference on Education and Training in Law and Psychology in which (1) graduate training programs in clinical psychology (n = 71, or the responding 47% of all programs surveyed) reported that 86% offered at least one practicum placement in which students could gain clinical forensic experience; (2) predoctoral psychology internships (n = 79, or 31% of those surveyed) reported offering at least some forensic training in 70 (89%) of these sites; and (3) postdoctoral forensic psychology fellowships (n = 10) described intensive forensic training during the fellowship year(s), but are highly competitive and typically accept only one or two trainees per year.

can result in bias.[8] Some factors are situational influences that could incline an evaluator in the direction of a given finding (e.g., a preexisting personal or professional relationship with a litigant, a financial interest in the outcome beyond usual professional fees). The beliefs and values of the individual evaluator are also important, if they might significantly influence that individual in the direction of a given finding (e.g., opposition to certain kinds of punishment, fear or anger at a certain kind of defendant or litigant based on prior experience, or an overwhelming personal reaction to the nature of the crime), or might interact with situational influences (e.g., the perception that a good deal of money can be made by providing findings favorable to a litigant whose attorney has retained the forensic clinician, and a willingness to provide such favorable findings even if doing so involves distorting, ignoring, or selectively emphasizing certain data).

ETHICS

It is difficult for a clinician to assume a forensic role with an individual when there has been a preexisting relationship between them. In this case the reasoning begins with the "dual role" problem described in the ethics codes of psychology and psychiatry. Mental health professionals are strongly discouraged from performing two separate professional roles simultaneously with a client. Dual-role relationships in the context of forensic evaluation will be discussed in detail in the next chapter.

The *Ethical Principles of Psychologists* (APA, 1992) addresses problems of dual role relationships and impartiality in the forensic context under Forensic Activities:

> In most circumstances, psychologists avoid performing multiple and potentially conflicting roles in forensic matters. When psychologists may be called on to serve in more than one role in a legal proceeding—for example, as consultant or expert for one party or for the court and as a fact witness—they clarify role expectations and the extent of confidentiality in advance to the extent feasible, and thereafter as changes occur, in order to avoid compromising their professional judgment and objectivity and in order to avoid misleading others regarding their role. (p. 1610)

[8]A related concept, "objectivity," refers to the tendency to use data that have been gathered using psychometrically reliable procedures. This can be contrasted with judgment that relies heavily on subjective impressions in gathering the information on which the decision is based. These definitions of impartiality and objectivity are consistent with those provided by others (e.g., Greenberg & Brodsky, in press). An additional concept addresses the way in which data (objective or subjective) are combined; this may be through a systematic approach, with weightings of different elements derived and refined empirically, or an approach that combines and weighs data without relying on a defined system (Sawyer, 1966).

Further elaboration is provided in the area of prior relationships:

> A prior professional relationship with a party does not preclude psychologists from testifying as fact witnesses or from testifying to their services to the extent permitted by applicable law. Psychologists appropriately take into account ways in which the prior relationship might affect their professional objectivity or opinions and disclose the potential conflict to the relevant parties.

The *Specialty Guidelines for Forensic Psychologists* (Committee on Ethical Guidelines for Forensic Psychologists, 1991) addresses the issue of impartiality in several different ways. First, in the section on Relationships, it is stressed that "prior and current personal or professional activities, obligations, and relationships that might produce a conflict of interest" are to be clarified during initial consultation with the legal representative of the party seeking services (p. 658). Potential conflicts of interest inherent in dual relationships are noted, and their effects minimized, in the following way:

> Forensic psychologists avoid providing professional services to parties in a legal proceeding with whom they have personal or professional relationships that are inconsistent with the anticipated relationship.... When it is necessary to provide both evaluation and treatment services to a party in a legal proceeding ... the forensic psychologist takes reasonable steps to minimize the potential negative effects of these circumstances on the rights of the party, confidentiality, and the process of treatment and evaluation. (p. 659)

Under the Methods and Procedures section, the issue of impartiality is addressed somewhat differently:

> In providing forensic psychological services, forensic psychologists take special care to avoid undue influence upon their methods, procedures, and products, such as might emanate from the party to a legal proceeding by financial compensation or other gains. As an expert conducting an evaluation, treatment, consultation, or scholarly/empirical investigation, the forensic psychologist maintains professional integrity by examining the issue at hand from all reasonable perspectives, actively seeking information that will differentially test plausible rival hypotheses. (p. 661).

On the topic of "contingent fees," it is clearly indicated that

> Forensic psychologists do not provide professional services to parties to a legal proceeding on the basis of "contingent fees," when those services involve the offering of expert testimony to a court or administrative body, or when they call upon the psychologist to make affirmations or representations intended to be relied upon by third parties. (p. 659)

The *Principles of Medical Ethics with Annotations Especially Applicable to Psychiatry* (American Psychiatric Association, 1998) does not address the issue of impartiality in evaluations directly or indirectly. There is no section of these *Principles* that is devoted primarily to assessment or forensic work of any kind, however.

The *Ethical Guidelines for the Practice of Forensic Psychiatry* (AAPL, 1995) devotes much of an entire section ("Honesty and Striving for Objectivity") to the issue of objectivity:

> Forensic psychiatrists function as an expert within the legal process. Although they may be retained by one party to a dispute in civil matter or the prosecution or defense in a criminal matter, they adhere to the principles of honesty and they strive for objectivity. Their clinical evaluation and the application of the data obtained to the legal criteria are performed in the spirit of such honesty and efforts to attain objectivity. Their opinion reflects this honesty and efforts to attain objectivity. (p. 3)

In the Commentary in this Section, it is further noted that

> It is the responsibility of forensic psychiatrists to minimize such hazards (to unintended bias and the danger of distortion of opinion) by carrying out their responsibilities in an honest manner striving to reach an objective opinion.
>
> Practicing forensic psychiatrists enhance the honesty and objectivity of their work by basing their forensic opinions, forensic reports and forensic testimony on all the data available to them. They communicate the honesty of their work, efforts to attain objectivity, and the soundness of their clinical opinion by distinguishing, to the extent possible, between verified and unverified information as well as between clinical "facts," "inferences" and "impressions."
>
> ... Honesty, objectivity, and the adequacy of the clinical evaluation may be called into question when an expert opinion is offered without a personal examination.... it is the position of the Academy that if, after earnest effort, it is not possible to conduct a personal examination, an opinion may be rendered on the basis of other information. However, under such circumstances, it is the responsibility of the forensic psychiatrist to assure that the statement of their opinion and any reports of testimony based on this opinion clearly indicate that there was no personal examination and the opinion expressed is thereby limited.
>
> ... Contingency fees, because of the problems that these create in regard to honesty and striving for objectivity, should not be accepted. On the other hand, retainer fees do not create problems in regard to honesty and striving for objectivity and, therefore, may be accepted.
>
> Treating psychiatrists should generally avoid agreeing to be an expert witness or to perform an evaluation of their patients for legal purposes because a forensic evaluation usually requires that other people be interviewed and testimony may adversely affect the therapeutic relationship. (p. 3)

LAW

Any witness in a court of law must take an oath to tell "the truth, the whole truth, and nothing but the truth" prior to testifying. The "whole truth" suggests that information and conclusions should be presented to incorporate both supportive and nonsupportive data. Since forensic evaluation reports may provide the basis for testimony in some cases, but serve as evidence even when testimony is not provided, it is reasonable to assume that this obligation to convey the truth should apply to reports as well as testimony.

The value placed on "impartiality" may vary for different roles that a forensic clinician or a behavioral scientist can play in the course of the forensic evaluation. First, the forensic clinician can function as an evaluator—someone who will (1) perform an assessment after receiving an order from the court or a request from one of the parties, (2) submit a report, and (3), if necessary, testify about the results of the evaluation. If the order comes from the court, then the role can be described as that of "court-appointed expert."

Second, if the request is made by one of the parties in the litigation, the forensic clinician's role is that of "defense/prosecution/plaintiff's expert." There is no meaningful difference between the first and second roles in the expectation of impartiality in FMHA assessment, report-writing, and testimony; the most important difference concerns to whom the results are communicated, and who controls whether these results are introduced in litigation.[9]

Third, a psychologist or psychiatrist may also testify as a behavioral scientist, and address questions raised by the case that may be answered by the scientific literature, without reference to the characteristics of the litigant.[10] Impartiality is highly valued as part of the roles of evaluator or scientist as expert, which have the associated assumption that the expert will be able (and willing) to provide accurate information to the court; such impartiality is enhanced when the expert has no apparent reason for distorting such information.[11]

[9]In most jurisdictions, procedural and evidentiary law allows the party requesting the FMHA provided in the "defense/prosecution/plaintiff's expert" role to review the evaluation results and decide whether they will be introduced in litigation, when the evaluation is authorized by the court in this role. Of course, litigants who can afford to do so are always free to retain their own evaluative experts, who would again function in this role. Both of these circumstances should be distinguished from the evaluation that is requested by a party but ordered by the court, with the stipulation that results be communicated to both parties and the court simultaneously. The latter is an example of a court-ordered evaluation, as discussed in this chapter.

[10]The role of scientist is one that may be played by researchers who are not clinicians. Such researchers may testify regarding various aspects of social, cognitive, developmental, and human experimental psychology, or regarding biological, genetic, or pharmacological issues in psychiatry, for example.

[11]For certain forensic issues, there are scientific positions that are strongly debated, and those representing them might not appear "impartial." Research on recovered memories is a good example. However, the same kind of analysis might be applied to determining the credibility attached to such testimony. If a psychologist or psychiatrist, testifying as a scientist, could acknowledge that the question is strongly debated and describe the studies in support of each position, then we might consider that person reasonably impartial even if his position was strongly in one direction or another. However, when such testimony not only reflected a strongly held position but failed to acknowledge important arguments and data favoring the opposite position, then impartiality would seem to be insufficient.

Fourth, the mental health professional can be a *consultant*, who *assists* an attorney. Since the primary purpose of the expert's role in this process is to assist the attorney rather than present information to the court, impartiality is less important and probably not necessary.[12] Nonetheless, impartiality in this context remains valuable. A consultant can best assist an attorney by maintaining a balanced viewpoint, which increases the likelihood of seeing issues that can help the other side. In seeing such issues, the consultant can help the attorney anticipate challenges to the evidence and strategies that the attorney plans to use.

A final possible role for a mental health professional is that of *fact witness*. A fact witness is not considered to be an "expert witness." The law's definition of an "expert" is typically one who is qualified, by virtue of knowledge, skill, experience, training, or education, to provide opinions to the court (*Federal Rules of Evidence*, Rule 702). In contrast, a fact witness is allowed to testify only to direct observations, and is not permitted to express an opinion or conclusion in the way that an expert witness can. However, whether a clinician serves as an expert in a given case should depend not only on whether that clinician meets the enumerated criteria for expertise. It should also depend on the *role* assumed by the clinician *in this particular case*. For example, a clinician who has worked with a couple and their child in family therapy and is asked to provide testimony regarding a custody issue with the children in that family should find it difficult to be objective in this case due to the preexisting therapeutic relationship. In such a case, if testimony cannot be avoided altogether (through attempts to clarify with the family, the attorney, and the court about the nature of the therapeutic relationship and the need to preserve it, and through referral to other mental health professionals who could perform a forensic assessment on the child custody issue in question), then the treating clinician could choose to testify only as a fact witness. This would involve testimony only about the clinician's observations from therapy and those involved, and avoid drawing any conclusions regarding the fitness of the respective parents or the best interest of the child, as the latter are components of the legal decision that is before the court.

Empirical

There is very little empirical research on the role of impartiality in FMHA. This is unfortunate, given the importance attached to the perfor-

---

[12]For reasons described in this book and also discussed at length elsewhere (Committee on Ethical Guidelines for Forensic Psychologists, 1991; Greenberg & Shuman, 1997; Heilbrun, 1995), these roles usually should not be combined in a single case.

mance of forensic clinicians and the perception (at least among the general public) that some experts are for sale to the highest bidder. However, it is not surprising, given how difficult it would be to do such research. One study (Kennedy, Kelley, & Homant, 1985), designed to test this "hired gun" hypothesis, surveyed 501 psychiatrists and 501 clinical psychologists and received responses from 26% of those surveyed. As reported by the respondents, prior "defense experience" correlated highly ($r = .78$) with prior "prosecution experience," leading the authors to suggest that clinicians could not readily be classified as working primarily for the defense or the prosecution. One problem with this study was the low return rate, which limits the generalizability of these findings. A second problem is that this correlation does not fairly test the "hired gun" hypothesis. A preferable way of doing so would involve the use of the ratio of

$$\frac{\text{Evaluations yielding favorable findings to the referring source}}{\text{Total number of evaluations}}$$

(comparable to Colbach's "Contrary Quotient," discussed in the next subsection). Given that social desirability would clearly affect the reporting of these numbers by clinicians, it would be preferable (although far more difficult) for researchers to examine products (e.g., reports or testimony) rather than self-reported descriptions.

STANDARD OF PRACTICE

Dual-role relationships are not conducive to high quality forensic evaluations. One of the important reasons for this is the absence of impartiality associated with having a previous or present therapeutic relationship with the individual to be evaluated, making it more difficult to perform a forensic evaluation without preexisting inclinations. Moreover, therapeutic assessment cannot substitute for FMHA. Forensic assessment is sufficiently different from therapeutic assessment so that even a good therapeutic assessment will not necessarily provide a reasonable basis for drawing conclusions relevant in forensic assessment. One implication of such differences is that therapeutic and forensic assessments do not yield results that can be used interchangeably. For both ethical and "effectiveness" reasons, therefore, it is better for a clinician who cannot avoid involvement in litigation with a current or former patient to assume the role of fact witness, in which the absence of impartiality will not be problematic in the same way. This preserves the preexisting therapeutic relationship, helps ensure the accuracy of the information that is provided to the court, and avoids potential dual-role ethical problems (Greenberg & Shuman, 1997; Heilbrun, 1995).

One possible *a priori* test of an evaluator's potential impartiality in a given case would capitalize on the dichotomous nature of legal decision-making, and involve a two-part question in which the expert should ask: (1) what would be the effect on me if the outcome of the case were A, and (2) what would be the effect on me if the outcome were B? Any clear imbalance in the answers to these two questions would suggest that impartiality will be difficult to achieve in that case.

A second test of impartiality has also been proposed to measure how well a forensic clinician has managed the pressures that can be exerted by the referring sources, anxious to have a favorable opinion from the expert. This test uses the "Contrary Quotient," a fraction whose numerator is defined by the number of times the clinician has reached an opinion unfavorable to the referring source and the denominator the total number of times an opinion has been requested, yielding a percentage estimate (Colbach, 1981). This is a more relevant measure of impartiality than the simple count of "how many times the expert has testified for the (defense, prosecution, plaintiff)." Using the latter measure can be misleading because an expert may be asked to testify more often by one side than another; moreover, the expert may provide an opinion favorable to the side that has requested it in only a fraction of the cases in which any involvement was requested, and simply never testify in the others. The frequency of testimony can be a misleading indicator for two reasons, then: (1) It may not accurately reflect the number of times the expert's findings have favored the requesting party (report findings may be accepted by the court without testimony on stipulation of both parties) and (2) it fails to incorporate the times an expert has reached findings that are not favorable to the referring party, and thus not been asked to testify in that case.[13]

An example regarding how these two measures could yield different results is useful. Assume that a forensic clinician was involved in evaluating 100 individuals on the issue of criminal responsibility, and that all of these referrals came from the defense (most from the public defender's office). Assume further that, under the legal standards of that state, only the defense received a copy of the results unless and until the defendant filed notice of intent to rely on the defense of insanity. Finally, assume that 10 of these reports described results supportive of a defense of insanity at the time of the offense and the remaining 90 would not support a defense argument for insanity. In this example, if the forensic clinician testified for the defense in all 10 of the cases in which results were supportive of

---

[13]The contrary quotient is less applicable in cases in which the referring party is the court, and a report will be written and testimony possibly given regardless of the expert's findings.

insanity, then she would have returned an "unfavorable" result to the referring source far more often than a "favorable" one (9/1 ratio under the first test), but testified for the defense more often than for the prosecution (10 versus 0 times, under the second test). A good test of impartiality must therefore incorporate the frequency of referrals from each side to be accurate.

There is another consideration as well. If the court or a state agency in this example were conscientious about collecting data on the frequency of recommended outcomes for such referrals, then the clinician reading these results over several years would be aware that 5–10% of referrals for sanity evaluations resulted in a recommendation for insanity in states that track this information (Warren & Fitch, 1993). She should not be troubled by her own base rate of 10%, therefore, as it is reasonably consistent with the results of the evaluations of all forensic clinicians over several years (and hence the best available estimate of the "true" base rate for insanity among referred defendants). However, if this clinician were recommending to referring attorneys that 50 of the 100 defendants she evaluated be considered insane, then this could represent a problem with objectivity that would not be measured well by either of the previous tests. This might suggest the need for a two-part test of impartiality: (1) a reasonable balance between favorable and unfavorable results rendered to referring sources and (2) reasonable consistency with available base rates.

For the role of consultant, impartiality is not required (although it may be helpful), and this principle would not apply to the same extent. However, when a forensic clinician performs an evaluation that yields a report and possibly testimony, or a behavioral scientist reports on the "state of the science" relevant to a legal issue, then impartiality *is* important.[14] Most applicable ethics codes, in emphasizing this, leave it to the individual to determine what is involved in "impartiality."[15] There is an emerging view

[14]A large part of the controversy over works by Ziskin and Faust (Faust & Ziskin, 1991; Ziskin & Faust, 1988) stems from a misunderstanding about how they should most appropriately be considered. Since these works were developed to assist attorneys and do not aspire to impartiality, they should properly be considered "consultations" rather than "science" or "learned treatises." However, the responsibility for some of this misperception may be attributed to the authors, who have published these ideas in *Science* (Faust & Ziskin, 1988) and made insufficiently clear that they should be considered as advocacy rather than science.

[15]The terms *impartiality* and *objectivity* are often used interchangeably in the literature. This may reflect the reality that either impartiality (defined here as relative freedom from bias) or objectivity (defined as tending to rely on data collected in a certain way, rather than global judgment or impressions), when impaired, can adversely affect the substantive accuracy of conclusions from FMHA.

in the professional literature that dual-role relationships in forensic assessment (as in many other professional activities) are to be avoided, but clearly the absence of requisite impartiality is not the only concern about such dual-role relationships. Nonetheless, given the value of impartiality in the forensic context, it should be viewed as one important influence on the way in which forensic assessment is done.

If the forensic clinician or behavioral scientist plays a role in which impartiality is important, then it is that individual's responsibility to ensure that personal values or circumstances do not preclude such impartiality. When this happens in a single case, then the solution is straightforward: decline the referral and provide the names of colleagues who would not have the same conflict on this case. When it encompasses a class of cases,[16] then the clinician should consider avoiding any involvement in such cases.

DISCUSSION

The impartiality of a clinician involved in FMHA is valued highly on ethical grounds, and the value is implicitly recognized in law. However, the classification of this principle must be conditional, since the importance of impartiality may vary according to the role played. Because of the importance of impartiality on ethical grounds, it seems appropriate to classify this as an *established* principle *for the roles of court-appointed evaluator* and for *defense, prosecution, or plaintiff-requested evaluator who will testify (not consult).* For the role of *scientist*, the importance of impartiality is unclear, as there is some argument that the court should be able to hear about the results of scientific studies or theories that may be strongly debated within the scientific community. Impartiality as a principle in the role of scientist in FMHA, therefore, will be considered to be *neither established nor emerging.* Impartiality seems comparably unimportant for the role of consultant. Litigation preparation requires that an attorney be aware of the range and quality of all relevant evidence. However, the results of the mental health professional's consultation will be communicated informally to the attorney, rather than through testimony. Consequently, there is less demand for

---

[16]A recent example of such a class of cases might involve personal injury litigation resulting from repressed memories of sexual abuse. Because of the strong polarization of the field on the issues of the frequency and validity of such memories, and the possibility that they can be "implanted" through certain therapeutic techniques, many clinicians have adopted a strong stance, either "pro" or "con," in this debate. Such clinicians would probably find it very difficult to evaluate a single case of "repressed memory" without their position affecting the outcome of their evaluation.

impartiality in the communication of results, since this communication may be combined with recommendations for presentation of this material as evidence. For the role of the consultant, therefore, this principle will again be considered *neither established nor emerging*. It is important to note that there is little research on the concept of impartiality—its meaning, impact, or correlates—in FMHA. This deficit must be addressed. Finally, it should be added that fees (particularly contingent fees) are a potentially important source of bias that will be discussed in detail later in this chapter, in the principle "Clarify Financial Arrangements."

CLARIFY ROLE WITH ATTORNEY

Determining the purpose of the forensic evaluation is a vital step in conducting the evaluation and presenting its results properly. Attorneys are frequently the source of referrals for such evaluations and a constant presence throughout, so it is important that the forensic clinician clarify expectations in a given case from the beginning.

The four possible roles for mental health professionals in the forensic assessment context—court-appointed, defense/prosecution/plaintiff's expert, consultant, and fact witness—were discussed in the previous section. The first question involves which of these roles will be assumed by the forensic clinician in the immediate case. Having already determined the relevant forensic issues and whether the evaluation of these issues is within his area of expertise, the forensic clinician is then able to discuss with the attorney which of these roles will be assumed.

ETHICS

The APA *Ethical Principles* (1992) addresses the issue of role selection in two sections. First, it is noted that

> When a psychologist agrees to provide services to a person or entity at the request of a third party, the psychologist clarifies to the extent feasible, at the outset of the service, the nature of the relationship with each party. This clarification includes the role of the psychologist (such as therapist, organizational consultant, diagnostician, or expert witness), the probable uses of the services provided or the information obtained, and the fact that there may be limits to confidentiality. (p. 1602)
>
> If there is a foreseeable risk of the psychologist's being called upon to perform conflicting roles because of the involvement of a third party, the psychologist clarifies the nature and direction of his or her responsibilities, keeps all parties appropriately informed as matters develop, and resolves the situation in accordance with this Ethics Code. (p. 1602)

Second, under role clarification in Forensic Activities:

> In most circumstances, psychologists avoid performing multiple and potentially conflicting roles in forensic matters. When psychologists may be called on to serve in more than one role in a legal proceeding—for example, as consultant or expert for one party or for the court and as a fact witness—they clarify role expectations and the extent of confidentiality in advance to the extent feasible, and thereafter as changes occur, in order to avoid compromising their professional judgement and objectivity and in order to avoid misleading others regarding their role. (p. 1610)

The *Specialty Guidelines for Forensic Psychologists* (Committee on Ethical Guidelines for Forensic Psychologists, 1991), however, does not address the matter of initial role clarification directly. It does describe an "initial consultation with the legal representative of the party seeking services" (p. 658), in which the forensic psychologist is obliged to inform that party of considerations that might affect the decision to contract with the psychologist. These considerations include fee structure, prior and current relationships that might produce a conflict of interest, areas of competence and the limits of competence, and the known scientific bases and limitations of the procedures that would be employed. While there is no specific reference to the issue of role clarification, one can assume that additional factors can be discussed during initial consultation; such factors could include role clarification.

The *Principles of Medical Ethics with Annotations* (American Psychiatric Association, 1998) does not describe the issue of role clarification with the attorney directly. However, Section 2 ("A physician shall deal honestly with patients and colleagues, and strive to expose those physicians deficient in character or competence, or who engage in fraud or deception") states that:

> Psychiatric services, like all medical services, are dispensed in the context of a contractual arrangement between the patient and the treating physician. The provisions of the contractual agreement, which are binding on the physician as well as on the patient, should be explicitly established. (p. 3)

The *Ethical Guidelines for the Practice of Forensic Psychiatry* (AAPL, 1995) does not address the matter of initial role clarification, either directly or indirectly.

LAW

When the role has been determined, there are several immediate consequences. A primary consideration is whether "impartiality" or "assisting the attorney" will be paramount. A related consideration involves how the findings will be communicated: whether a written report will be generated, whether findings will be discussed with the attorney prior to writing the report, and whether the attorney will have the authority to decline such a report.

Some attorneys do not recognize a clear distinction between the "impartial evaluator" (often termed "objective evaluator") and "defense assistant" roles. The failure to distinguish these roles is apparent in *Ake v. Oklahoma* (1985), in which the Court described the role of the "defense expert" in litigation as follows:

> Without a psychiatrist's assistance to conduct a professional examination on issues relevant to the insanity defense, to help determine whether that defense is viable, to present testimony, and to assist in preparing the cross-examination of the State's psychiatric witnesses, the risk of an accurate resolution of sanity issues is extremely high. (p. 69)

Despite the Court's language in *Ake*, however, there are good arguments against combining the roles of objective evaluator and consultant. The fact finder should be able to expect that expert witnesses called by either side will provide accurate, balanced testimony. This is more difficult for an expert when the roles are combined, suggesting that one tells the truth, but only in a way that benefits the individual on whose behalf you are testifying. The obvious problem produced by this blending of roles will be apparent to the courts in many instances, creating a related credibility problem for the expert. When courts perceive such a credibility problem, this produces genuine difficulty for the FMHA field *regardless of the accuracy of this perception*. This comment pertains mostly to the *substance* of an expert's testimony, that is, the expert has a responsibility to describe findings that are inconsistent with, as well as those supportive of, the conclusions that have been reached.

It has less to do with the *style* of the testimony, however. It would not preclude an expert from testifying firmly and vigorously about conclusions, assuming that expert has reached such conclusions based on a thorough evaluation and considered the relevant information in an impartial and objective fashion. It is this impartiality that is at risk, however, when the expert agrees to serve as both evaluator and consultant. It is not reasonable to expect that an expert can alternate consistently between the goals of "evaluating and presenting the results of this evaluation impartially" (albeit vigorously) and "helping the client with the case." Yet this is precisely what would need to occur if the mental health professional were to effectively play both roles simultaneously.

In criminal law, one important consideration in *Estelle v. Smith* (1981) was the failure of the court and the psychiatrist to clarify his role as involving the evaluation of both a pretrial issue (competence to stand trial) and a postconviction issue (future dangerousness). If this had been clarified in advance through a court order specifying both issues and provided to the defendant through notification of the nature of the evaluation, then it might not have been necessary for the U.S. Supreme Court to establish the need for a warning about the right to remain silent as part of mental health evaluation in the context of capital sentencing. When the role is clarified *and* documentation for that role established through court order, then forensic mental health testimony is unlikely for a defendant who (like Mr. Smith, the defendant in this case) does not initiate or attempt to introduce mental health evidence.

If the clinician assumes the role of the impartial evaluator doing a court-ordered evaluation, then typically several steps will follow. Often these steps are specified in the relevant statutes or administrative code of the jurisdiction. It usually means that the forensic clinician will write a report describing the results of the evaluation, submit the report to the court and both attorneys,[17] and be prepared to testify about these results if subpoenaed by either side. In many jurisdictions, the clinician assumes this role on receipt of a court order specifying the legal issue(s) to be evaluated. When this happens, then "role clarification" has already occurred and usually further discussion is not necessary. The report can be submitted to the court, the defense, and the prosecution, unless the relevant legal authority (e.g., the court order, statutes, administrative code, or case law) indicates otherwise.

The role of the *defense expert* can be more complex. The clinician must strive for impartiality in the evaluation process when a report and possible testimony are expected. In some jurisdictions, however, the defense can veto the writing of a report by the defense expert if the obtained results are not favorable. If this occurs, there should be no further expectation that the forensic clinician would provide expert testimony. In such cases, it would not seem problematic for the forensic clinician subsequently to assume the role of consultant, assisting the defense in the preparation of its case, and providing strategies for the cross-examination of opposing experts. It would be contraindicated to change roles in the opposite direction, however, moving from consultant to impartial evaluator. Once the forensic

---

[17]Variations in the practice of submitting court-ordered evaluations occur between jurisdictions. In some states (e.g., Massachusetts), the forensic clinician submits the court-ordered report to the court, and the court provides it to the attorneys. On the issue of sanity at the time of the offense, some states (e.g., Massachusetts, Virginia) do not allow the prosecutor to receive a report containing a description of this issue unless the defense has filed notice of intent to rely on the defense of insanity.

clinician has committed to assisting the attorney, it would be very difficult to return to the "balanced" stance required for impartial evaluation and testimony.

EMPIRICAL

No empirical research has been located on the topic of clarifying the forensic clinician's role in advance in relation to the referring attorney.

STANDARD OF PRACTICE

On the question of role selection and clarification, Emery and Rogers (1990) have observed that behavior therapists face several role choices about their involvement in child custody litigation. They identify "evaluator," "mediator," and "therapist" as three possibilities, and discuss the advisability of defining a single role "from the outset" and remaining in that role throughout.

A somewhat different view is offered by Halleck (1980). Although he emphasizes the importance of initially clarifying a number of issues with the attorney (e.g., the legal issue, the fee, and the place and conditions of examination), he also describes how multiple roles (such as consultant and impartial evaluator) can be played until the time of testimony, when he recommends that only one role, impartial evaluator, be assumed. During testimony, Halleck emphasizes that it is crucial for the expert to be impartial and provide relevant information to the court. This is consistent with my comments earlier in this section. Where Halleck and I diverge on this issue (cf. Emery & Rogers, 1990, as well) is in his view that the roles of both consultant and impartial evaluator can be simultaneously performed prior to testimony.

DISCUSSION

It would seem reasonable to clarify one's role initially in any professional circumstance, including forensic assessment. Yet explicit role clarification is not needed for many of the professional functions performed by psychologists and psychiatrists, because of the implicit assumptions shared by clinician and patient. In FMHA, however, the implicit assumptions made in treatment cases may not apply at all, or to the same extent. The blurring of roles, or the assumption of multiple roles, are among the most frequent bases for ethics complaints against psychologists in custody cases, for example. It should be apparent that role clarification is important in FMHA, and helpful to the forensic clinician (in conceptualizing *which* role is to be played) as well as to the court, attorneys, and individual(s) being evaluated.

However, it should also be clear that the sources of authority that are relevant to this principle are not consistent in this regard. This principle has mixed or indirect support in both ethical and legal areas. No empirical research was located on this topic. There is some disagreement among those discussing the need for role clarification as part of standard of practice. Thus, this principle will be classified as *emerging* at present. It remains an area in which important conceptual and empirical work is needed in coming years, if the field is to reach a better consensus on whether this principle should be established.

CLARIFY FINANCIAL ARRANGEMENTS

As part of the initial agreement of evaluation details, it is important to determine who will pay for the forensic clinician's services, and at what rate. Most independent clinicians and agencies have a standard hourly rate or a sliding scale for professional services. If this rate differs by type of service (e.g., therapy versus forensic evaluation), then the clinician should be prepared to explain the reason for this difference. Additionally, some forensic clinicians charge a higher rate for testimony than for other components of forensic evaluation services. A convincing explanation for this practice should also be prepared, as this information can be elicited during cross-examination to impugn the expert's impartiality.

Under some circumstances, it may be preferable to have the fee arrangements (as well as other provisions relevant to the forensic evaluation) addressed in a written document. This is not necessary when the responsibility for payment rests with the court, following the completion of a court-ordered evaluation. It can become more important in cases in which the forensic clinician is privately retained, either as an evaluator or as a consultant, and there is need for a clear, written agreement.

Such an agreement should address several areas. These include (1) the nature of services to be provided by the forensic clinician, (2) the estimated hours and time period, and the provisions if the services cannot be per- formed within these estimates, (3) the hourly rate for services, and whether the rate will differ for different services (see earlier discussion), (4) who will be responsible for payment, (5) any special financial consid- erations (such as whether reimbursement of fee and expenses will be interim or only on final completion of all services, or whether an escrow account will be established), and (6) the anticipated products (e.g., verbal consultation, report, testimony).

It is possible to have compensation provided for performing FMHA as part of a job with a court clinic, community mental health center, or hospital. This kind of compensation is beyond the scope of the principles being described in this principle, as salaried positions do not require the clarification of financial arrangements for FMHA on a case by case basis. Other than to salary, there are three major sources of reimbursement for a forensic evaluation: the court itself, the referring attorney, and the individual who is being evaluated. Each will be discussed in this section.

ETHICS

In the section entitled "Fees and Financial Arrangements," the *Ethical Principles of Psychologists* (APA, 1992) indicate that

> As early as is feasible in a professional or scientific relationship, the psychologist and the patient, client, or other appropriate recipient of psychological services reach an agreement specifying the compensation and the billing arrangements. (p. 1602)

The *Specialty Guidelines for Forensic Psychologists* (Committee on Ethical Guidelines for Forensic Psychologists, 1991) allude to the issue of fee clarification in two ways. During initial consultation with the legal representative of the party seeking services, the forensic psychologist is obligated to inform the party of a number of factors that might affect the decision to contract with the psychologist. The first consideration on the list of factors is "the fee structure for anticipated services" (p. 658). It should also be noted that forensic psychologists

> do not provide professional services to parties to a legal proceeding on the basis of "contingent fees" (p. 659)

and

> who derive a substantial portion of their income from fee-for-service arrangements should offer some portion of their professional services on a pro bono or reduced fee basis where the public interest or the welfare of clients may be inhibited by insufficient financial resources. (p. 659)

The *Principles of Medical Ethics with Annotations* (American Psychiatric Association, 1998) provides a framework within which the initial discussion of fee with an attorney can occur. In Section 2, in which physicians "shall deal honestly with patients and colleagues," there are several relevant subsections:

> Psychiatric services, like all medical services, are dispensed in the context of a contractual arrangement between the patient and the treating physician. The provisions of the contractual arrangement, which are binding on the physician as well as on the patient, should be explicitly established.

It is ethical for the psychiatrist to make a charge for a missed appointment when this falls within the terms of the specific contractual agreement with the patient ....

An arrangement in which a psychiatrist provides supervision or administration to other physicians or nonmedical persons for a percentage of their fees or gross income is not acceptable; this would constitute fee-splitting. In a team of practitioners, or a multidisciplinary team, it is ethical for the psychiatrist to receive income for administration, research, education, or consultation. This should be based upon a mutually agreed upon and set fee or salary, open to renegotiation when a change in the time demand occurs. (p. 3)

The *Ethical Guidelines for the Practice of Forensic Psychiatry* (AAPL, 1995) assesses fees under the section on Honesty and Striving for Objectivity. In the Commentary in this section, it is observed that

Contingency fees, because of the problems that these create in regard to honesty and efforts to obtain objectivity, should not be accepted. On the other hand, retainer fees do not create problems in regard to honesty and efforts to obtain objectivity and, therefore, may be accepted. (p. 3)

LAW

There is a useful discussion of the compensation of court-appointed experts in the *Reference Manual on Scientific Evidence* (Federal Judicial Center, 1994). In criminal cases, [*Federal Rules of Evidence* 706(b); 18 U.S.C. Sec. 3006(e), 1988] permits payment of experts' fees from public funds.[18] In other litigation contexts, however, the court appoints an expert with the expectation that a report and/or testimony will possibly result, but the expert's compensation is paid by the parties involved in the litigation, in a manner directed by the court. Under Rule 706(b), court-appointed experts are entitled to "reasonable compensation" in "whatever sum the court may allow." The federal court also has the discretion to order a single party to pay in advance the full cost of appointing an expert (*McKinney v. Anderson*, 1991; *Helling v. McKinney*, 1991). Most judges require parties in civil litigation to split the expert's fee (Cecil & Willging, 1994), with some courts having expert fees split equally between the parties (*United States v. Michigan*, 1987; *Unique Concepts, Inc. v. Brown*, 1987) and others basing the percentage paid on the outcome of the case (*In re Fleshman*, 1987).

The mechanisms for paying experts in the federal court system reflect some variability in the amount and approach to compensation, typically subject to the court's discretion. For these reasons, it is important to clarify

[18]In criminal cases in which the United States is a party, the source of this payment is the Department of Justice, not the U.S. Courts (*In re Payment of Court-Appointed Expert Witness*, 1980).

the fee arrangements in advance of services being delivered. It seems reasonable to expect that this pattern of variation in reimbursement according to the nature of the case and subject to the court's discretion will be observed in other jurisdictions, except for those specifying a fixed amount for a specific kind of evaluation. When such *fee specification* is in effect in a given jurisdiction, then fee clarification is largely unnecessary.

EMPIRICAL

No research is available at present on the issues of fee clarification, fee setting, or the impact of professional fees on the process of FMHA.

STANDARD OF PRACTICE

When the forensic clinician assumes the role of court-ordered evaluator, then compensation is typically authorized by the court when the evaluation is completed. The amount authorized can vary considerably between states, and even between different jurisdictions within the same state (Grisso, Cocozza, Steadman, Fisher, & Greer, 1994).[19] Often there is an accepted rate for such evaluations. If the rate is fixed under statute or administrative code, then it requires no further clarification. Billing in excess of this fixed rate should be done only with prior authorization from the court, however, regardless of the time invested in the evaluation. The failure to obtain such prior authorization can result in significant problems in reimbursement in the requested amount. Possible outcomes under this circumstance have included the refusal of the court to authorize any payment beyond what is statutorily prescribed, eventual authorization but after lengthy delay and written justification, and the judge's perception that the forensic clinician is inexperienced, dishonest, or greedy.

It becomes more complex when billing is done according to time rather than for a prescribed total. Judges rely on their experience with such evaluations to determine an "acceptable range" for reimbursement, but the limits of this range may be unstated. They become known when the clinician bills beyond this range, however. For some judges, the upper limits of this range can be low. Conversely, some clinicians may present a

[19]In Florida, for example, where pretrial criminal forensic evaluations are conducted primarily by independent practitioners, the reimbursement for an evaluation of trial competence in Miami is $150; in Tampa, it is $300 in the city and $400 in the adjoining counties. In Virginia, by contrast, most of the pretrial criminal forensic evaluations are done by community mental health centers or at a forensic unit in a centrally located state hospital. The rate at which such evaluations are reimbursed varies according to the legal issue being assessed: trial competence ($200), sanity at the time of the offense ($300), or both ($400).

bill that is unreasonably high, given the demands of the particular case. This kind of circumstance can require further fee clarification. For a variety of reasons, the question of fee amount may be most appropriately discussed with attorneys who often appear before this particular judge, and other forensic clinicians who have performed evaluations for this court.

The second possible source of funding for forensic evaluation is the attorney. This is the usual source when the evaluator assumes the role of defense expert[20] (in the criminal context), or is retained to conduct an evaluation on behalf of the plaintiff or defendant (in civil litigation). Important questions to be discussed during "fee clarification" in such cases include the forensic clinician's hourly rate, the anticipated time involved, when the work can be conducted, whether there will be special provisions for billing for travel and "waiting" time, and whether testimony time will be billed at the same rate as other time.

It is not unusual for clinicians to bill at a higher rate for time associated with testimony than for the other activities involved with forensic mental health assessment. Some of the reasons that have been cited for this practice include the added stress of testimony (particularly cross-examination), the inconvenience of having to adjust one's schedule to be available for testimony, and the creation of a financial incentive to courts to accept a written report rather than in-person testimony. There is no clear legal impediment to this practice, except in states that provide a flat expert witness fee regardless of the duration of the testimony.

However, there may be ethical difficulties with charging a higher rate for an activity that is clearly an integral part of the forensic evaluation. Such a practice could create an incentive for the forensic clinician to engage in more frequent testimony. Just as contingency reimbursement is ethically unacceptable because it creates a financial incentive for the clinician to reach a given conclusion, the practice of billing at a higher rate for testimony could be seen as an incentive to testify more often. Increasing the probability that a forensic clinician will be called to testify can be done in a number of ways: A report that is short or vague, a comment to an attorney about information that is not provided in the report, or a willingness to provide case consultation as well as testimony are only a few. For reasons discussed throughout this book, each of these actions is problematic for reasons beyond artificially increasing the probability of testimony in a given case.

---

[20]In some states, the implementation of *Ake v. Oklahoma* (1985) has resulted in a statutory provision for the appointment of a defense expert at state expense. In such jurisdictions, the forensic clinician functioning as a defense expert in a given case would be reimbursed through the court rather than the defense attorney's office.

There is also the related problem of the perception of courts, attorneys, and juries, as well as the media and the general public, regarding this practice. Forensic mental health professionals are already burdened with the media-enhanced public perception that they are "hired guns," available to the highest bidder, whose primary activity is to provide testimony in high-profile cases. In this context, it is difficult to provide a coherent rationale to a judge or jury for why an already-substantial professional rate would need to be increased. None of the reasons that have been described—greater stress or inconvenience for the clinician, or the desire to avoid testimony—seem convincing. One risk in charging higher rates for testimony involves the possibility that the judge, jury, or general public will conclude that the reason for the higher rate is, simply, that the professional can charge it with impunity. Even worse, they could conclude that the testimony is "bought." When a forensic clinician does not have a good explanation for this practice, it may affect her credibility adversely.

When cases are referred by the attorney, it is important that it be understood, either through oral or written agreement, that the responsibility for payment is with that attorney. Funding for the expert's evaluation may be obtained by the attorney from another source (e.g., public funds provided under court order for a defense evaluation in a death penalty case, or payment from the attorney's client in a child custody dispute). However, it should not become the forensic clinician's responsibility to seek this payment.[21] It should be authorized (if a court order is necessary) or deposited in escrow (if the attorney's client is paying) before the evaluation is begun, unless the forensic clinician is confident that the fee will be paid regardless of the results of the evaluation. Fees and reimbursement procedures should be established through the initial consultation between the mental health professional and the attorney in such cases (Blau, 1984b; Halleck, 1980).

To do otherwise—to make the forensic clinician responsible for collecting the fee—would create a clear conflict between the need to be impartial and the need to be paid. When it is perceived that favorable findings are linked with subsequent reimbursement, it becomes much more difficult for the clinician to remain balanced. In a related vein, the use of third party reimbursement from the client's insurance company, promised to the forensic clinician in anticipation of the evaluation's completion, is problematic for two reasons: (1) The client may be reluctant to submit

---

[21]In some states, the administrative rules provide for payment to defense experts in criminal cases through a procedure that is similar to payment for other court-ordered evaluations. Under these circumstances, it may not be necessary to have the attorney guarantee payment.

authorization for payment or (2) the company may refuse to authorize payment because mental health evaluation for "court purposes" is not reimbursable under the policy.

Finally, a financial arrangement in which the forensic clinician provides evaluation and possibly testimony on a "contingent" basis, with the amount of the fee dependent on the outcome of the case, is both unethical (see Ethics, this principle) and strongly discouraged by those describing indicated forensic practice (Blau, 1984b; Shapiro, 1991). A clear and powerful conflict of interest is created by such an arrangement for clinicians who must remain impartial in their evaluation.

When a mental health professional or behavioral scientist serves as a consultant in a given case, with the primary purpose of assisting the attorney, a contingency fee arrangement is not necessarily as problematic. It is always important for the consulting mental health professional to provide accurate information to the attorney. If working under a contingency arrangement would tend to make it more difficult for the consulting mental health professional to provide accurate information, from an impartial stance, then it would still be undesirable. It might be argued that effective consultation involves giving accurate, comprehensive information, and also enhances the likelihood of winning. Considered from this perspective, a contingency fee arrangement for case consultation may not be problematic.

Discussion

There is consistent, strong support from the areas of Ethics and Standard of Practice for the importance of clarifying financial arrangements. Legal authority provides some support for fee clarification, although typically it would be handled through procedural rule or administrative code (particularly in jurisdictions with specified fees for given evaluative tasks). No empirical research is yet available in this area, but the literature on standard of practice consistently reflects the importance of initial fee clarification. The way in which the fee is structured may depend on the role being played by the forensic clinician; a contingency fee arrangement, for example, which would be ethically prohibited for the role of defense or plaintiff s expert, might not be problematic in the role of consultant. This principle appears *established*.

FMHA is a "quasi-public" process. In certain cases, some members of the public are personally exposed to the results of FMHA in the course of observing or participating in litigation. Far more are exposed indirectly, through media coverage of certain cases. A forensic clinician's fee may be the subject of questions during testimony, and the public perception that testimony can be "bought" or "influenced"[22] through financial means remains a source of concern for the integrity of FMHA. At present, however, the levels of reimbursement for FMHA appear less regulated than for other kinds of mental health services.

This may change. It would not be surprising to see courts, agencies, and other consumers of FMHA services contracting on a large scale within the foreseeable future with companies providing "managed forensic assessment" services. At present, however, it remains primarily the responsibility of professional disciplines and individual providers to clarify fees through setting them at reasonable levels and willingly describing them, both at the initial stage of agreement regarding FMHA and at subsequent stages in this process.

OBTAIN APPROPRIATE AUTHORIZATION

Authorization is always needed to begin a forensic evaluation, and there are several times in the evaluation process when additional authorization may be necessary. In some cases, the initial authorization is obtained through a signed order from the court. If the evaluation is being conducted on a court-ordered basis, such an order provides the forensic clinician with the legal authority to proceed. Such orders are also routinely copied to attorneys involved in the case, thereby formally documenting the ordering of the evaluation. If the evaluation is being performed at the request of the attorney for one of the parties involved in litigation, then authorization may not be required from the court—assuming that the status of the work (at least initially) is attorney work product.

ETHICS

The *Ethical Principles of Psychologists* (APA, 1992) does not directly address the nature of the authorization to be obtained prior to conducting a forensic assessment. There is indirect reference to the authorization in the section under Forensic Activities, as follows: "In performing forensic roles,

---

[22]The issue of whether expert mental health testimony can be "bought" or "influenced" actually contains two separate questions. The possibility that a mental health professional would fabricate results, or greatly distort their meaning, in exchange for money obviously exists, but hopefully is relatively rare. What is undoubtedly more frequent, and hence more problematic for the legal system and the mental health professions, is the influence of financial considerations on the way in which FMHA is conducted and communicated. More open discussion of this issue, as well as empirical research, is greatly needed.

psychologists are reasonably familiar with the rules governing their roles" (p. 1610). The *Specialty Guidelines for Forensic Psychologists* (Committee on Ethical Guidelines for Forensic Psychologists, 1991) discusses the issue of authorization more directly, and in some detail. In the section on Relationships, there is a description of various ways in which a forensic evaluation might be authorized:

> via contract with the "legal representative of the party seeking services" (p. 658)

or

> in situations where the client or party may not have the capacity to provide informed consent to services or the evaluation is pursuant to court order, the forensic psychologist provides reasonable notice to the client's legal representative of the nature of the anticipated forensic service before proceeding. If the client's legal representative objects to the evaluation, the forensic psychologist notifies the court issuing the order and responds as directed (p. 659)

or

> after a psychologist has advised the subject of a clinical forensic evaluation of the intended uses of the evaluation and its work product, the psychologist may not use the evaluation work product for other purposes without explicit waiver to do so by the client or the client's legal representative. (pp. 659–660)

The *Principles of Medical Ethics with Annotations* (American Psychiatric Association, 1998) does not address the nature of the authorization to be obtained prior to a forensic evaluation being conducted. The *Ethical Guidelines for the Practice of Forensic Psychiatry* (AAPL, 1995), however, describes several forms of possible authorization:

> The informed consent of the subject of a forensic evaluation is obtained when possible. When consent is not required, notice is given to the evaluee of the nature of the evaluation; in particular situations, such as court-ordered evaluations for competency to stand trial or involuntary commitment, consent is not required. In such a case, the psychiatrist should so inform the subject and explain that the evaluation is legally required and that if the subject refuses to participate in the evaluation, this fact will be included in any report or testimony.... If the evaluee is not competent to give consent, substituted consent is obtained in accordance with the laws of the jurisdiction. (p. 2)

It is also observed in the *Ethical Guidelines* that, in criminal cases, ethical considerations preclude forensic evaluation before legal counsel has been obtained.

LAW

If the evaluation is being conducted on a "defense expert" or "prosecution expert" basis, or the forensic clinician otherwise has been retained to conduct an evaluation for an attorney (e.g., in a personal injury or child custody case, or when retained privately as a defense expert in a criminal case), then the authorization is not necessarily provided by the court. In the criminal context, in states with a statutory provision (consistent with *Ake v. Oklahoma*, 1985) for the appointment of a defense expert, the appointment may be a court order specifying this role. However, the agreement to perform the evaluation may also be made directly with the attorney; authorization in such cases may be verbal or written, depending on the preference of the parties involved.

The appropriate authorization from the individual being evaluated again depends on the role of the evaluator. In court-ordered forensic evaluations in criminal cases, there may be a Fifth Amendment right to refuse to answer certain questions or to participate at all in certain kinds of evaluations (e.g., capital sentencing, see *Estelle v. Smith*, 1981; Slobogin, 1982, 1984). If the forensic clinician is conducting a court-ordered or prosecution-requested evaluation of sentencing in a capital case, therefore, it may be appropriate to inform the defendant that he or she has a legal right to remain silent. It "may" be appropriate because this issue is not settled; the U.S. Supreme Court has held that the introduction of psychiatric evidence by the prosecution in capital cases, when this evidence was originally obtained for another purpose, does not necessarily violate the defendant's Fifth Amendment privilege against self-incrimination (*Buchanan v. Kentucky*, 1987). Jurisdiction-specific law should be reviewed for more specific guidance.

In many jurisdictions there are explicit protections in criminal cases against the use of material obtained in a forensic evaluation for any purpose other than deciding the legal issue that triggered the evaluation.[23] If there is such protection, then the individual being evaluated on a court-ordered basis typically does not have a legal right to refuse participation. The question of the forensic clinician's ethical obligation to both inform the defendant and obtain consent to participate in an evaluation has been discussed at length elsewhere (Committee on Ethical Guidelines for Forensic Psychologists, 1991; Melton et al., 1997). Under these circumstances, the initial ethical duty is better described as "notification of purpose" than "informed consent." The defendant may refuse to participate following this notification. In such cases, the evaluator may be ethically obligated to ask the defendant about the reasons for such a refusal, allow the defendant

---

[23]In Florida, for example, the *Florida Rules of Criminal Procedure* bars the use of material obtained in an evaluation of trial competence from admission at the guilt phase of a trial, unless this evidence is introduced by the defense.

the opportunity to consult with counsel, and describe the possible consequences of refusing to participate—including sending a report that is less
thorough than it would have been with full participation (Melton et al.,
1997). However, there is no ethical obligation to halt the entire evaluation
absent a consent, as would be the case for a research subject or a clinical
care patient.

This changes, however, if the forensic clinician is performing an evaluation that has been ordered by the court on a "defense expert" basis (in
the criminal context), or initiated independently by the representing attorney (for either criminal or civil litigation). In such cases, the individual is
not legally compelled to proceed, and therefore an informed consent is
needed in order to proceed. Two similar steps should be taken if an individual refuses to participate in the evaluation under this circumstance—
asking about the individual's reasoning and allowing time for discussion
with counsel. However, it is preferable for the attorney, not the evaluator,
to explain the consequences of such a refusal. The forensic clinician simply
proceeds no further in the event of such a refusal, unless the client agrees
to participate.

When records or other documented third party information are
sought, then two kinds of authorization are possible. Hospitals, schools,
prisons, employers, and independent mental health professionals are gov-
erned by internal policies, and usually statutes or administrative code, on
the release of information. These requirements can typically be met in two
ways: through the signed consent of the individual being evaluated or
through a court order for their release.

EMPIRICAL

No studies have been located that are relevant to the role of the
authorization obtained prior to beginning a forensic evaluation.

STANDARD OF PRACTICE

One source of guidance for standard of practice for evaluations in the
criminal context is contained in the ABA's *Criminal Justice Mental Health
Standards* (1989). There it is noted that the authority for initiating a pretrial
mental health evaluation in criminal cases should reside with the court or
the defense attorney, except in cases in which the sole purpose of the
evaluation involves diverting the defendant from the criminal process or
determining whether emergency mental health treatment or habilitation is
warranted. Initiation of evaluations relevant to decisions at other stages in

the criminal justice process (e.g., sentencing, commitment of insanity acquittees, transfer of mentally ill inmates) is likewise to be controlled by the court or the attorney.

This approach has been incorporated in forensic evaluation training programs in various states (Fein et al., 1991; Florida Mental Health Institute, 1989; Institute of Law, Psychiatry, and Public Policy, 1995). It is consistent with the recommendations offered in standard texts on FMHA (e.g., Grisso, 1988; Melton et al., 1987; Roesch & Golding, 1980; Shapiro, 1991). It is also consistent with recommendations made by the APA's Task Force on the Role of Psychology in the Criminal Justice System (Monahan, 1980). This group concluded that there may be multiple clients for the different services delivered within the criminal justice system, and it is important to specify the "client(s)" for any particular service. This applies to FMHA, and the principle of obtaining appropriate authorization, in the following sense: When the specific FMHA "client" has been identified, then the forensic clinician can see more clearly how (and from whom) authorization should be obtained.

DISCUSSION

The principle appears to be *established*. Despite the absence of empirical studies in which the issue of formal authorization has been examined, there appears to be strong and consistent support for this principle among legal, ethical, and practice sources of authority. The nature of the required authorization can vary according to the forensic issues being evaluated and the role assumed by the forensic clinician. It is useful to distinguish between circumstances in which there is a legal demand or a legal right to refuse participation from those in which there is no such demand or right; notification of purpose is applicable in cases in which the evaluation is legally compelled, while informed consent applies better when the evaluation is not legally compelled.

The nature of the authorization needed in FMHA is linked to the initial notification (specifically whether it includes a request for consent). Evaluators who are unclear about the required authorization, and deliver an inaccurate notification (involving a request for consent when none is needed, or describing a process that does not require consent when it actually *does*) can create a number of difficulties. A defendant who is incorrectly told that his consent is required for a court-ordered evaluation, and subsequently informed (correctly this time) that a report can be sent to the court regardless of whether he consents, may understandably become confused and angry. A parent involved in child custody litigation, who is mistakenly notified that her consent is not required in order to proceed with the evaluation that has been requested by her husband's attorney, might become more defensive and suspicious, as well as angry when the mistake is corrected. The importance of obtaining appropriate authorization, linked with providing accurate initial notification, cannot be over-emphasized.

3

Defining the Evaluator's Role

The initial stage of the forensic evaluation process has now been discussed. The relevant forensic issue has been identified and determined to be within the forensic clinician's area of expertise, the fee and role with the attorney have been clarified, appropriate authorization to proceed has been obtained, and relevant sources of information have been identified. When this stage has been completed, there are still several principles that are applicable to the "preparation" stage of the evaluation. Two of those principles will be discussed in this chapter: avoiding the dual-role relationships of therapist and forensic evaluator, and determining the role to be played in forensic evaluation if the referral is accepted. Four possible roles for mental health professionals in legal proceedings were described in the last chapter: court-appointed, defense/prosecution/plaintiff's expert, consultant, and fact witness. The focus in the present chapter will be on the first three, which are clearly forensic, when the discussion addresses FMHA roles.

AVOID DUAL-ROLE RELATIONSHIPS
OF THERAPIST AND FORENSIC EVALUATOR

A dual-role relationship in FMHA is one in which two roles are assumed by a mental health professional in the context of a single case. There are several circumstances under which this might occur. The first involves the combination of a professional role (e.g., therapist, consultant, or forensic evaluator) with a personal or vocational role (e.g., spouse, lover, family member, friend, co-worker, or business associate). A second possibility involves the circumstance in which both roles are professional, most often a treatment role combined with a forensic evaluator role (e.g., a therapist serving as a forensic expert for a current therapy client). Finally, there is a third possibility: the assumption of a second role within a forensic case (e.g., consultant), either concurrent with the role of forensic evaluator or after it has been completed The first and second kinds of dual roles will be discussed in this section, and the third will be addressed in the section that follows the present one.

ETHICS

The *Ethical Principles of Psychologists* (APA, 1992) addresses dual-role relationships as follows: "Psychologists make every effort to avoid dual relationships that could impair their professional judgment or increase the risk of exploitation" (p. 393). More detail is provided under "Multiple Relationships":

(a) In many communities and situations, it may not be feasible or reasonable for psychologists to avoid social or other nonprofessional contacts with persons such as patients, clients, students, supervisees, or research participants. Psychologists must always be sensitive to the potential harmful effects of other contacts on their work and on those persons with whom they deal. A psychologist refrains from entering into or promising another personal, scientific, professional, financial, or other relationship with such persons if it appears likely that such a relationship reasonably might impair the psychologist's objectivity or otherwise interfere with the psychologist's effectively performing his or her functions as a psychologist, or might harm or exploit the other party.

(b) Likewise, whenever feasible, a psychologist refrains from taking on professional or scientific obligations when preexisting relationships would create a risk of such harm.

(c) If a psychologist finds that, due to unforeseen factors, a potentially harmful multiple relationship has arisen, the psychologist attempts to resolve it with due regard for the best interests of the affected person and maximal compliance with the Ethics Code. (p. 1601)

Dual relationships are discouraged, although not ruled out, under the *Ethical Principles of Psychologists*. Important considerations include whether the dual relationship might impair the psychologist's objectivity or otherwise diminish her effectiveness, or whether the dual relationship might harm or exploit the other party.

The *Specialty Guidelines for Forensic Psychologists* (1991) also discusses dual-role relationships. They indicate that "[f]orensic psychologists recognize potential conflicts of interest in dual relationships with parties to a legal proceeding, and they seek to minimize their effects" (p. 659). The language in the *Guidelines* generally discourages dual-role relationships of either the "professional–personal" or the "therapeutic–forensic" variety. In particular:

1. Forensic psychologists avoid providing professional services to parties in a legal proceeding with whom they have personal or professional relationships that are inconsistent with the anticipated relationship, and

2. When it is necessary to provide both evaluation and treatment services to a party in a legal proceeding (as may be the case in small forensic hospital settings or small communities), the forensic psychologist takes reasonable steps to minimize the potential negative effects of these circumstances on the rights of the party, confidentiality, and the process of treatment and evaluation. (p. 659)

One "reasonable step" would involve ongoing assurance that clients are informed of their legal rights and of the other elements in the "notification of purpose" that is given prior to beginning any forensic service. This information can change, depending on the role being played by the forensic clinician and the legal issues being evaluated:

Forensic psychologists have an obligation to ensure that prospective clients are informed of their legal rights with respect to the anticipated forensic service, of the purposes of any evaluation, of the nature of procedures to be employed, of the intended uses of any product of their services, and of the party who has employed the forensic psychologist. (p. 659)

One circumstance suggested by the *Specialty Guidelines*, under which a forensic clinician might play more than one role in the course of forensic services, is when resources are limited (as might be the case in a small forensic hospital setting or a small community). This might seem inconsistent with the conclusion that simultaneously playing both assessment and treatment roles in the same case is inherently problematic.

However, it is not necessarily inconsistent. The crucial consideration is the initial understanding regarding both evaluation and treatment. In some specialized settings (a forensic hospital, for example), the purposes for commitment are reasonably clear. A defendant who is committed as Incompetent for Trial is to be evaluated and treated to help her toward sufficient improvement in the areas rendering her Incompetent for Trial, and to return her to court when this has occurred.[1] Under such circumstances, it is possible to inform the individual that treatment and evaluation will be provided to help her improve and determine whether she has, respectively. If such notification is given, then there would seem to be no ethical problem with the same individual providing both therapy and evaluation services.[2]

---

[1]Questions about how these areas of deficit are described in relation to the "ultimate legal issue," in this case competence to stand trial, are part of a larger controversy within the forensic assessment field on whether, and to what extent, the ultimate issue should be addressed by evaluators in reports and testimony. This controversy will be discussed in detail later in this book.

[2]There are other reasons why it is preferable to separate assessment and treatment, even when treatment is provided to address a primary goal such as restoring trial competence. It is clearer for both the therapist and the patient, and both can probably adjust better within a role that is more sharply defined. However, there is one important justification for combining these roles. When the primary goal of treatment is the restoration of trial

The *Principles of Medical Ethics with Annotations Applicable to Psychiatry* (American Psychiatric Association, 1998) addresses dual-role relationships of the professional–personal kind. A specific instance of a dual-role relationship (sexual activity with a patient) is described as unethical, and it is also observed that the

> psychiatrist should diligently guard against exploiting information furnished by the patient and should not use the unique position of power afforded him/ her by the psychotherapeutic situation to influence the patient in any way not directly relevant to the treatment goals. (p. 3)

Finally, it is noted that

> Psychiatric services ... are dispensed in the context of a contractual arrangement between the patient and the treating physician. The provisions of the contractual arrangements ... should be explicitly established. (p. 3)

The *Ethical Guidelines for the Practice of Forensic Psychiatry* (AAPL, 1995) also addresses the dual-role issue, although this particular language is not used and the focus is on dual relationships of the professional–professional kind. Two specific examples of dual-role conflicts and the desirable approach to avoiding each are provided. First, when describing the need for notifying the evaluee about the purpose of the assessment, the *Guidelines* explicitly states that the psychiatrist should indicate that he or she is not the evaluee's "doctor" and should take care to avoid "slippage and [any] treatment relationship [that] may develop in the mind of the examinee" (p. 1). Second, when a treatment relationship between psychiatrist and patient already exists:

> Treating psychiatrists should generally avoid agreeing to be an expert witness or to perform an evaluation of their patients for legal purposes because a forensic evaluation usually requires that other people be interviewed and testimony may adversely affect the therapeutic relationship. (p. 3)

LAW

No legal authority on this principle was located.

EMPIRICAL

There is not a great deal of empirical research that could be located on the impact of dual or multiple roles on the FMHA process. There is

---

competence through improved mental and emotional functioning *as quickly as reasonably possible*, then the association of ongoing forensic assessment in conjunction with treatment can facilitate and quicken this improvement. Therapists may set treatment goals more broadly than necessary when working with individuals who are incompetent for trial, and ongoing assessment of the areas directly relevant to trial competence can serve to remind both therapist and patient of which areas of functioning are most relevant for therapeutic work.

evidence from one study that attorneys involved in child custody litigation have historically favored using treating therapists as forensic experts in such cases. In a survey of 92 attorneys who had handled at least 10 divorce cases involving custody of minor children, it was reported that the most important considerations rated by attorneys when deciding whether to involve a mental health professional was whether that professional (1) was willing to testify in court and (2) was already working with the family (Felner, Rowlison, Farber, Primavera, & Bishop, 1987).

It is possible that attorneys' views have changed during the time since the publication of this study, however. In a more recent survey of 166 Canadian lawyers who devoted at least 10% of their time to divorce cases involving minor children (Lee, Beauregard, & Hunsley, 1998), the "availability of good assessors" was the single item relevant to the characteristics of mental health professionals, and it was not explicitly indicated that the use of currently treating professionals was desirable.[3] Taken together, the data from these two studies provide some basis for understanding the views of attorneys regarding dual roles in child custody cases that may be communicated to mental health professionals: good child custody assessors are desirable, and using currently treating professionals may be seen as one of the best sources of good assessors.

There is also evidence, however, that performing the dual roles of therapist and child custody evaluator in a single case is associated with the risk of ethics complaints. Glassman (1998) reported that from 1990 to 1994 ethics complaints related to child custody evaluations accounted for 7–10% of all ethics complaints to the APA. Based on Glassman's recommendations for avoiding such ethics complaints, it may be inferred that dual roles and related problems (e.g., failing to explain the loss of confidentiality associated with a custody evaluation role, failing to adequately explain the other differences between the roles and hence securing informed consent) are directly associated with many such ethics complaints.

STANDARD OF PRACTICE

The professional literature provides reasonable support for not blending the roles of therapeutic and forensic clinician in the same case, particularly when there is no good justification for doing so. There is very limited discussion of the professional–personal kind of dual-role problem as it might apply to FMHA.

Several commentators have advocated a fairly strict separation of

[3]The results of this study cannot be interpreted as strong support for the possibility that attorneys are currently less inclined to use treating professionals in child custody FMHA, however, because it was unclear from the study whether attorneys responding to the survey were asked directly about this point.

roles between therapeutic and forensic functions for mental health professions (Greenberg & Shuman, 1997; Heilbrun, 1995), and the proposal has
even been made to "bar treating mental health professionals from the
courtroom" on cases in which they have been involved therapeutically
(Shuman, Greenberg, Heilbrun, & Foote, 1998). There appears to be mixed
support for this position in the professional literature. One argument holds
that therapists need to be aware of three potential roles that mental health
professionals can play with individuals involved in child custody litigation: evaluator, mediator, and therapist (Emery & Rogers, 1990). While
noting that such roles overlap somewhat in function, and that, on occasion,
the same mental health professional may play more than one role, the
authors also conclude that it is preferable for the therapist to define a single
role from the outset and maintain it throughout (Emery & Rogers, 1990).
This position is consistent with one of the recommendations made by
Glassman (1998) for practices to avoid ethics complaints in child custody
evaluations. He observes that "changing roles from therapist to custody
evaluator will most likely be interpreted as an ethics violation" and the
"custody evaluator should preferably be unknown to the parties prior to
appointment" (p. 123).

    Playing multiple roles in the same case is also problematic because of
the differing expectations of clinician and evaluee that are associated with
each role. These expectations are communicated in different ways for
therapeutic and forensic roles. For example, it is important that the expert
understand, and clearly communicate to all clients, the nature and limitations of privileged communication (Blau, 1984b). However, if the mental
health professional initially plays a therapeutic role, and subsequently
adopts a forensic role in the same case, then any initial notification of
purpose will no longer apply. Changing this notification may be problematic, because there are important differences between "informed consent,"
which typically applies in treatment contexts, and "notification of purpose," which is applicable under many circumstances in which forensic
assessment is performed.[4] Thus, it would be inappropriate to provide a
comparable kind of notification, premised on similar facts and assumptions. Even if circumstances allowed providing a second notification comparable to the first, however, there are other problems with changing this

---

[4]The most important of these differences is the role of choice in the decision about participation. When the informed consent doctrine applies, there is usually a choice about whether to
accept or refuse the intervention; the decision must be made in a knowing, intelligent, and
voluntary way. When there is no meaningful choice about participation, then it remains
important that the person understand the purpose of the evaluation and the limits of
confidentiality. However, the "intelligent" aspect of decision-making is less important, and
the "voluntary" component clearly does not apply.

notification. First, the initial notification may have been done informally (or not at all) in the treatment context, requiring that any subsequent notification address explicitly certain issues that have been heretofore implicit. Second, the next notification, and the associated decision about participation in the forensic context, may be influenced by the trust between patient and therapist, and as a result the patient may be insufficiently attentive to the risks involved in forensic proceedings. Third, when role boundaries are loose, the clinician may be asked to perform tasks that are not only beyond the scope of the initial therapeutic role, but also beyond the scope of the forensic evaluator role. Finally, the failure to be clear about the limits of expertise can lead to the public perception that a forensic clinician is unrealistic, naive, or dishonest. To the extent that these problems would limit fully informed notification of purpose, or decision-making that is knowing, intelligent, and voluntary, then Blau's position would discourage changing the notification.

A different position on this issue has been advanced by Halleck (1980):

> A psychiatrist can also find himself in an expert role through unanticipated circumstances. Sometimes a patient already in treatment may ask the psychiatrist to help him with a legal problem by testifying as to his mental status. The problem may have little to do with the patient's treatment needs and in some instances the patient may be helped by honoring his request. (p. 196)

The *Criminal Justice Mental Health Standards* (1989) also offer some support for the possibility of playing multiple roles in the forensic assessment process. Standard 7-3.11, on Expert Witness Qualifications, indicates that there are two ways in which sufficient knowledge in a given case may be gained:

> forensic training or an acceptable substitute therefor, relevant to conducting the specific type(s) of mental evaluation actually conducted in the case, and relevant to the substantive law concerning the specific matter(s) on which expert opinion is to be proffered;

or

> has had a professional therapeutic or habilitative relationship with the person whose mental condition is in question. (p. 132)

None of the positions just described would support the frequent or indiscriminate practice of playing both therapeutic and forensic roles in the same case. Even when it is argued, as Halleck does,[5] that these roles can

[5]It may be inaccurate to suggest that Halleck advocates blending these roles. Since Halleck (1980) observes that a psychiatrist may "testify to ... mental status" (p. 196) as a fact witness rather than an expert, it is possible to avoid assuming a forensic role even when testifying about a patient in treatment. Alternatively, the psychiatrist could carefully limit her testi-

be occasionally blended, there are certain conditions that must be met (e.g., informed consent, accurate communication of loss of confidentiality, "the patient may be helped") before this is considered.

There is an emerging view in child custody evaluation about the desirability of limiting the participation of forensic clinicians to a single role in a given case. According to the *Guidelines for Child Custody Evaluations in Divorce Proceedings* (APA, 1994):

> Psychologists generally avoid conducting a child custody evaluation in a case in which the psychologist served in a therapeutic role for the child or his or her immediate family or has had other involvement that may compromise the psychologist's objectivity. This should not, however, preclude the psychologist from testifying in the case as a fact witness concerning treatment of the child. In addition, during the course of a child custody evaluation, a psychologist does not accept any of the involved participants in the evaluation as a therapy client. Therapeutic contact with the child or involved participants following a child custody evaluation is undertaken with caution.
>
> A psychologist asked to testify regarding a therapy client who is involved in a child custody case is aware of the limitations and possible biases inherent in such a role and the possible impact on the ongoing therapeutic relationship. Although the court may require the psychologist to testify as a fact witness regarding factual information he or she became aware of in a professional relationship with a client, that psychologist should generally decline the role of an expert witness who gives a professional opinion regarding custody and visitation (see Ethical Standard 7.03) unless so ordered by the court. (p. 678)

This language also emphasizes the avoidance of any "other involvement" (such as a prior personal or vocational relationship) that might decrease impartiality, indicating that dual-role relationships of the professional–personal kind are to be avoided in child custody evaluation.

DISCUSSION

There is limited consistency on this principle between different sources of authority. Ethical standards and guidelines are consistent in their recognition that dual-role relationships of the professional–personal and therapeutic–forensic kind are to be avoided when possible. There is

---

mony to questions related to mental status, and avoid areas related more directly to the ultimate legal issue being decided. For example, when a psychiatrist testifies about one of the parents in a child custody case who is currently in treatment with her, she might confine her responses to questions about diagnosis, treatment response, and treatment compliance, but decline to answer questions about that individual's abilities as a parent or the best interests of the child, on the grounds that she had not performed the forensic evaluation necessary to address such questions. Neither of these approaches would involve much blending of therapeutic and forensic roles, and both could fit comfortably within Halleck's "testify to ... mental status" dictum.

less support for the stronger position that such relationships are to be avoided absolutely, except for specific examples such as sexual intimacies with clients that are not particularly applicable to FMHA. The law is largely silent on this principle, although the *Criminal Justice Mental Health Standards* does describe a therapeutic relationship as providing one basis for expert testimony. Although there is some diversity of opinion in the area of standard of practice, the majority of the literature is inclined against blending personal–professional or therapeutic–forensic roles in a single case. There is sufficient support to conclude that this principle is *established*.

DETERMINE THE ROLE TO BE PLAYED WITHIN FORENSIC ASSESSMENT IF THE REFERRAL IS ACCEPTED

This principle involves the identification of the specific role that the evaluator will assume in a given forensic case. Two major points will be made. The first is that it is undesirable to blend the roles of court-appointed, defense/prosecution/plaintiff's expert, or consultant in a single case. The second is that there may be an exception to this first point under one particular circumstance: The roles of *impartial evaluator* and *consultant* will be considered as they might be combined in a single case.[6]

ETHICS

The *Ethical Principles of Psychologists* (APA, 1992) does not address the issue of dual roles within FMHA specifically, so it is necessary to consider the language that is applied to dual roles more generally. The *Ethical Principles* begins with the undesirability of dual roles when the result of playing two roles is potentially harmful: "Psychologists make every effort to avoid dual relationships that could impair their professional judgment or increase the risk of exploitation" (p. 393). Additional comments are provided regarding multiple relationships:

(a) ... Psychologists must always be sensitive to the potential harmful effects of other contacts on their work and on those persons with whom they deal. A

---

[6]Possible roles for the clinician in legal proceedings such as "advocate" and "fact witness" cannot be combined readily, and will not be considered in this discussion. The "hired gun" role (Wasyliw, Cavanaugh, & Rogers, 1985) does not appear to be a separate forensic role that can be distinguished using ethical, legal, empirical, and standard of practice criteria. Rather, it appears to be a version of the impartial evaluator role, in which the clinician's motivation and work quality differ. The "ivory tower" role (Wasyliw et al., 1985) is not sufficiently similar to the kind of forensic activity being considered in this book to treat it as a separate category.

psychologist refrains from entering into or promising another personal, scientific, professional, financial, or other relationship with such persons if it appears likely that such a relationship reasonably might impair the psychologist's objectivity or otherwise interfere with the psychologist's effectively performing his or her functions as a psychologist, or might harm or exploit the other party.

(b) Likewise, whenever feasible, a psychologist refrains from taking on professional or scientific obligations when preexisting relationships would create a risk of such harm.

(c) If a psychologist finds that, due to unforeseen factors, a potentially harmful multiple relationship has arisen, the psychologist attempts to resolve it with due regard for the best interests of the affected person and maximal compliance with the Ethics Code. (p. 1601)

These points are more applicable to circumstances in which the request for services within a second role is difficult to anticipate. Since forensic clinicians will almost always make decisions and conduct planning with the litigant's attorney, rather than with the litigant, the next question concerns what services an attorney might request. Such requests can be anticipated more readily through training and experience.

The *Ethical Principles* provides a broad framework for considering dual roles according to potentially harmful consequences. In the case of FMHA, the "harm" could occur in the damage to integrity of the forensic clinician, the FMHA process, and the justice system if a consultant, who was retained to help win the case, were subsequently asked to become an impartial expert in the same case and testify about what is true.

The *Specialty Guidelines for Forensic Psychologists* (1991) notes that "[f]orensic psychologists avoid providing professional services to parties in a legal proceeding with whom they have personal or professional relationships that are inconsistent with the anticipated relationship" (p. 659). In the present context, since impartiality and credibility are important for the roles of court-appointed and defense/prosecution/plaintiff's expert, respectively, it is likely that any combination of either of these two roles with the role of consultant could both (1) diminish the impartiality and credibility and (2) thereby lessen the effectiveness with which the forensic clinician could conduct FMHA.

Under one circumstance, however, the blending of some roles within the forensic context may occur. The nature of such circumstances is not addressed in the *Ethical Principles*, but explicit guidance is available from the *Specialty Guidelines*. The first step is the nature of the understanding between the forensic psychologist and the legal representative of the party seeking services:

During initial consultation with the legal representative of the party seeking services, forensic psychologists have an obligation to inform the party of factors that might reasonably affect the decision to contract with the forensic psychologist. These factors include ... prior and current personal or professional activities, obligations, and relationships that might produce a conflict of interest. (p. 658)

After this step, which involves a full notification of the interests that might create conflicts in the course of the forensic evaluation, there is another consideration for the evaluator:

Forensic psychologists recognize potential conflicts of interest in dual relationships with parties to a legal proceeding, and they seek to minimize their effects. (p. 659)

One circumstance in which the roles of plaintiff's expert and consultant might be combined without problems is illustrated in the following example. The clinician is retained by the plaintiff's attorney in a personal injury case to perform an impartial evaluation that could result in testimony. The clinician, having performed a thorough evaluation, informs the attorney that the overall pattern of findings will apparently not be helpful to the plaintiff's case. Under such circumstances, it is likely that the attorney would instruct the evaluating clinician not to write a report. Further, it is likely that the attorney would indicate that these results will not be used in litigation. Following this, it is possible for the clinician to assume the broader role of consultant, which would involve advising the attorney about the strengths and weaknesses of reports written by other clinicians involved in the case, reviewing the scientific and professional literature for relevant studies and standards, and offering other advice relevant to the case. Whether this could be accomplished without ethical difficulty would depend on whether (1) the new arrangement was acceptable to the plaintiff, his attorney, and the clinician, after each clearly understood its parameters, and (2) there was agreement that *under no circumstances* could the clinician return to the role of impartial evaluator *in this case*.

The *Principles of Medical Ethics with Annotations* (American Psychiatric Association, 1998) does not directly address the desirability of blending forensic roles. It does consider this principle indirectly, by indicating that psychiatric services are dispensed in the context of a contractual relationship. Since the provisions of such a relationship should be "explicitly established," the initial agreement between attorney and psychiatrist should include the roles that are to be played by the latter. If there is any change from the original agreement suggested later in the process, then such a change in roles should also be a matter of explicit discussion and agreement.

The *Ethical Guidelines for the Practice of Forensic Psychiatry* (AAPL, 1995) addresses only one particular aspect of this principle:

Psychiatrists should clarify with a potentially retaining attorney whether an initial screening conversation prior to a formal agreement will interdict consultation with the opposing side if the psychiatrist decides not to accept the consultation. (p. 2)

This represents a small but important part of the role distinction, as it suggests that any involvement (however limited) as an evaluator on behalf of one litigant's attorney may bar participation in the same case on behalf of the opposing attorney.

LAW

One of the landmark decisions concerning psychiatric assistance to the defense was set forth in an Oklahoma death penalty case. In *Ake v. Oklahoma* (1985), the U.S. Supreme Court held that when a defendant has made a preliminary showing that sanity at the time of the offense is likely to be a significant factor at trial, then due process requires that a state must provide a defendant access to a psychiatrist's assistance, if the defendant cannot afford one otherwise. In some jurisdictions, this right has since been extended to include access to a psychiatrist *or* a psychologist under these circumstances (see, e.g., *Funk v. Commonwealth*, 1989).

In the course of the *Ake* decision, the Court addressed the issue of multiple roles played by forensic clinicians in the same case. In particular, the Court noted that

without a psychiatrist's assistance to conduct a professional examination on issues relevant to the insanity defense, to help determine whether that defense is viable, to present testimony, and to assist in preparing the cross-examination of the State's psychiatric witness, the risk of an inaccurate resolution of sanity issues is extremely high.

When the State at a capital sentencing proceeding presents psychiatric evidence of the defendant's future dangerousness, the defendant, without a psychiatrist's assistance, cannot offer an expert's opposing view, and thereby loses a significant opportunity to raise in the jurors' minds questions about the State's proof of an aggravating factor. In such a circumstance, where the consequence of error is so great, the relevance of responsive psychiatric testimony so evident, and the State's burden so slim, due process requires access to a psychiatric examination on relevant issues, to a psychiatrist's testimony, and to assistance in preparation at the sentencing phase. (p. 1097)

It is clear from the *Ake* decision that the Court did not envision separating the roles of defense expert and consultant. The functions of "professional examination" and "testimony" (associated with a defense expert role) as well as "assistance in preparing the cross-examination of the State's psychiatric witness" and other trial preparation assistance (associated with a consultant role) are clearly enumerated. The Court also makes it very clear that these functions are to be performed by the same individual:

> We consider, next, the interest of the State. Oklahoma asserts that to provide Ake with psychiatric assistance on the record before us would result in a staggering burden to the State. We are unpersuaded by this assertion. Many States, as well as the Federal Government, currently make psychiatric assistance available to indigent defendants, and they have not found the financial burden so great as to preclude this assistance. This is especially so when the obligation of the State is limited to provision of one competent psychiatrist, as it is in many States, and as we limit the right we recognize today. (pp. 1093-1094)

Thus, to the extent that the question of multiple roles and evaluators is considered at all, the Court uses a financial argument that, for Oklahoma (like other states[7]), providing a single psychiatrist to assist the defense in capital cases like *Ake* will not present an overwhelming burden. However, there is no discussion of potential problems presented by having one mental health professional assume the dual roles of impartial evaluator and defense consultant; indeed, there is no indication that the Court perceives them as different roles. Thus, there may be little or no recognition among legal professionals that "evaluator" and "consultant" are different roles for forensic clinicians, and that there may be ethical problems in combining them in a single case.

EMPIRICAL

No studies were located that would provide data on the frequency with which specific roles are identified and assumed in the FMHA process, or the extent to which a single role is maintained throughout the overall process. This would be extraordinarily difficult to study in practice, as it would involve the observation of multiple documents (e.g., court orders, letters, reports), verbal interactions (e.g., conferences and telephone calls between attorney and forensic clinician), and work products (e.g., reports, testimony in depositions, hearings, and trials). Almost certainly, it would be necessary to study this principle through surveying attorneys, judges,

---

[7]When *Ake* was decided in 1985, the federal jurisdiction plus the following states were cited in an *Ake* footnote as providing "psychiatric assistance to indigent defendants": Alabama, Alaska, Arizona, Arkansas, California, Colorado, Connecticut, Delaware, Florida, Idaho, Illinois, Indiana, Iowa, Kansas, Kentucky, Louisiana, Maine, Massachusetts, Michigan, Minnesota, Mississippi, Missouri, Montana, Nebraska, Nevada, New Hampshire, New Mexico, New York, North Carolina, Ohio, Oregon, Pennsylvania, Rhode Island, South Carolina South Dakota, Tennessee, Texas, Utah, Washington, West Virginia, and Wyoming.

and/or forensic clinicians, or performing analogue studies with graduate students and law students.

STANDARD OF PRACTICE

There is no apparent consensus within the literature regarding blending different forensic roles within the same case. Different positions have been advanced. The first position is that only a single forensic role should be assumed within a given case. The primary justification for this position involves the probable interference of one role with the clinician's ability to fulfill the other role with quality and integrity; a second reason involves the understanding between the forensic clinician and the individual being evaluated. The notification of purpose, delivered before the clinician begins the evaluation, should describe the nature of this evaluation and the ways in which it will (or might) be used. When the evaluation is used for purposes not cited in the notification, then the original understanding is no longer applicable. Particularly if this occurs against the defendant's wishes or best interests, it can lead to complications on both ethical and legal grounds.

Intermediate positions have been advanced by others. Wasyliw, Cavanaugh, and Rogers (1985) have provided a detailed description of possible forensic roles that can be played by mental health professionals; these roles are described in terms of *purpose* and *use of data*. They identify the following roles: (1) *hired gun* (whose purpose is financial or other self-interest and who distorts data to support an opinion), (2) *advocate* (whose purpose is support of an adversary position and who selects data supportive of this position), (3) *impartial expert* (who evaluates the case by reviewing all data and then forming an opinion based on those data rather than the side soliciting their services), (4) *consultant* (who evaluates the applicability of data and reviews the comprehensiveness and generalizability of research as it relates to particular legal issues), and (5) *ivory tower* (involving the evaluation of public policy by commenting on the relevance of scientific inquiry and knowledge to public policy issues). They conclude that these roles may not be mutually exclusive.

Another intermediate position has been advanced by Rachlin (1988), in the wake of *Ake v. Oklahoma*. He argued for a reconsideration of roles within the forensic context, noting that

> *Ake* ... raises issues relative to the proper role of the psychiatric expert. The Supreme Court's decision, although not introducing a new ethical topic, appears to be favoring a more adversarial posture, at least within certain parameters. I suggest that impartiality, independence, and advocacy need not be mutually exclusive concepts and that some of our traditional beliefs about what

part we should play in criminal law may have to be modified and expanded. (Rachlin, 1988, p. 25)

Finally, the broadest approach to role boundaries is advanced by Halleck:

> Sometimes the psychiatrist as an expert witness may feel that his testimony helps to support a social position which he firmly advocates. Here the expert witness is in the happy position of being able to make money and further his moral and political beliefs at the same time. (Halleck, 1980, p. 195)

Halleck further argues that multiple roles can be played up to the time when the mental health professional begins to testify, but that role considerations change at this time:

> The psychiatrist who is committed to using the expert witness role to help initiate social change may up to this point (pre-testimony) allow himself similar indulgence (helping the "cause of his employer"). Once the psychiatrist is sworn in, however, and takes the witness stand, he should cease to view himself as an adversary. At this point he becomes a servant of the court. ... When he takes the witness stand the psychiatrist becomes a person committed to the process of truth seeking no matter how the truth may conflict with his own ideologies. ... He should never make any effort to embellish his testimony in a manner which leads to even minor distortions of information. (Halleck, 1980, pp. 198-199)[8]

The standard of practice may vary somewhat according to the feasibility of role separation. As Hess (1998) has noted, there are three important principles that may be tested to their limits in small communities: confidentiality, competence, and conflicting interests. One of the recurring threats to role separation involves having too few forensic clinicians (and other parties to litigation) available, when "attorneys, parties in the case, bailiff and clerks, and jurors ... are ... someone's Little League coach, school teacher, or banker" (p. 112).

The *Criminal Justice Mental Health Standards* (ABA, 1989) offers guidance on the approach to role selection in FMHA. Under Standard 7-1.1, the

---

[8]It should be noted that Halleck's position in this matter seems inconsistent with one of the premises of this book: Testimony provided in the role of impartial expert, which Halleck describes here, should be based on the results of a forensic evaluation performed within the same role. To suggest that a mental health professional may be concerned with "helping to initiate social change" or "helping the cause of his employer" up to the time that he begins his testimony, but only view himself as a truth-seeking servant of the court during such testimony, gives insufficient weight to the "impartial evaluation as foundation for objective testimony" principle which will be discussed at greater length in a subsequent chapter. Also, it does not seem to account for the ways in which clinicians' opinions can be influenced through trying to "help the cause of the employer"—once having played the role of consultant in the forensic context, it may be difficult or impossible to assume the role of impartial truth-seeker.

roles of scientist, consultant, evaluator, and therapist are described; the "nature and limitations" of each respective role should be clarified at the outset with all appropriate parties in cases in which a given role may involve "differing and sometimes conflicting obligations and functions." If a single role is selected at the outset, and the forensic clinician is careful to limit her participation to activities within that role, then the need for ongoing clarification of role definition will be very limited. For example, if a forensic clinician agrees to perform a child custody evaluation at the request of the court, and limits her participation in the case to the interviews, testing, document review, and observation that are needed to write a thorough report and provide testimony, then it may only be necessary to offer limiting statements whenever the possibility of alternative roles arise.

However, there is also the circumstance involving the simultaneous assumption of the role of consultant and that of court-appointed expert or defense/prosecution/plaintiff's expert. For example, assume that a forensic clinician participates in a trial in the role of evaluator, having performed a court-ordered FMHA of the defendant's sanity at the time of the offense. To what extent might it be acceptable for the clinician to also provide consultative advice to the attorney, not only how best to present his own testimony, but also how to cross-examine opposing experts? This question is most likely to arise at the stage in which the attorney is preparing for a hearing or trial. Hence, the important question is whether the "additional role" of consultant can be added without compromising the integrity of the original evaluator's role. It may work acceptably when experts and attorneys for both sides agree to this additional role.[9] Without such agreement by all parties, however, there is significant potential for ethical and procedural difficulties with these multiple roles. One of the significant differences between the roles involves emotional commitments: The impartial evaluator's commitment is to the truth, while the consultant's commitment is to the cause or issue at hand (Hess, 1998). This difference in orientations must be considered as well if there is to be a successful shift from the role of impartial evaluator to that of consultant. However, the change from evaluator to consultant *when the forensic clinician is no longer*

---

[9]Common sense should prescribe limits on the role of consultant under these circumstances, however. There is the real potential that being a member of an attorney's "team," with the goal of winning the case, will interfere with the evaluator's demand for presenting testimony in a balanced fashion. There is the further danger that this loss of impartiality will be perceived by the judge or jury. To guard against either, it is advisable under such circumstances to limit contact with the attorney to formal, private meetings, and to avoid activities (e.g., sitting at the attorney's table, passing notes, socializing) that increase the risk of actual or perceived loss of impartiality.

playing the role of evaluator means that only one role is being played at a time, and that the emotional difficulty of alternating the goals of "winning" and "impartiality" is less problematic.

Discussion

The legal precedent in this case, *Ake*, would suggest that simultaneous multiple roles within FMHA do not create conceptual difficulty. This is a single case, however, in which role definition was only a very minor part. No relevant empirical studies were located. Much of the analysis of this principle, therefore, is influenced by the existing literature in ethics and standard of practice. The practice literature provides a range of positions, with most adopting a stance advocating no dual-role involvement whatsoever, or an intermediate stance recommending limited, carefully explained involvement. Different sources of ethics authority are consistent in their emphasis on role specificity: It is important to select a single role when playing multiple roles is potentially harmful. In the context of FMHA, the "harm" that occurs is more likely to be to the integrity of the forensic clinician, the FMHA process, and the justice system than to the litigant (whose legal circumstances *could* be harmed through dual roles being played by the forensic clinician, but they could also be helped). Simultaneously playing the roles of impartial evaluator and consultant, as envisioned in *Ake*, could result in a lessening of impartiality and credibility. The immediate loss of credibility (from among the judge and the attorneys) may be handled if the court and both attorneys agree to these dual roles. Both impartiality loss and the broader lessening of credibility (from a larger society, particularly in high-profile cases in which the forensic clinicians are seen as both experts and advocates) remain problematic, however.

Further complicating this issue is the consideration of playing the roles of impartial expert and consultant, but sequentially rather than simultaneously. It is possible to move from the role of impartial evaluator to consultant, as long as all parties understand and agree on the ramifications of this change, and the forensic clinician is successful in managing the shift in emotional commitments. However, simultaneously performing these roles, or attempting to return to the impartial role after having served as a consultant, is particularly problematic because the required striving for impartiality within the evaluator role may be unduly influenced by the nature of the consultant role. This appears to be an *emerging* principle, of great complexity, and with limited relevant law and no apparent empirical research for guidance.

The choice about single versus multiple roles in forensic assessment is very important for the practitioner, with ramifications that can go well beyond a single case. With the exception noted in the last paragraph, the selection of a single role always makes the clinician's participation "cleaner," in the sense that this role and its associated demands are the entire focus of the participation. Moreover, this encourages forensic clinicians to think clearly about their role from the beginning, and to avoid being "drawn into" forensic roles that were not in the initial understanding. It should also be noted that playing multiple roles often creates complications, increases complexity, and may engender conflicting loyalties. It may also result more frequently in dissatisfaction among individuals who are evaluated, and increase the likelihood of ethics complaints and other actions against clinicians.[10] Clinicians should thus be exceedingly cautious in circumstances that might yield dual-role participation, and avoid assuming more than one forensic role in a single case whenever possible, with the exception noted in the last paragraph.

[10]One of the most frequently reported sources of dissatisfaction with forensic clinicians is in the area of child custody evaluations, when the clinician is perceived by one of the parents as biased in favor of the other. Having a previous or ongoing therapy relationship with one or both of the parents might understandably contribute to the perception that a mental health professional is biased against the parent not "favored" by the results of the evaluation.

4

Using a Model

The next consideration in the forensic evaluation process involves the use of a model to guide the entire FMHA process. Some information in forensic assessment is collected directly from the individual being evaluated, while other data are obtained from collateral sources. However, the importance of thoroughness (see, e.g., Shapiro, 1991) creates the demand to consider a good deal of information, typically from different sources, in the course of most forensic evaluations.

This demand for thoroughness creates several challenges for the forensic clinician. Other principles in this book will cover a number of these challenges: determining the relevance and accuracy of varying sources of information, assessing how each source contributes to broader conclusions, clarifying the reasoning associated with transforming raw data and information into conclusions, and communicating these conclusions so that they are clear, but their contributing data are not obscured. The use of a model in forensic assessment is relevant to each of these principles in several ways. In this chapter, I will discuss how a model can facilitate the implementation of other principles described in this book.

A model for FMHA has potentially broad applicability to the forensic assessment process. It is relevant to the selection of data sources, the identification of specific legal issues, and the determination of the relationship between clinical symptoms and legally relevant functional deficits. It can also serve to clarify communication and reasoning. A forensic assessment model can function as a blueprint, from which case-specific plans and procedures can be derived.

SELECT AND EMPLOY A MODEL TO GUIDE DATA GATHERING, INTERPRETATION, AND COMMUNICATION

A forensic assessment model can be selected and used in a given case to help guide the forensic clinician in the important areas of data gathering, data interpretation, and communication of results. The use of a model in forensic evaluation has received relatively little attention in the literature. Only two general models, developed in the context of civil commitment (Morse, 1978a,b) and for a range of criminal and civil competencies (Grisso, 1986a), have been located. Each will be described and discussed. Other models (e.g., Bonnie, 1992, for competence to stand trial, and APA, 1994, for child custody), have been described as well, and will be considered as they apply to more specific kinds of FMHA.

Morse (1978a,b) has observed that the structures of different mental health laws are fundamentally similar in their focus on three broad questions: (1) the existence of a mental disorder, (2) the functional abilities related to the tasks that are part of the relevant legal question, and (3) the strength of the causal connection between the first and the second areas. This model was constructed from the observation that courts most frequently ask mental health professionals questions related to these areas: (1) Does the person have a mental disorder? (2) Is the person's legally relevant behavior caused by or the product of mental disorder rather than the product of the person's free choice? and (3) How will the person behave in the future? (Morse, 1978a,b).

Grisso (1986a) has also developed a model for forensic evaluations of legal competencies. It consists of six characteristics shared by "legal competencies." These characteristics are termed functional, contextual, causal, interactive, judgmental, and dispositional. *Functional* abilities are those that "an individual can do or accomplish, as well as to the specific knowledge, understanding, or beliefs" that are relevant to the particular legal competency (p. 15). *Contextual* describes the "general environmental context, which establishes the parameters for defining the relevance of particular functional abilities for the legal competency construct" (p. 18). *Causal* inferences "explain (how) an individual's functional abilities or deficits (are) related to a legal competency" (p. 20). The *interactive* characteristic of the model asks "Does this person's level of ability meet the demands of the specific situation with which the person will be (was) faced?" (p. 23). The *judgmental* aspect addresses whether the "person–context incongruency is of a sufficient magnitude to warrant a finding of legal incompetency and its disposition consequences" (p. 26). Finally, the *dispositional* aspect of the judgment refers to the consequences of a finding of incompetence, which may give the state "the authority to act in some way toward the individual" (p. 27).

The model described by Morse has several advantages. It is simple, as it includes the elements that are most commonly cited by courts and commentators (clinical condition, functional capabilities, and relationship between the two). It describes the implications for data-gathering directly: the need to obtain information about mental health symptoms or intellectual deficits, and the importance of capabilities that are specifically relevant to elements of the legal test. It addresses the reasoning task as well; the forensic clinician, in describing how the clinical characteristics affect the functional abilities, is asked to describe the strength of this causal connection, and the reasons for her conclusions about this strength. Finally, it facilitates communication of the results of the forensic evaluation. Both in the written report and in testimony, applying this model makes it easier for the clinician to describe her data and reasoning to attorneys and judges.

However, Morse's model may not account for some important influences in the process of forensic assessment. There are two elements in the Grisso model that are not present in Morse's: context and interaction. The variable of "situation" has long been recognized as an important influence on behavior (Bem & Allen, 1974; Bem & Funder, 1978; Steadman, 1982). Grisso's *context* relates directly to the influence of situation in the competence construct. The influences contained within the contextual variable— the nature of the charges, the choice of plea and the subsequent determination of whether charge disposition will result from a trial or a plea bargain, the characteristics of the attorney who represents the defendant— might play an important part in explaining why the same defendant could justifiably be adjudicated competent to stand trial in one situation, but not another.

This is consistent with a recent theoretical reformulation of the construct of criminal competence (Bonnie, 1992), in which competence is not treated as a single, open-textured construct. Rather, Bonnie describes two related but separable constructs: a foundational concept of competence to assist counsel and a contextualized concept of decisional competence. This reformulation has the advantages of (1) providing a useful explanatory framework for settled features of existing law, (2) clarifying questions on which the law is unsettled, (3) exposing similarities between criminal competencies and other competencies (thereby linking heretofore discrete literatures in law and behavioral sciences), and (4) providing a framework for defining "psycho-legal abilities" that are encompassed by each of the two competency constructs. Bonnie argues strongly that contextual variables linked with the defendant's capacities to consider and decide on a plea, and the associated circumstances resulting from discrete plea decisions, should be considered as part of the trial competence construct.[1]

If context *is* considered, then the importance of the other Grisso variable not described by Morse—interaction—must be considered as well. As framed by Grisso, the issue of interaction addresses whether the person's abilities meet the demands of the context with which that person will be faced. Interaction is weighed by considering the difference between the "needed" and the "observed" levels of legally relevant abilities. When the "needed" level is lower, then a correspondingly lower level of "observed" abilities would be sufficient to allow the individual to proceed. However, when the "needed" abilities level is higher, the level of "observed" abilities must also be higher in order for the individual to be considered competent. This means that a greater range of overall abilities (moderate to high) would be acceptable when the "needed abilities" demand is lower, while a smaller ranger (only higher) of abilities would be seen when the "needed abilities" demand is higher. Like the statistical technique analysis of variance, the "interaction" is thus defined by a "difference in differences."

However, the notions of context and interaction can be difficult to convey in written communication or testimony. This is not because the idea that a person's capacities might be adequate for one context but not another (e.g., he has the capacity to make A's in high school but not college) is hard to grasp; indeed, it is a fairly commonsense idea. What seems to be difficult at times, however, is determining whether a given judge will consider context to be important in the same way that symptoms and abilities are important. When context is not treated by the court to be a "variable" relevant to the evaluation, then neither context nor its interaction with personal capacities can be a meaningful part of the court's decision. For example, the observation that a defendant's capacity in a given area (e.g., capacity to communicate) might be adequate under some circumstances (e.g., with minor charges and an attorney willing to pa-

[1]Bonnie's formulation is not consistent with the U.S. Supreme Court's decision in *Godinez v. Moran* (1993), in which the court held that there should be a single standard for competence to stand trial rather than discrete standards depending on context (e.g., in a case in which a defendant wished to represent himself in an extremely serious case, versus wished to plead guilty as part of a plea bargain in a relatively minor case). The *Godinez* decision, however, makes it conceptually more difficult to apply a higher standard in a case like that of Colin Ferguson, a mentally disabled defendant who represented himself in the shooting of passengers on a Long Island train in a trial that was widely viewed as a "charade" (see, e.g., Perlin, 1996, for a fuller discussion).

tiently "coach"[2] the defendant) but not adequate under others (e.g., with charges necessitating testimony as part of the preferred defense, or with an attorney committed to only advising rather than "coaching" the defendant) would be considered only in terms of the level of the defendant's communication ability in both instances.

As another example, consider a child custody case in which the court was weighing a shared custody arrangement for parents with two children: one a well-adjusted 14-year-old boy actively involved with friends and a number of school activities and the other a developmentally disabled 8-year-old boy who required an extraordinary amount of supervision and who reacted very badly to even minor changes in his environment. Assume further that the father's work often kept him at his office until early evening, while the mother's employment allowed her to be at home by the time the children returned from school. In this case, the needs of the older boy might be met comparably well by each parent, and a shared custody decision might therefore be indicated. However, the needs of the younger boy might be met much better by remaining in the mother's home than through a shared custody arrangement in which he spent half of the week at his father's new home.

This example might also be considered by using a particular model described in the *Guidelines for Child Custody Evaluations in Divorce Proceedings* (APA, 1994). This model might be described as a specific adaptation of the more general Grisso model:

> The focus of the evaluation is on parenting capacity, the psychological and developmental needs of the child, and the resulting fit. In considering psychological factors affecting the best interests of the child, the psychologist focuses on the parenting capacity of the prospective custodians in conjunction with the psychological and developmental needs of each involved child. This involves (a) an assessment of the adults' capacities for parenting, including whatever

---

[2]I've informally observed that attorneys vary a good deal in how they represent defendants with severe mental illness, and in their preferences regarding what the client needs to be able to do. Assessment reports and testimony about defendants who have been adjudicated incompetent, committed and treated in a forensic hospital, and responded favorably to treatment so they appear appropriate for reconsideration as competent usually emphasize how the defendant's continuing deficits can be managed. Further, such reports and testimony may advise the attorney how to best communicate with his client. Some attorneys incorporate these suggestions easily, and are comfortable with a "coaching" style—active involvement with advising, restating options, directing communication, and generally helping the defendant in a number of ways. Other attorneys feel obligated to avoid such tactics, sometimes for reasons of stylistic preference and other times because of the ethical demand that the attorney only advise, but not "become," the client. One contextual variable concerns which of these styles seems to better characterize the attorney.

knowledge, attributes, skills, and abilities, or lack thereof, are present; (b) an assessment of the psychological functioning and developmental needs of each child and of the wishes of each child where appropriate; and (c) an assessment of the functional ability of each parent to meet these needs, including an evaluation of the interaction between each adult and child.

The values of the parents relevant to parenting, ability to plan for the child's future needs, capacity to provide a stable and loving home, and any potential for inappropriate behavior or misconduct that might negatively influence the child also are considered. Psychopathology may be relevant to such an assessment, insofar as it has impact on the child or the ability to parent, but it is not the primary focus. (p. 678)

In this particular model, there is no prong that includes only clinical symptoms or functioning. Rather, the areas of functional criteria (parenting capacity and psychological/developmental needs of the child) are described directly, in terms that could be affected by clinical functioning (but also by a variety of other influences). Moreover, the "resulting fit" between parenting capacity and children's needs describes both the interaction and the context from the Grisso model. In the example from the last paragraph, given the differing needs of the two children, the "fit" between each parent and each child was different, so that the recommendation for custodial arrangement might be different between the two children.

It would be easier to describe context by providing *separate* constructs for different legal competencies. This would allow the evaluator to use different criteria for the varying legal standards, rather than interpreting the same criteria differently according to the features of the case. The application of Bonnie's (1992) reconceptualization would clearly be facilitated by separating competence to stand trial from competence to plead guilty, for example, with the contextualized area of decisional competence varying according to the defendant's preference for plea. If this were an option, then context would be less important, since it would have been considered by separating the legal competencies. If legal competencies were considered separately, then a simpler model (such as Morse's) that does not explicitly consider context might be preferable.

The law does allow for separate consideration of some forms of legal competence. Civil competencies (e.g., guardianship, competence to consent to treatment, competence to consent to research, testamentary capacity) pertain to different circumstances *and* can clearly be considered in the context of such circumstances. For example, the following have been proposed as functional criteria relevant to competence to make treatment decisions: (1) expressing a choice, (2) understanding information relevant to treatment decision-making, (3) appreciating the significance of that information for one's own situation, and (4) reasoning about treatment options (Grisso & Appelbaum, 1998a,b). This proposal reflects an awareness that there is sufficient flexibility in the legal standard to consider the specific decision that must be made, because courts have not attempted to define a more uniform standard across situations. Such flexibility, and contextual relevance, has been restricted for criminal competencies by *Godinez v. Moran* (1993), which is discussed in the Law section of this principle.

In trying to determine whether a general model is appropriate, and under what circumstances, it is useful to compare their common elements. Both Morse and Grisso describe a *functional* component (what a litigant must be able to do in order to satisfy a legal standard) and a *causal* component (the extent to which the functional behavior is affected by relevant influences such as clinical condition). After these common elements, however, the models diverge in several ways. The Morse model specifies "mental disorder" as the general area in which mental health law is concerned as the possible cause of functional deficits in the context of a forensic evaluation. Grisso's model, in contrast, does not provide a specific area that would influence functional abilities. While it clearly includes mental disorder, it also could incorporate a broader range of possible influences. These might include, for example, being naive or uninformed about the legal process, or having insufficient developmental maturity to appreciate one's rights or make rational decisions. The basic elements of mental disorder, functional abilities, and the causal connection between the two can thus be recognized in both models, although in Grisso's the first element is neither explicit nor limited to mental disorder. After such "common ground" between the models has been identified, it seems clearer that these three elements, at least, should be included in any model that is used in forensic assessment.

ETHICS

There is little direct support from sources of ethics authority for the use of a model in forensic assessment. There is some indirect support— that is, using a model is *one way* in which several ethical principles can be satisfied. This would only be true if the model is a good one, however. To the extent that a model facilitates *conceptualization, organization*, and *communication* of *legally relevant information*, it is useful. When a model fails to meet these purposes (or, worse, when it detracts from them), then its usefulness is lost and the reasons for applying it are no longer persuasive. The value of different models has been reviewed earlier, but subsequent discussion of various kinds of support for using a model *is premised on the assumption that the model is both useful in broad terms and appropriate to the nature of the forensic issues.*

In the *Ethical Principles of Psychologists and Code of Conduct* (APA, 1992), it is noted that "psychologists rely on scientifically and professionally derived knowledge when making scientific or professional judgments or when engaging in scholarly or professional endeavors" (p. 1600). Using a good model can clarify the knowledge being relied on in making observations and drawing conclusions. Both of the general models discussed in this chapter contain a "causal" component, requiring the evaluator to describe the connection between the clinical characteristics and the functional abilities in a given case. More specifically, the *Ethical Principles* stipulates that possible involvement in legal proceedings creates a responsibility on the part of the psychologist "to create and maintain documentation in the kind of ... quality that would be consistent with reasonable scrutiny in an adjudicative forum" (p. 1602). The most important forms of documentation and communication are the report and expert testimony. Using a model can help to clarify the relationship between clinical characteristics and functional attributes. The resulting enhancement of organization and communication should improve the "quality ... consistent with reasonable scrutiny" described in this section of the *Ethical Principles*.

Consistent with this, and elaborated more specifically, is the following standard from the *Specialty Guidelines for Forensic Psychologists* (1991):

> Forensic psychologists have an obligation to document and be prepared to make available ... all data that form the basis for their evidence or services. The standard to be applied to such documentation or recording *anticipates* that the detail and quality of such documentation will be subject to reasonable judicial scrutiny; this standard is higher than the normative standard for general clinical practice. (p. 661)

Under this standard, good documentation in the forensic context is expected, and "all data" are considered under what is to be documented. Reasoning is not mentioned explicitly in this paragraph, although the expectation that the forensic psychologist examines the issue "from all reasonable perspectives, actively seeking information that will differentially test plausible rival hypotheses" (p. 661) suggests that both data and reasoning should be provided to the court.

Neither the *Principles of Medical Ethics with Annotations* (APA, 1998) nor the *Ethical Guidelines for the Practice of Forensic Psychiatry* (AAPL, 1995) addresses this principle, either directly or indirectly.

LAW

Within the structure of mental health law is embedded the three elements of Morse's model: mental disorder, functional demands, and causal connection between the two. These three elements were originally discussed by Morse in the context of civil commitment, and may be seen in the structure of civil commitment statutes throughout the United States.[3] A similar structure may also be seen in the commitment criteria for individuals in the criminal justice system. The model commitment criteria for individuals acquitted by reason of insanity are described in the *Criminal Justice Mental Health Standards* (ABA, 1989) as follows:

> the acquittee (i) is currently mentally ill or mentally retarded; and, as a result, (ii) poses a substantial risk of serious bodily harm to others. (Standard 7-7.4, p. 418)

How would the use of a model affect the admissibility of forensic mental health assessment evidence under the two major evidentiary standards—*Frye* and *Daubert*—currently applied to expert testimony in the United States? While a model serves to *organize* procedures, techniques, and their results, it does not *provide* them. Hence, the effect of using a model is not likely to be identified as such admitting expert mental health evidence. Rather, the consequences of using a model—conceptualization, organization, and communication of legally relevant material—would likely affect the weight of the evidence being provided, if not its admissibility.

Under the 1923 *Frye v. United States* decision, the standard for admissibility of expert evidence was described in terms of "general acceptance":

> Just when a scientific principle or discovery crosses the line between the experimental and demonstrable stages is difficult to define. Somewhere in this twilight zone the evidential force of the principle must be recognized, and while courts will go a long way in admitting expert testimony deduced from a well-recognized scientific principle or discovery, the thing from which the deduction is made must be sufficiently established to have gained general acceptance in the particular field in which it belongs. (p. 1014)

Does using a model help a court determine whether particular FMHA evidence is "generally accepted" in the field? To the extent that using a model makes it clearer to the court (1) what sources of information are related to which conclusions and (2) the evaluator's reasoning about these relationships, then the *Frye* standard is consistent with using a model.

Presuming that *Daubert* applies to FMHA evidence, there are two ways in which *Daubert's* influence on such evidence might be considered. The first involves the specific techniques used in the overall assessment:

[3]This appears as applicable in 1996 as it did in 1978, when Morse published his lengthy treatise on mental health law (Morse, 1978a). Civil commitment statutes typically begin with a "threshold issue" (mental disease or defect), connected to the functional legal test (usually danger to others or danger to self, either through self-harm or incapacity to care for self) by language such as "as a result of" or "due to." In Pennsylvania, for example, an individual must have a "severe mental disability" that results in a "clear and present danger to self or others" [50 Pa.Con.Stat.Ann., sec 301(b), with further definitions of "danger to self" and "danger to others" provided].

the interview(s) with the litigant, the review of collateral documents, the interviews with third parties, and the use of specific psychological tests or medical procedures. Each of these techniques could be analyzed using the criteria set forth in *Daubert*. If a technique were held to be inadmissible under these criteria, then the court could exclude either the entire testimony, or that part based on the nonadmissible technique.

The implications of *Daubert* have also been considered more broadly (e.g., Walker & Monahan, 1996). If the "scientific" method described in *Daubert* were considered as *an approach to gathering knowledge* rather than merely the particular tools or products of science, then the court could analyze FMHA by considering whether the assessment in a given case had used scientific reasoning. The question would then be whether the forensic clinician had formulated the issues being evaluated in terms of testable hypotheses, and whether these hypotheses had been tested. For these questions, the use of a model could help the court answer these questions. For example, one straightforward way of formulating a hypothesis (similar to the null hypothesis) would be as follows: "Relevant clinical characteristics were not present in the defendant at the time of the alleged offense, and hence could bear no causal relationship to his behavior." A second version of the null hypothesis could be stated: "The defendant's clinical symptoms, although actively experienced around the time of the alleged offense, bore little or no causal relationship to his behavior, which was instead more strongly influenced by other factors." An alternative hypothesis might be the following: "The clinical characteristics of the defendant directly and strongly influenced his behavior at the time of the offense, so that it was very difficult for him to understand the wrongfulness of his behavior."

Framing hypotheses in this way is facilitated by the use of a model containing the elements of clinical characteristics, functional behaviors, and causal connection. The procedures used by the evaluator to assess each hypothesis, the evidence that is supportive and nonsupportive of each, and the reasoning about such hypothesis-testing and its subsequent conclusions are all clearer under a model that promotes an explicit description of each.

In an important case relevant to several kinds of criminal competencies— those relevant to disposition of charges under *Godinez v. Moran* (1993)—the U.S. Supreme Court considered the question of whether there is a different standard from general competence to stand trial contrasted with the decisions that must be made in the course of disposing of charges (most often, competence to plead guilty, and other decisions relevant to Fifth and Sixth Amendment rights such as that of dismissing one's attorney, which occurred in the *Godinez* case). Reversing a Ninth Circuit finding that a different and higher standard was applicable to a defendant's decision to waive constitutional rights and plead guilty,[4] the U.S. Supreme Court in *Godinez* held that the decision to plead guilty does not represent a separate competence, although the court should ensure that the decision to waive any constitutional right on the part of the defendant is "knowing and voluntary."

The Court's holding in *Godinez* is relevant to the use of a model in one important way. First, the role of "context" is considerably diminished as part of competence to stand trial if a similar standard is applied to defendants choosing to plead guilty and those preferring to plead not guilty. It is clear that the process for charge disposition is considerably different for defendants making choices for a negotiated plea and a trial, respectively. There has been discussion of the "higher standard" necessary for waiving constitutional rights set forth by the *Sieling v. Eyman* (1973) decision (see Melton et al., 1997), although it would perhaps better be described as a different standard: The cognitive demands for factual awareness and reasoning may be higher for a plea of guilty, but the behavioral demands for impulse control, stress tolerance, and the capacity to work with counsel throughout a trial are more prominent for a plea of not guilty. This difference, however, is less important under *Godinez*. By the promulgation of a more unified standard for trial competence, the Court has reduced the sensitivity to the different contexts created by trial versus negotiated plea, respectively. Using a model (such as Grisso's) in which context is explicitly considered must be done in light of the legal emphasis (or lack thereof) on context. After *Godinez*, the "context" in Grisso's model would be weighed less heavily in the evaluation of a defendant's trial competence. This point is particularly relevant to the kind of model that might be used (that is, one incorporating the use of context), although less relevant to the broader question of whether a model should be used.

Empirical

No empirical evidence is available on the use of a model in forensic assessment.

Standard of Practice

Except for the original discussions by Morse (1978a) and Grisso (1986a) on the structure of mental health law and the use of a model in

---

[4]This is consistent with other Ninth Circuit decisions on this issue (see, e.g., *Sieling v. Eyman*, 1973).

forensic assessment, respectively, there is very little literature on the use of such a model. Indirect assessment of a model's value may be obtained by determining how well it assists the forensic clinician in performing an evaluation that is consistent with conventional measures of forensic quality.

One such set of quality measures has been offered by Petrella and Poythress's (1983) study of the interdisciplinary differences in forensic evaluations. They used seven measures of quality in rating forensic evaluation reports: (1) examiner used proper legal criteria, (2) ultimate opinion clearly stated, (3) adequate basis for opinion is stated, (4) clinical characterization of defendant, (5) psychiatric jargon versus plain language, (6) information needed to assist court, and (7) overall quality. These criteria represent a reasonably well-accepted set of standards for forensic practice (with the exception of the "ultimate opinion clearly stated," around which there is continuing controversy). How might they be affected when a model is used in forensic assessment, particularly when the criteria for a good model discussed earlier in this chapter—*conceptualization, organization,* and *communication* of *legally relevant information*—are applied?

First, a good model should increase the likelihood that the forensic clinician will use proper legal criteria. The functional legal characteristics that are components in both the Grisso and Morse models are derived directly from the relevant legal test. Requiring that the evaluator describe explicitly the relevant legal characteristics, as a model does, should make the evaluator more conscious of the relevant legal criteria (if they are known to her), or more inclined to determine what they are (if she is not aware of them).

Because expressing an ultimate issue remains somewhat controversial, and is discussed elsewhere in this book, it will not be considered in the present discussion. The next "criterion of quality" used by Petrella and Poythress is whether an adequate basis for the opinion is stated (consistent with conceptualization, organization, communication, *and* relevance, noted earlier). How might a good model improve the basis of the opinion being given? There are at least two possibilities: (1) by requiring that the observed clinical characteristics be discussed in relation to the functional legal demands, and thereby (2) increasing the relevance of the information that is obtained, and the discussion about it, by framing this discussion in concepts that are of most interest to the court.

A good model would probably not improve the clinical characterization of the defendant, except perhaps by encouraging a focus on areas that are relevant to the functional legal criteria. However, there seems to be nothing about the use of a model that would increase the amount or the quality of the clinical information obtained during FMHA. While a model may not be dramatically useful in promoting the use of plain language over psychiatric jargon—a forensic clinician inclined to use technical language in a report could do so with or without a model—using a model does provide a structure for certain kinds of information, which cannot be communicated as effectively with technical jargon as with plain language.

A good model does have significant potential for improving "information needed to assist the court." The use of such a model will promote better conceptualized and more tightly organized material that is directly relevant to the forensic issues underlying the immediate legal decision(s). In this respect, the use of a good model helps to bridge the chasm between legal practice and the behavioral sciences. This analysis would suggest, therefore, that a model does have the potential to improve the quality of FMHA evaluations on certain dimensions that are generally accepted as good practice.

DISCUSSION

Although the literature contains relatively little about the use of models in forensic assessment, there is a good deal of evidence from different areas that the use of a good model simplifies and clarifies. Simplicity and clarity are important in deciding which model to employ; a complex discussion should be avoided when it is not needed. Thus, Morse's model would seem preferable when the litigant's functional abilities are either so limited, or so good, that the contextual considerations would have virtually no impact on the recommendation. However, for those individuals whose functional abilities are not so clearly strong or weak, the incorporation of context becomes more important. Under these circumstances, a model incorporating context (such as Grisso's) would be preferable. Context is useful when recommendations are conditional, which may occur not only with competencies but across a wider range of forensic issues (e.g., risk assessment, fitness to parent, capacity to work).

This discussion has considered the application of a model in FMHA in a contingent way. It should be added that the use of a poor model would probably result in forensic assessment and testimony that is *even worse* than using no model at all. When ideas or methods are flawed, conceptually or empirically, there is the potential to mislead the decision-maker who incorporates information based on such ideas or methods. When a model promotes an organizational structure that distracts or needlessly complicates the material, or encourages the use of jargon or otherwise obscures communication, then it poorly serves all involved. Finally, if a model promotes the use of standards that are not relevant to the legal decision or its underlying constructs, there is the potential for significantly misinforming the decision-maker. It is fair to conclude that a model has the potential to *improve or diminish* the quality of FMHA, depending on the characteristics of the model itself.

There is a fair amount of indirect support for using a good model, and no apparent contraindicating considerations, from the ethics, law, and standard of practice sources reviewed. No empirical evidence is apparently available on this issue. Therefore, the use of a model in FMHA would seem better classified as an *emerging* principle.

III

Data Collection

5

Selection

This chapter addresses principles that can help the forensic clinician in selecting the sources of information to be used in the forensic assessment. The first two principles involve the significance of multiple sources of information and the importance of relevance and reliability. Following this, several principles applicable to the various domains of information (history, clinical characteristics, and legally relevant behavior) will be considered. Finally, the principle addressing response style (which is relevant to both selection of sources of information and their subsequent interpretation) will be discussed.

USE MULTIPLE SOURCES OF INFORMATION FOR EACH AREA BEING ASSESSED

There is typically a variety of potential sources of information from which to select, including the self-report of the individual(s) being evaluated, obtained through clinical interview and via psychological testing and structured interview. There is also comparison to the groups with whom a psychological test has been normed and validated, allowing the clinician to consider the responses of the individual taking the test in the broader context of existing norms. Information based on others' observation of the individual being evaluated can be obtained from (1) those who frequently observe and interact with the individual (e.g., family members, friends, employers, teachers, nurses, aides) and (2) those who have had the opportunity to observe particularly relevant behavior (e.g., victims of or witnesses to a criminal offense). Documented records in areas such as mental health, medical, criminal, school, vocational, and military functioning are another source of potentially valuable information in FMHA.

ETHICS

The *Ethical Principles of Psychologists and Code of Conduct* (APA, 1992) does not provide commentary that directly addresses the issue of multiple sources of information. Some language relevant to this principle is that

> Psychologists' assessments, recommendations, reports, and psychological di-
> agnostic or evaluative statements are based on information and techniques
> (including personal interviews of the individual when appropriate) sufficient
> to provide appropriate substantiation for their findings. (p. 1603)

One of the important considerations related to the use of multiple sources of information is the question of whether there is personal contact with the individual being evaluated.[1] The *Ethics Code* is clear about the desirability of such contact, although it is not described as essential in all cases:

> Except as noted ... below, psychologists provide written or oral forensic reports
> or testimony of the psychological characteristics of an individual only after
> they have conducted an examination of the individual adequate to support
> their statements or conclusions.
>   When, despite reasonable efforts, such an examination is not feasible,
> psychologists clarify the impact of their limited information on the reliability
> and validity of their reports and testimony, and they appropriately limit the
> nature and extent of their conclusions or recommendations. (p. 1610)

The *Specialty Guidelines for Forensic Psychologists* (1991) addresses the issue of multiple sources of information in several ways. It stresses the importance of "examining the issue at hand from all reasonable perspectives, actively seeking information that will differentially test plausible rival hypotheses" (p. 661). It emphasizes the need for psychologists to "corroborate critical data that form the basis for their professional opinion" (p. 662). One of the most promising approaches to "corroborating" findings from one source is to compare them with findings from an independent source.[2] On the question of whether personal contact is a necessary part of FMHA, the *Guidelines* states:

---

[1]While the desirability of the evaluator's having personal contact with the individual undergoing FMHA may seem self-evident, there are some circumstances under which such contact is not possible. These include, for example, an individual refusing to participate in a court-ordered evaluation, or being unavailable to participate (e.g., as in postmortem reconstruction of psychological states; see Schneidman, 1981; but cf. Poythress, Otto, Darkes, & Starr, 1993; Otto, Poythress, Starr, & Darkes, 1993, for problems in the application of the psychological autopsy in forensic contexts).

[2]In this context, "corroboration" could have two different meanings. The first involves the consistency between two sources of information. The second meaning refers to gauging the accuracy of the information from the first source by using information from the second source. These two definitions correspond to the scientific constructs of reliability and validity, which are related in the following sense: higher reliability (more consistency) does not necessarily yield greater validity (more accuracy), but lower reliability (less consistency) does mean that at least one of the sources of information is less accurate.

> Forensic psychologists avoid giving written or oral evidence about the psychological characteristics of particular individuals when they have not had an opportunity to conduct an examination of the individual adequate to the scope of the statements, opinions, or conclusions to be issued. Forensic psychologists make every reasonable effort to conduct such examinations. When it is not possible or feasible to do so, they make clear the impact of such limitations on the reliability and validity of their professional products, evidence, or testimony. (p. 663)

The *Principles of Medical Ethics with Annotations* (American Psychiatric Association, 1998) does not address the use of multiple sources of information directly or indirectly. Nor does the *Ethical Guidelines* (AAPL, 1995) provide direct commentary on the use of multiple sources of information, but it describes the importance of "distinguishing, to the extent possible, between verified and unverified information as well as between clinical 'facts,' 'inferences' and 'impressions'" (p. 3). The *Guidelines* also notes that "[h]onesty, objectivity, and the adequacy of the clinical evaluation may be called into question when an expert opinion is offered without a personal examination" (p. 3), adding that

> it is the position of the Academy that if, after earnest effort, it is not possible to conduct a personal examination, an opinion may be rendered on the basis of other information. However, under such circumstances, it is the responsibility of forensic psychiatrists to assure that the statement of their opinion and any reports of testimony based on those opinions clearly indicate that there was no personal examination and opinions expressed are thereby limited. (p. 3)

LAW

Depending on whether the rules of evidence governing expert mental health testimony derive from *Frye* (1923) or *Daubert* (1993), there are somewhat different criteria for judging the legal standard applicable to the use of multiple sources of information in FMHA. Under the *Frye* standard, the question would turn on whether using multiple sources of information is "generally accepted." *Daubert* adds the criterion of scientific validity to "general acceptance in the field," raising the additional question (to be discussed in this section) about whether the use of multiple sources of information increases the accuracy of the conclusions reached in the course of an evaluation.

In a review of the 276 appellate decisions citing *Daubert* as of March 1996, there was no holding in which the court had applied *Daubert* criteria to some of the sources of information for FMHA: the interview, document review, third-party observations, or third-party interviews (Heilbrun, 1996). There is one case in which *Daubert* was cited; the Federal Court of Appeals in New Jersey recognized the importance of assessing the validity of each of the methods that were contributing to the overall conclusions

(*Waldorf v. Shuta*, 1996). This finding was consistent with the use of multiple sources (and critical evaluation of each) as part of forensic assessment.

EMPIRICAL

Relatively little empirical data are available to assess the sources of information that are used in FMHA. In a study on the use of various kinds of information in evaluations of defendant competence to stand trial and/or sanity at the time of the alleged offense in Florida (Heilbrun & Collins, 1995), it was observed that the clinical interview was virtually always used. The use of psychological testing (most frequently the Minnesota Multiphasic Personality Inventory, or MMPI, and the Wechsler Adult Intelligence Scale-Revised, or WAIS-R) was seen more often in reports done in the community than in reports generated while the defendant was hospitalized. However, it still was not as frequent as the use of various kinds of third-party information: (1) previous mental health evaluations (81% of hospital reports, 30% of community reports), (2) arrest report (95% of hospital reports, 48% of community reports), and (3) interview with hospital or jail staff (70% of hospital reports, 17% of community reports). It appears that most of the hospital evaluators used multiple sources (since almost all used all three of these). When the Florida sample was compared with data from Virginia, it was observed that third-party information was also used at high rates: (1) information about the offense (87% of Virginia community reports, 68% of Virginia hospital reports), (2) mental health records (50% of Virginia community reports, 35% of Virginia hospital reports), and (3) victim/witness statements (2% of Florida community reports, 36% of Virginia community reports, 1% of Florida hospital reports, 18% of Virginia hospital reports) (Heilbrun, Rosenfeld, Warren, & Collins, 1994).

A national survey of forensic psychologists and psychiatrists (about 80% of whom were board-certified) regarding procedures used in criminal forensic evaluations (Borum & Grisso, 1996) reflected participants' ratings of importance of various areas and sources of information in evaluations of competence to stand trial, and sanity at the time of the offense. These areas and sources of information included: (1) psychiatric history, (2) mental health records, (3) current mental status, (4) observations by the examiner and others from other settings, (5) information from the police, and (6) psychological testing. These areas were all rated as either "essential" or "recommended" by the majority of both psychiatrists and psychologists, for both trial competence and criminal responsibility evaluations, with the exceptions of information from the police for trial competence evaluations (only 44% of psychologists rated this as either essential or recommended) and psychological testing for criminal responsibility (only 29% of psychologists rated it as recommended, and none rated it essential). These studies suggest that both use of and recommendations for information from multiple sources are endorsed by significant numbers of mental health professionals involved in FMHA.

Recent research in risk assessment provides a good illustration of the broader forensic principle regarding multiple sources of information. According to Monahan (1981), one of the difficulties seen in most of the violence research performed in the 1970s and early 1980s was that much undetected violence may have occurred. When researchers use insensitive outcome measures (e.g., rearrest, rehospitalization), then confidence in the accuracy of the violence outcome rate is undermined. This problem was addressed by the MacArthur Research Network in a long-term study of violence and mental disorder done between 1988 and 1997 (Monahan & Steadman, 1994; Steadman et al., 1998). Multiple measures of violence outcomes were obtained, including regularly scheduled self-report and concurrent interviews with a previously identified collateral observer. Research using this approach found higher rates of identified participants who had behaved violently when a collateral informer is used, as opposed to simply asking for self-report (Lidz, Mulvey, & Gardner, 1993; Mulvey, 1992; Mulvey & Lidz, 1993; Steadman et al., 1998). Presumably one of the reasons for this involves the use of an outcome measure that is more sensitive because it included a collateral description of violent behavior. Otto (1994) has observed that multiple sources of information to determine violence outcome have been used to improve accuracy of research outcomes and can guide clinical evaluations, to the extent that they are shaped by violence research.

Response style is another area in which multiple sources of information are important. This will be discussed in detail later in this chapter. For present purposes, however, consider the approaches to assessing response style and the associated sources of information covered in the most recent edition of Rogers's (1997b) edited work on malingering and deception. These include psychological tests (multiscale inventories, projective measures, and intellectual and neuropsychological instruments) as well as specialized measures such as drug-assisted interviews, polygraphy, hypnosis, and structured interviews.[3] While the empirical support for these different approaches varies, it is clear that there are several different approaches that could be used in assessing response style in a given case, providing the evaluator with the opportunity to gauge the consistency of several different measures.

---

[3]The noteworthy exception to the comprehensive coverage of approaches relevant to malingering described in this book are those approaches in which third parties describe their observations of the individual being assessed.

This is one example of the multitrait–multimethod matrix (Campbell & Fiske, 1959), a powerful tool for assessing validity at a quantitative or commonsense level (see Meier, 1994, for a review of the literature in this area). The approach has had a significant impact on the field of psychological measurement generally. Its particular influence on FMHA is described by Grisso (1986b), who noted the importance of collecting several measures of any given behavior, trait, or symptom to enhance accuracy.

An appropriate note of caution in this regard has also been sounded, however (Faust, 1989). The assumption that clinicians can effectively integrate "all the data" to produce more valid conclusions can be problematic for two reasons. First, different sources of information may have different levels of validity; their indiscriminant combination can actually produce a *less* accurate conclusion than would result from relying on fewer sources with uniformly higher validity. Second, the problem of data combination—determining how to weigh different sources of information optimally—is better addressed through actuarial approaches than clinical judgment (a point to be discussed later in this chapter in more detail, under the "Assess Relevant Clinical Characteristics" principle). These problems are best addressed through attention to the validity of each measure (when known), and proceeding with caution when combining measures with different (or unknown) levels of validity.[4]

STANDARD OF PRACTICE

Multiple measures may serve two purposes: (1) to enhance accuracy in measuring a given trait, symptom, or behavior and (2) to check "hypotheses" that may have been generated, in part, by observations stemming from one or more of the measures. Both of these purposes will be discussed.

[4]Critical thinking and common sense can help with this problem. The validity of a procedure may be "unknown" when the procedure (1) *cannot* be tested scientifically (e.g., the role of the "clinical interview" in FMHA, when such interviews are used for multiple purposes across a variety of forensic issues and legal questions), (2) *has not* been tested scientifically (e.g., the role of the clinical interview in evaluating a defendant's risk for future violent behavior, which could be tested under controlled conditions that would isolate the contribution of such an interview—but this has not yet been done), or (3) has been tested scientifically, with mixed or inconclusive results that may be exacerbated by methodological flaws in some of the studies (e.g., the role of specialized sexual offender treatment in reducing the risk of further sexual offending). Further, there is a difference regarding information obtained *from the individual* versus observations made *of the individual* during the interview. Finally, the value of the clinical interview may vary according to the extent to which the interviewer is informed about the individual, and can therefore point out inconsistences and ask for clarification (as contrasted with simply asking for information).

The multitrait–multimethod matrix (Campbell & Fiske, 1959) noted in the last section can serve as a powerful validity indicator, at both a quantitative and a commonsense level. Some commentators (Elwork, 1984; Grisso, 1986b) have stressed the importance of the multitrait–multimethod approach in forensic practice, involving the collection of several measures of any given behavior, trait, or symptom to enhance accuracy. Related points have been made by others: There are different constructs underlying any given legal issue, for which multiple measures are needed (Blau, 1984a), and the overreliance on one or two measures is a potential source of error in FMHA (Podboy & Kastl, 1993).

Brodzinsky (1993) has observed that some sources of information, such as psychological tests, may be applied routinely and uncritically to certain legal questions—child custody litigation, for example—due to perceived pressures (e.g., "the other side's expert is using them") or misunderstandings (e.g., lawyers and judges assuming that psychological tests measure aspects of the person or situation that cannot be uncovered through other procedures). As an alternative or adjunct to psychological testing, several sources of information are recommended. These include self-report questionnaires to assess relevant attitudes, behaviors, abilities, or styles, and a multi-source, multimethod assessment strategy within the context of a functional–contextualistic framework consistent with that described by Grisso (1986a).

The importance of multiple sources of information may also be seen in the *Guidelines for Child Custody Evaluations in Divorce Proceedings* (APA, 1994), which recommends that the psychologist use multiple methods for gathering data (clinical interviews, observation, psychological assessment, potentially relevant reports, and interviews with family and friends, for example). The *Guidelines* recommends corroboration of an observation from at least two sources and the documentation of such corroboration. The notes of caution about effectively integrating multiple sources of data through optimal combination and weighting (Faust, 1989; Meehl, 1954; Sawyer, 1966) should be considered carefully, however, so that forensic clinicians are attentive to validity indicators and cautious about clinical approaches to data combination.

The second purpose for multiple sources of information in FMHA is to "check" hypotheses that may explain the observed findings on forensic issues. In a 1990 APA symposium on forensic assessment, the discussant (David Faust) consistently emphasized problems of validity[5] for diag-

---

[5]Validity problems in social science differ in important ways from those in legal decision-making, however. The accuracy of a construct's measurement cannot be assessed in a social science context without a clearly defined, well-operationalized outcome measure. In law,

nosis, psychological testing, and clinical interviewing when applied to forensic issues. During the period for questions that followed the symposium, he was asked by David Shapiro, "In forensic evaluation, shouldn't we regard the results of these various measures as *hypotheses to be verified?*" This question succinctly summarized the second major purpose for obtaining multiple measures: Independently obtained information on a second measure about the same construct can be used to support (or refute) hypotheses that may have been generated by the results of the first measure. Thus, impressions from a psychological test in the forensic context should most appropriately be treated as hypotheses subject to verification through other psychological tests, history, medical tests, and third-party observations (Heilbrun, 1992). It should be added that an important component of this "verification" is consistency. To the extent that a forensic clinician can observe consistent accounts of behavior, reported by multiple sources, in a direction that would be expected based on a given hypothesis, we may have increased confidence in the accuracy of that hypothesis.

      This role of hypothesis-testing, and the related value of multiple sources of information, are noted in their application to child custody evaluation (Bricklin, 1992), where it was observed that the role of interview data should be to "set up hypotheses, not to reach definite conclusions" (p. 256). Ackerman and Kane (1998) also describe the importance of multiple sources of information in child custody evaluations, although in somewhat more detail. They suggest that child custody FMHA include school records (may provide information regarding whether a child has performed better in the custody of one parent or the other), medical records (which may provide information about possible child abuse), and arrest histories (if any) for both parents. In addition, Weissman (1991) has described the following as essential sources in child custody evaluation: (1) clinical, child custody oriented, mental status and biohistorical interviews of the parties and the minor child(ren), (2) psychological testing of the parties and the minor child(ren), and (3) assessment/observation of the interaction between respective parties and the minor child(ren). The following sources, although not considered essential by Weissman, are described as important in this context: (1) assessment of significant others, (2) contacts with relevant collaterals, (3) case-related documents and records, and (4) case-specific empirical data and theoretical concepts.

      The importance of hypothesis formulation, and the role of third-party

---

however, the "accuracy" of a decision may be measured in a far more diffuse way (e.g., consistency with settled law, with "facts" established through rules of evidence, or with community standards). Hence, standard measures of psychometric validity do not translate in straightforward fashion into legal "reliability."

information in helping to develop hypotheses, are also described by Gutheil (1992) in the context of litigation regarding claims of therapist–patient sexual misconduct. He discusses the importance of the *pattern* of responses, rather than a single positive finding in one category, and cites the importance of considering this information from a balanced perspective that incorporates the possibility of false accusations and considers response style.

Many other commentators have observed that any source of information should not be used in isolation in forensic cases, but combined with history, medical findings, and observations of behavior made by others (Melton et al., 1997; Shapiro, 1984, 1991). This appears as applicable in forensic evaluations in the area of personal injury (Matarazzo, 1990) as in the criminal context.

DISCUSSION

The use of multiple sources of information in FMHA is supported indirectly by ethics sources through the emphasis on "testing plausible rival hypotheses" and "distinguishing between verified and unverified information." Legal decisions concerning the admissibility of various measures have generally been limited thus far to considering psychological tests and specialized measures. Several empirical studies support the use of different sources of input and multiple measures in FMHA. This is theoretically consistent with the multitrait–multimethod matrix (Campbell & Fiske, 1959), which is influential in contemporary FMHA. A number of commentators have stressed that standard of practice considerations involve such multiple measures, both for enhancing accuracy and for testing hypotheses. When appropriate caution about combining measures of unknown validity is exercised, it seems clear that this principle should be considered *established*.

USE RELEVANCE AND RELIABILITY (VALIDITY) AS GUIDES FOR SEEKING INFORMATION AND SELECTING DATA SOURCES

Obtaining information and selecting different sources of such information in FMHA should be guided by relevance to the forensic issues and validity of the different sources. Although multiple sources of information are important in FMHA, there must be selectivity exercised regarding the choice of sources of information. If a given source has little or no accuracy, then it cannot increase the overall accuracy of the evaluation of forensic issues, and will decrease it if given much weight. This has been discussed for over 40 years in the context of "clinical versus statistical prediction" (Dawes, Faust, & Meehl, 1989; Faust, 1989; Meehl, 1954). However, the selection criteria in the forensic context are usually broader than the "predictive validity" criterion used in establishing the superiority of actuarial measures over clinical judgment. Rather, it is proposed that *relevance* and *reliability*, two important components of the law of evidence, be applied toward the selection of FMHA measures.

Relevance to the forensic issue is a judgment that can be made qualitatively, by describing the logical basis for a connection between a mental health construct (e.g., severe mental illness) and certain forensic issues (e.g., capacities to consider information in a knowing and intelligent way). It could also be described quantitatively, by citing empirical evidence about the strength of the relationship between these constructs in a research sample.

The issue of reliability, which can be applied to FMHA under the *Federal Rules of Evidence* and *Daubert* (1994), is more complex. There are different forms of reliability (test–retest and internal consistency, primarily) and validity (construct, predictive, convergent, and discriminant, for instance) that could be of interest to the court as they apply to a given measure. However, one of the particular criteria cited in *Daubert* concerns the "error rate" of the measure. To obtain this information, there must have been research with a "correct" outcome against which the accuracy of the particular measure can be calibrated. This design is particularly hard to implement in legal settings, given the difficulty in operationalizing an uncontaminated outcome[6] (see Grisso & Appelbaum, 1996; Kapp & Mossman, 1996; Roesch & Golding, 1980). For this principle, the criteria of reliability and relevance will be applied toward the selection of sources of information in FMHA.

---

[6]The issue of the appropriate outcome variable has shifted somewhat during the last two decades. As has been discussed at length (Roesch & Golding, 1980), the use of judges' decisions against which to validate an instrument or measure of a legal question is usually not appropriate, given that judges may not be accurate in their judgments about human behavior, they may not agree with other judges, and such decisions are not made independently of the evidence given by mental health professionals (which may be, in turn, related to the use of the measure). Nor is it appropriate to use the conclusion based on the results of the instrument to validate components of that instrument. There has been a trend during the last 25 years, however, toward the measurement of relevant constructs (what are called *forensic issues* in this book) rather than legal questions/conclusions, seen in earlier works such as Grisso (1981) and particularly in more recent research such as that done by the MacArthur Network and Mental Health and Law (Appelbaum & Grisso, 1995; Grisso, Appelbaum, Mulvey, & Fletcher, 1995; Grisso & Appelbaum, 1995, 1998a,b).

ETHICS

The *Ethical Principles of Psychologists and Code of Conduct* (APA, 1992) address the issues of validity and relevance in several ways. First, it is noted that psychological test construction should incorporate "scientific procedures and current professional knowledge for test design, standardization, validation, reduction or elimination of bias, and recommendations for use" (p. 1603). Further, caution is to be exercised in the application of tests to special populations:

> Psychologists attempt to identify situations in which particular interventions or assessment techniques or norms may not be applicable or may require adjustment in administration or interpretation because of factors such as individuals' gender, age, race, ethnicity, national origin, religion, sexual orientation, disability, language, or socioeconomic status. (p. 1603)

Finally, it is emphasized that forensic assessments, recommendations, and reports should be "based on information and techniques ... sufficient to provide appropriate substantiation for their findings" (p. 1610).

On the issue of "reliability," the *Specialty Guidelines for Forensic Psychologists* (1991) stresses the importance of using "current knowledge of scientific, professional and legal developments" in selecting data collection methods and procedures for an evaluation (p. 661). With respect to "relevance," it is noted that

> forensic psychologists avoid offering information from their investigations or evaluations that does not bear directly upon the legal purpose of their professional services and that is not critical as support for their product, evidence, or testimony, except where such disclosure is required by law. (p. 662)

Although it is not stated directly, this clearly implies that relevance should be important in the selection as well as the communication stage of the evaluation process, and that evaluators should select approaches and tests whose results allow communication of data relevant to the legal issue guiding the evaluation.

Neither the *Principles of Medical Ethics with Annotations* (American Psychiatric Association, 1998) nor the *Ethical Guidelines for the Practice of Forensic Psychiatry* (AAPL, 1995) addresses this principle directly or indirectly.

LAW

Consistent with Rule 702 in the *Federal Rules of Evidence*, the U.S. Supreme Court, in *Daubert* (1993), underscored *relevance* and *reliability* as the most important criteria for acceptance of scientific evidence in federal jurisdictions. The Court considered Rule 702 in terms of relevance (*Dau-*

bert, 1993, p. 2796), in that there must be "a valid scientific connection to the pertinent inquiry as a precondition to admissibility," as well as reliability, in that the expert's assertion must be based on scientific evidence and "supported by the appropriate validation" (p. 2795) (Fisher, 1994). The focus is on evaluation of a particular method or technique, which may present additional considerations in qualifying experts in forensic assessment, going beyond credentials to consider methods in a particular way (Thames, 1994).

In theory and occasionally in practice, *Daubert* does apply to FMHA. However, the frequency of its application, judging from a review of appellate cases, is limited. Of 276 cases citing *Daubert* between 1993 and 1996, only 12 applied even indirectly to FMHA (Heilbrun, 1996). The admissibility of techniques such as interview, document review, and third-party interviews or observations was not cited. Only one case addressed the use of any psychological test; it was held that the Child Behavior Checklist was not admissible for the evaluation of mentally retarded clients, because it had not been normed on that population (*Gier v. Educational Service Unit No. 16*, 1994). For specialized techniques, two courts held that evidence based on penile plethysmography was not admissibile because that technique was insufficiently reliable (*State v. Spencer*, 1995; *U.S. v. Powers*, 1995). Several kinds of diagnostic testimony, including DSM-IV-based diagnosis as well as syndrome testimony (e.g., Rape Trauma Syndrome, Battered Woman's Syndrome, Child Sexual Abuse Accommodation Syndrome), were held admissible with respect to the experience of symptoms or state of mind, but not on the question of whether the alleged event "actually occurred" (*Isely v. Capuchin Province*, 1995; *State v. Alberico*, 1993; *State v. Foret*, 1993; *State v. Martens*, 1993; *Steward v. State*, 1995; *Tungate v. Commonwealth*, 1995; *U.S. v. Brown*, 1995).[7] Finally, profile testimony was not admissible on the question of whether the alleged sexual offender fit a "sex offender profile" (*State v. Cavaliere*, 1995). Although relevance and reliability are criteria, courts have not seemed inclined to use these criteria to limit many of the bases for FMHA evaluation and testimony. This is true even since *Daubert*, which arguably gives courts the latitude to exclude techniques on grounds of scientific reliability as well as general acceptance.[8]

---

[7]In this respect, *Daubert* does not change the law of evidence regarding expert mental health testimony, which has never been admissible to prove the occurrence (or nonoccurrence) of an act.

[8]*Daubert* gives trial court judges far more discretion to consider expert mental health evidence than they have apparently used, at least to date. A good example is the use of the clinical interview, unsupported by other sources of information, as a basis for drawing

EMPIRICAL

There is apparently no available research that specifically tests "relevance" and "reliability" as criteria considered by courts in their acceptance of, or preference for, particular approaches. However, a broader view of the development of FMHA during the last two decades reveals a strong emphasis in these areas, with the development of specialized techniques (what Grisso, 1986, has called Forensic Assessment Instruments, or FAIs) to assess forensic issues. As an example, consider the evolution of the assessment of the capacities to understand and assist in one's criminal defense, and its relationship to the legal question of competence to stand trial.

The development of instruments to assist in the evaluation of constructs relevant to competence to stand trial has undergone several transitions. Prior to the *Dusky* (1960) decision, in which the legal criteria of "understand and assist" were described, the forensic assessments of trial competence were not guided by existing legal criteria that could increase their relevance, nor were they enhanced by instruments whose psychometric properties and outcome research could be used to gauge their empirical value. After *Dusky*, it was still over a decade until the Competency Screening Test and the Competency to Stand Trial Assessment Instrument were developed (Laboratory of Community Psychiatry, 1973), although some work focusing on legal relevance had been done several years earlier (Robey, 1965). Both the test and the assessment instrument represented important advances, as they were developed with the recognition of the legal question and the included forensic issues, but also validated through empirical research and amenable to description of their psychometric properties.

The next important transition in the assessment of forensic issues relevant to trial competence came with the expansion of the clinical criteria that were assessed in a structured way as part of the evaluation, and the requirement that the evaluator explicitly rate the relationship between clinical symptoms and functional legal deficits. This was seen in the development of the Interdisciplinary Fitness Interview (IFI; Golding, Roesch, &

---

conclusions regarding mental status and functional capacities. There is good scientific evidence to suggest that the clinical interview, when used in this fashion, is limited in both reliability and validity—yet no appellate court has yet focused on this "core" clinical procedure. One possible explanation is that courts are less critical in their scrutiny of clinical procedures that are "generally accepted" in the field, in effect emphasizing the *Frye* portion of the *Daubert* criteria, *regardless of the empirically established value of such procedures*. A second possible explanation is that considering each procedure described in each FMHA (not simply those that are unfamiliar to the court) would take so much time that court schedules would be seriously disrupted.

112

CHAPTER 5

Schreiber, 1984) and its revised version (Golding, 1993). The psychometric reliability of the original instrument was good (kappa coefficients for agreement between raters ranging between .40 and .58 on the legal items, and between .48 and .91 on psychopathological symptoms, and 97% agreement between interviewer pairs consisting of one mental health professional and one attorney on the legal question of competency). Norms and validation data for large samples of defendants are not available for the IFI and IFI-R, however.

The third important step in the incorporation of relevance and reliability into FAI development may be seen in the research of the MacArthur Research Network on Mental Health and Law. The work done by the MacArthur Network in the area of trial competence began with the "theoretical reformulation" of the competence construct into adjudicative and decisional components (Bonnie, 1992), with the former emphasizing the more traditional *Dusky* capacities of understanding and assisting in one's defense, but the latter area focusing more specifically on the important question of the individual's capacity to make a knowing and intelligent choice regarding plea. Based in part on this distinction, the Network has developed both a research tool for the measurement of capacities relevant to trial competence (the MacArthur Structured Assessment of Competencies of Criminal Defendants, or MacSAC-CD; Hoge, Bonnie, Poythress, Monahan, Eisenberg, & Feucht-Haviar, 1997) and a clinical-forensic tool for use by mental health professionals in the assessment of forensic issues relevant to trial competence (the MacArthur Competence Assessment Tool–Criminal Adjudication, or MacCAT-CA; Otto et al., 1998). The focus of both is on the measurement of forensic issues that are relevant to the broader legal question of trial competence, rather than the measurement of or conclusion regarding the defendant's competence to stand trial.

The changes occurring in this area may be understood by considering them according to the criteria of relevance and reliability. A major shift in relevance occurred with the introduction of assessment that explicitly considered the legal standard; a second shift may be seen in the emphasis on measuring the relevant included constructs rather than the broader legal question. When considered in this way, some of the most difficult problems that have plagued behavioral science research in legal contexts are greatly diminished. The measurement of psychometric reliability and validity using criteria such as the decision made by the court has always been problematic because courts' decisions (1) often are not independent of the mental health evidence that would affect a given measure and (2) are also influenced by concerns that are political, moral, and reflect community values. By focusing on measuring the forensic issues rather than predicting the ultimate legal decision, researchers can provide empirical evidence on reliability and validity that are not affected by political and moral considerations to a comparable extent.

Research and instrument development of this kind also leads more easily to report-writing and testimony that focuses on specific capacities than on the ultimate legal issue. This trend may be observed in the recent development of instruments in other areas, such as (1) the capacities to make treatment decisions, as measured by the MacArthur Competence Assessment Tool–Treatment (Grisso, Appelbaum, & Hill-Fotouhi, 1997), (2) response style, as measured by the Structured Instrument of Reported Symptoms (Rogers, 1992; Rogers, Bagby, & Dickens, 1992), (3) violence risk assessment, as measured by the Violence Risk Appraisal Guide (Rice & Harris, 1995) or the Violence Prediction Scheme (Webster, Harris, Rice, Cormier, & Quinsey, 1994), (4) capacities relevant to competence to waive Miranda rights, as measured by the Instruments for Assessing Understanding and Appreciation of Miranda Rights (Grisso, 1998b), and (5) capacities relevant to child custody, such as self-concept, interpersonal relationship, and emotional/cognitive functioning, as measured by the Ackerman–Schoendorf Parent Evaluation of Custody Tests (ASPECT; Ackerman & Schoendorf, 1992).

STANDARD OF PRACTICE

In an earlier discussion of the use of psychological testing in forensic contexts, I offered pre-*Daubert* guidelines for selecting particular instruments (Heilbrun, 1992). Although the discussion focused primarily on psychological testing, the broader framework is applicable to the selection of other sources of information as well. Relevance to the legal issue and reliability (the test's psychometric properties, plus validation research base) were used as the major criteria for deciding whether a given test should be among the sources of information used in a given case. The nature of legal decision-making was discussed as a useful context in which this decision must be made. Two points about such decision-making are salient. First, there is flexibility in legal contexts that accommodates the political, moral, and community standards influences that differ between jurisdictions. Such flexibility is also evident for different legal questions; for example, the range of mental health testimony considered relevant in a capital sentencing hearing is much broader than that relevant to the question of sanity at the time of the offense.[9] Second, the "relevance" of mental

[9]This notion has been promoted by legal scholars (e.g., Slobogin, 1984; Wyda & Black, 1989) and supported by U.S. Supreme Court decisions (*Chambers v. Mississippi*, 1973; *Rock v. Arkansas*, 1987).

health information typically pertains to underlying constructs (in this book, termed *forensic issues*) rather than to legal questions. It is not as straightforward as asserting (as some have; see, e.g., Ziskin, 1981; Ziskin & Faust, 1988) that information sources such as psychological tests should be excluded because they are not directly applicable to the legal question. Finally, my discussion offered seven guidelines for test selection, including the test's reliability and relevance to the forensic issue.

Marlowe (1995) has also offered a set of criteria to be applied to the question of whether certain tests are appropriate for forensic use. These criteria include (1) support by a sufficient body of literature, (2) having items with adequate range that represent all relevant content domains, (3) standard administration procedures and justified norms yielding sound data, and (4) yielding valid expert reasoning linking data to conclusions. Both the Heilbrun (1992) and Marlowe (1995) discussions have been incorporated into an analysis of the application of testing to response style in juvenile evaluations (McCann, 1998), and could be applied as well to other forensic issues in the contexts of different legal questions.

DISCUSSION

Relevance and reliability are among the most important considerations for FMHA, both when considering it broadly and when structuring the contours of an individual evaluation. Even before *Daubert* was decided, relevance and reliability were important considerations in FMHA. This may be seen in several areas. Ethical sources of authority stress the validity and reliability of measures used for assessment, as well as attention to current scientific, professional, and legal developments. More specialized ethics sources also recommend the exclusion of information that does not bear directly on the legal purpose of the evaluation. Legal authority has stressed reliability and relevance. The developing empirical literature over the last three decades has clearly been shaped by the dual influences of legal relevance and scientific reliability/validity. The standard of practice literature has also emphasized the use in FMHA of sources relevant to the forensic issues, although there has been some move away from sources that may be oriented directly toward the legal question. This literature has also included some discussion of "reliability" as including not only psychometric reliability and validation, but also the kind of scientific thinking involved in operationalization and testing of hypotheses.

Since the *Daubert* decision, there has been even greater emphasis placed on reliability. Courts have been given broader latitude to use this criterion to admit or exclude specific components of FMHA, although (judging from appellate law) they may not exercise this discretion very frequently. The principle of considering relevance and reliability in selecting sources clearly appears to be *established*.

OBTAIN RELEVENT HISTORICAL INFORMATION

This principle concerns the collection of historical information on the person(s) being evaluated in FMHA, and the question of what historical information is relevant in a given case. The number of domains in which historical information is needed in forensic assessment is potentially large. Information about social, medical, mental health, and family functioning is routinely obtained in the course of therapeutic assessment, but other areas that are potentially relevant to constructs being assessed in FMHA include criminal, military, school, sexual, and vocational history. Relevance to the forensic issue(s) in the case is an important consideration in whether information from such domains should be gathered. Historical information is particularly important for assessing patterns of behavior, and understanding how a specific act in question may fit into the larger pattern of behavior in the person's life. It is also important in assessing response style and the genuineness of self-reported facts, characteristics, and symptoms. Finally, historical information can be essential when, in the course of a reconstructive evaluation, the forensic clinician must use history to provide direct information about relevant thoughts, feelings, and behavior of the individual.

Ethics

The *Ethical Principles of Psychologists and Code of Conduct* (APA, 1992) indirectly addresses the importance of history as follows:

> Psychologists' assessments, recommendations, reports, and psychological diagnostic or evaluative statements are based on information and techniques (including personal interviews of the individual when appropriate) sufficient to provide appropriate substantiation for their findings. (p. 1603; also p. 1610 under Forensic Activities)

The *Specialty Guidelines for Forensic Psychologists* (1991) indicates that

> forensic psychologists have an obligation to maintain current knowledge of scientific, professional, and legal developments within their area of claimed competence. They are obligated also to use that knowledge, consistent with accepted clinical and scientific standards, in selecting data collection methods and procedures for an evaluation, treatment, consultation or scholarly/ empirical investigation. (p. 661)

The "accepted clinical and scientific standards" cited here would include a history obtained and refined through multiple sources. In addition:

> As an expert conducting an evaluation, treatment, consultation, or scholarly/empirical investigation, the forensic psychologist maintains professional integrity by examining the issue at hand from all reasonable perspectives, actively seeking information that will differentially test plausible rival hypotheses. (p. 661)

Hypothesis generation and testing is facilitated by good historical information. In addition, history is directly relevant to the assessment of forensic issues in reconstructive evaluations.

Neither the *Principles of Medical Ethics with Annotations* (1998) nor the *Ethical Guidelines* (1995) addresses this principle.

LAW

The *Criminal Justice Mental Health Standards* (ABA, 1989) indicates that the contents of the written report should include the "clinical findings and opinions on each matter referred for evaluation" as well as the "sources of information and ... factual basis for the evaluator's clinical findings and opinions" (p. 109). The *Standards* does not indicate directly that historical information must be obtained. However, we may infer that when information from the individual's history serves as either a source of information or a factual basis for such "clinical findings and opinions," it is important to describe such history in some detail.

History is relevant to FMHA whenever there is a reconstructive aspect to the evaluation (e.g., personal injury, criminal responsibility) or whenever a prediction of future behavior or a response to possible intervention are requested. Consider the example of criminal sentencing evaluations. There are four broad areas regarding which mental health professionals may provide information in the context of sentencing: (1) *retribution*, which may involve issues related to *mens rea*,[10] or whether mental status abnormalities or significantly reduced mental capacity not caused by voluntary intoxication contribute to the commission of a nonviolent offense in a federal jurisdiction,[11] (2) *deterrence*, involving the question of whether and to what extent mental state will motivate future criminal behavior,[12] (3) *incapacitation*, in which there is consideration of the conditional probability

---

[10]Although legally responsible, does the defendant experience diminished ability to appreciate the nature, quality, or wrongfulness of the act? See *U.S. v. Coleman*, 1991.

[11]See, e.g., *U.S. v. Coleman*, 1991; *U.S. v. Ruklick*, 1991; *U.S. v. Speight*, 1989; *U.S. v. McMurray*, 1993.

[12]The impact of deterrence may possibly be diminished if mental illness or mental retardation contributed to the criminal conduct, and cannot be treated in a way that focuses on risk reduction (*State v. Jarbath*, 1989; *U.S. v. Coleman*, 1991), arguably increasing the need for incarceration (*Jones v. United States*, 1983).

of recidivism given the defendant's risk of future criminal behavior, needs in and amenability to risk-relevant rehabilitation, and necessary level of security during incarceration,[13] and (4) *rehabilitation*, where courts may consider particular conditions in a sentence when relevant to risk factors for reoffending as well as risk-relevant rehabilitation needs[14] (Appelbaum & Zaitchik, 1995). In each of these areas, the relevance of history is apparent, although the particular aspect of the person's history also varies according to the issue being weighed by the court.

EMPIRICAL

Empirical developments in the application of history to FMHA will be discussed in three contexts: (1) evaluating response style, (2) establishing a pattern of behavior to serve as a context for the forensic issues being assessed, and (3) using historical information to suggest and test hypotheses.

The literature on response style and its particular importance in FMHA will be discussed in detail in Chapter 7. It should be observed, however, that the veracity of self-reported symptoms and behaviors can be evaluated more accurately when good historical information is available about the individual's previous experience of such symptoms and behaviors. The empirical literature provides little support for the prospect that mental health professionals can detect dissimulation at greater than chance levels from observing cues normally available to interviewers (see, e.g., Ekman & O'Sullivan, 1991). Given this, it would be valuable to confirm, for example, that an individual describing the experience of auditory hallucinations and ideas of reference has (1) a history of psychiatric hospitalization accompanied by the prescription of psychotropic medications versus (2) no apparent contact of any kind with the mental health system, and behavior described by close observers as unremarkable with respect to mental health problems over a number of years.

The importance of history in establishing a pattern of behavior, and

---

[13]Some courts may be inclined to give longer sentences when the defendant's risk is higher, or rehabilitation amenability more limited (*Washington v. McNallie*, 1994; *Washington v. Pryor*, 1990). In high-risk cases, the sentence may involve incarceration rather than probation (*Idaho v. Snow*, 1991); conversely, "atypical" risk factors related to mental condition that decrease risk may result in a more lenient sentence (*U.S. v. Studley*, 1990).
[14]Such conditions have included supervised psychiatric treatment (*U.S. v. Poff*, 1991) and revocation of probated defendants who do not comply with imposed conditions of mental health treatment and monitoring (*Connecticut v. Villano*, 1993; *U.S. v. Gallo*, 1994), as well as the role of coercion in the compliance with such conditions (see, e.g., Committee on Government Policy, Group for the Advancement of Psychiatry, 1994; Dennis & Monahan, 1996).

serving as a source of information about the probability of certain kinds of future behavior, may be seen particularly in forensic issues that involve a prediction. One good example is violence risk assessment. The history of aggressive behavior has historically played an important role regarding violence risk (e.g., Megargee, 1982; Monahan, 1981). Even more important, the most promising research on violence risk in the mentally disordered has consistently included a measure of the individual's violence history (see, e.g., Borum, Swartz, & Swanson, 1996; Monahan & Steadman, 1994; Steadman et al., 1998). Every promising tool at present that is relevant to risk assessment includes a section or factor on history [see, e.g., the Psychopathy Checklist-Revised (Hare, 1991); the HCR-20 (Webster, Eaves, Douglas, & Wintrup, 1995); the Violence Prediction Scheme (Webster et al., 1994); the Violence Risk Appraisal Guide (Harris, Rice, & Quinsey, 1993)]. Research on violence or reoffense risk in other populations, such as the larger population consisting of those who are arrested in the juvenile or criminal justice system, has also yielded actuarial approaches to classification of risk that has included arrest history as an important feature (see OJJDP, 1995). In addition, there are tools such as the Youth Level of Service/Case Management Inventory (YLS/CMI; Hoge & Andrews, 1994) for juveniles that use both historical factors to assign *a priori* risk level and other risk factors that are potentially changeable through intervention that can assist in planning relevant intervention and monitoring.

STANDARD OF PRACTICE

Historical information is part of virtually every form of mental health assessment, whether forensic or not. History is described by ethics sources of authority (see previous section) as an integral part of mental health assessment within "accepted clinical standards." In forensic contexts, history facilitates hypothesis-testing, a crucial part of FMHA. A number of examples of such facilitation will be discussed in this section.

Relevant aspects of history can vary significantly across legal questions. Some have argued that competence to stand trial, for instance, requires relatively little personal history (Melton et al., 1997), although others have suggested that certain kinds of history are particularly important for competence to stand trial (CST)-relevant capacities (Grisso, personal communication).[15] However, other kinds of reports (e.g., personal

---

[15]Grisso has suggested that history in the following areas may be particularly important in the assessment of capacities relevant to competence to stand trial: (1) past experience in the justice system, (2) previous mental health diagnoses and treatment, relevant for questions of malingering and questions of restoration to competence, (3) past reactions to stress, as

injury, child custody, criminal responsibility, sentencing) more consistently require a detailed history. When a forensic issue is focused on the individual's present state and is relatively narrow in scope, then the history can be more focused. When the forensic issue is broader, or with potentially very serious consequences, however, then the history should be more extensive.

A good example involving broad forensic issues with serious consequences is capital litigation. Two issues that may arise in this context are sentencing recommendations and (rarely) competence for execution. The historical breadth that is often indicated in sentencing evaluation has been discussed in detail (see Appelbaum & Zaitchik, 1995), as has the role of history (and other factors) in the assessment of competence for execution (Heilbrun & McClaren, 1988). Other legal questions for which relevant history is particularly important to the included forensic issues include (1) reconstructive circumstances (e.g., sanity at the time of the offense, or any question involving capacities exercised at a prior time, such as competence to execute a will or competence to waive *Miranda* rights), (2) questions focused on changes subsequent to a certain event (e.g., personal injury), and (3) questions involving prediction (e.g., child custody, sentencing, juvenile waiver) (Melton et al., 1997).

The creation and testing of hypotheses regarding forensic issues can be facilitated with certain kinds of historical information. This may be illustrated in the context of an FMHA evaluation in the area of vocational disability, in which the forensic clinician is retained by an insurance company to evaluate an insured client to determine (1) the nature and severity of mental or emotional disorder currently experienced, (2) the impact of this disorder on the insured's capacity to work, and (3) if this capacity is impaired, what recommended course of intervention would be indicated.[16] Several hypotheses might be considered as part of such an evaluation. First, it is possible that the individual does not suffer from any significant mental or emotional disorder, but has fabricated such symptoms in an attempt to receive insurance benefits. Second, it is also possible that the individual does experience significant symptoms of disorder, but these symptoms would not be significantly disabling (at least for some kinds of employment). Third, it may be that there is both significant psychopathology and significant resulting disability, but both may respond favorably to a series of planned treatment interventions over a

related to capacity to manage the trial process, (4) previous occupational and educational achievement, potentially relevant for malingering, and (5) past family relations (potentially relevant with juveniles, at least, concerning whether parental support can compensate for deficits in capacities relevant to trial participation) (personal communication, 6-15-00).
[16]Insurance companies may refer to such evaluations as *Independent medical evaluations*.

specified time. Finally, it is possible that the clinical symptomatology has produced a vocational disability that is unlikely to respond to planned interventions and allow the individual to return to work in the near future. To help the evaluator distinguish among these possibilities, it would be important to have a detailed mental health history (including interventions and responses) as well as a detailed work history. In particular, to assess the impact of the clinical symptoms on the work performance, the evaluator must compare work performance and capacities before the onset of symptoms with those following symptom onset. Without such historical information, the evaluator would not be able to make such comparisons in any meaningful way.

DISCUSSION

There is reasonably strong support from ethics, law, empirical, and standard of practice areas regarding the importance of history in FMHA, although this support sometimes must be inferred because history is not mentioned specifically. Ethics sources of authority are the most direct, emphasizing that history is an integral part of mental health evaluation within "accepted clinical and scientific standards." Hypothesis-testing is discussed more in forensic specialized guidelines than the broader psychological and psychiatric ethical standards, suggesting that this particular use of history is more a forensic than a therapeutic assessment function. Legal standards emphasize the application of history to various legal questions, rather than stressing the broad importance of history, but this is consistent with the use of relevance as a guide for selecting various sources of information in FMHA. Standard of practice literature, using ethics and law as guides, also describes the use of history according to the nature of the forensic issues being evaluated. This principle would appear to be *established.*

Obtaining relevant history from multiple sources in FMHA helps the evaluator to assess patterns of behavior and provide a context for a single event, weigh response style and gauge the accuracy of self-reported factual information, and generate and test hypotheses. Familiarity with the history of an individual being assessed can enhance the "face validity" of an evaluation, which can be extremely important in forensic contexts (Grisso, 1986a). Such familiarity can serve as a valuable tool in protecting the evaluator from a certain line of cross-examination in a hearing or trial. Questions beginning with "Doctor, were you aware that ..." and completed with a specific historical fact that may seem inconsistent with the thrust of the FMHA results and testimony can be an effective cross-examination strategy with witnesses who are unfamiliar with seemingly relevant aspects of the individual's history. A series of admissions that the evaluator was *not* aware of these historical facts may create the impression (perhaps accurately) that the evaluator's conclusions are not well informed. Only when the evaluator *is* aware of most of these historical facts, and can truthfully reply that they were considered in the process of reaching the present conclusions, can the effectiveness of this strategy be limited.[17]

ASSESS RELEVANT CLINICAL CHARACTERISTICS IN RELIABLE AND VALID WAYS

This principle describes the importance of assessing clinical characteristics that are relevant to the forensic issues, in ways that are reliable and valid, in the course of FMHA. "Clinical characteristics" are symptoms of disorders of mental, emotional, or cognitive functioning that are recognized in an authoritative source such as the DSM-IV, regardless of whether they constitute a fully diagnosable disorder. This is a broad initial definition. The breadth of this initial category is partly a function of the law's broad definition of relevance; under evidentiary law, "relevance" makes a fact "more or less probable than it would be without the evidence" whose relevance is being weighed (F.R.E. 401).

In some contexts, clinical characteristics may be important to consider in a very broad sense (as in capital sentencing, when there may be relevance to mental illness, mental retardation, personality disorder, history of learning, academic dysfunction, vocational problems, substance abuse as well as dependence, response to previous traumatic events, and the like). At other times, they may also be considered much more narrowly (as in competence to stand trial, in which the clinical focus is typically severe mental illness, neurological dysfunction, or cognitive limitations). Developmental considerations are important when FMHA includes children

---

[17]A good awareness of historical facts can also protect the evaluator from the distorted impression such facts may create during cross-examination. An attorney who asks a forensic clinician on cross-examination in the course of a juvenile transfer hearing, "Doctor, were you aware that Sam was suspended from school twice during the last year for fighting?" would probably prefer a "yes" or "no" response to one incorporating more history, such as "Judging from Sam's description of his performance in different schools, my review of his school records and previous program records, and conversations with his mother and his teacher, Sam does poorly in a number of ways in a mainstream school. He seems to attend and perform much better in a program in which smaller classes are combined with behavioral interventions, skills training in anger management, and vocational training."

and adolescents, and the issue of the individual's role in a group may be important when FMHA is focused on areas such as child custody or capacity to work. Characteristics such as patience, impulse control, response to stress, and the like are important in those instances, such as child custody evaluation, when personality characteristics may be relevant as well.

One might ask why a separate principle is needed here, particularly since the following principle ("Assess Legally Relevant Behavior") might arguably apply to all symptoms, characteristics, and capacities that are relevant to the forensic issues being assessed. It is mainly for the sake of conceptual clarity, consistency with the structure of mental health laws, and at least one model of FMHA (Morse, 1978a) that a separate principle is described for the assessment of relevant clinical characteristics.

The issues of reliability and validity in assessing clinical characteristics will also be discussed. This discussion will consider the nature of the assessment measures (objective versus subjective) and how information can be combined (clinical versus actuarial). There is a literature that fairly clearly demonstrates the importance of objective measures and the superior accuracy of actuarial predictions when contrasted with clinical predictions. However, the application of this literature to FMHA must be considered in light of the reality that combining actuarial data is sometimes not possible, if no "formula" has been developed through validation research, and objective measures sometimes cannot be used because none have been developed for the specific purpose for which they are needed in a given FMHA. These considerations will be discussed in this section.

ETHICS

The *Ethical Principles of Psychologists and Code of Conduct* (APA, 1992) indicates that

> Psychologists who perform interventions or administer, score, interpret, or use assessment techniques are familiar with the reliability, validation, and related standardization or outcome studies of, and proper applications and uses of, the techniques they use … recognize limits to the certainty with which diagnoses, judgments, or predictions can be made about individuals … attempt to identify situations in which particular interventions or assessment techniques or norms may not be applicable or may require adjustment in administration or interpretation because of factors such as individuals' gender, age, race, ethnicity, national origin, religion, sexual orientation, disability, language, or socioeconomic status. (p. 1603)

This clearly refers to the most valid possible assessment of "clinical characteristics," broadly speaking. It is important to determine not only what areas will be assessed, but also the measures used to assess them and the psychometric properties of these measures. The *Ethics Code* also indicates that

> Psychologists' assessments, recommendations, reports, and psychological diagnostic or evaluative statements are based on information and techniques (including personal interviews of the individual when appropriate) sufficient to provide appropriate substantiation for their findings. (p. 1603)

This statement applies as well to "forensic assessments" (p. 1610). More applicable to the question of actuarial interpretation, it is noted that

> When interpreting assessment results, including automated interpretations, psychologists take into account the various test factors and characteristics of the person being assessed that might affect psychologists' judgments or reduce the accuracy of their interpretations. They indicate any significant reservations they have about the accuracy or limitations of their interpretations. (p. 1603)

The *Specialty Guidelines for Forensic Psychologists* (1991) notes the importance of personal contact with the individual being evaluated:

> Forensic psychologists avoid giving written or oral evidence about the psychological characteristics of particular individuals when they have not had an opportunity to conduct an examination of the individual adequate to the scope of the statements, opinions, or conclusions to be issues. Forensic psychologists make every reasonable effort to conduct such examinations. When it is not possible or feasible to do so, they make clear the impact of such limitations on the reliability and validity of their professional products, evidence, or testimony. (p. 663)

Without such contact, there is no opportunity to observe the individual's presentation, behavior, form of communication, capacity for attention and concentration, response to stress, and reaction to the evaluator, all of which are important to the accurate assessment of clinical characteristics. There is also no opportunity for direct questions that would yield responses about relevant clinical characteristics that cannot be observed (e.g., thoughts, fantasies) and are therefore difficult or impossible to infer through the behavioral observations offered by others. There is also less face validity to the evaluation.

The *Specialty Guidelines* also makes the following point, which is relevant to objective measures and actuarial judgment:

> Because of their special status as persons qualified as experts to the court, forensic psychologists have an obligation to maintain current knowledge of scientific, professional and legal developments within their area of claimed competence. They are obligated also to use that knowledge, consistent with accepted clinical and scientific standards, in selecting data collection methods and procedures for an evaluation, treatment, consultation or scholarly/empirical investigation. (p. 661)

The *Principles of Medical Ethics with Annotations* (1998) does not provide material on point. The *Ethical Guidelines* (AAPL, 1995) refers to the "clinical evaluation and the application of the data obtained to the legal criteria" (p. 3) and "the soundness of their clinical opinion" (p. 3). It is also observed that forensic psychiatrists

> communicate honesty of their work, efforts to attain objectivity, and the soundness of their clinical opinion by distinguishing, to the extent possible, between verified and unverified information as well as between clinical "facts," "inferences" and "impressions." (p. 3)

It should be noted that there is some explicit contrast between the approach to achieving reliability that is advocated by the AAPL's *Guidelines*, which appears to be more of the "hypothesis testing" than the "actuarial measures" approach that is apparent in the APA's *Ethical Principles*. The *Specialty Guidelines* explicitly endorses both as approaches to improving the validity of evaluations.

LAW

The structure of most law related to mental health contains reference to "mental disease or defect," "mental illness," and the like (Morse, 1978a,b). The *Criminal Justice Mental Health Standards* (ABA, 1989), in describing the contents of the written report of mental evaluations, include separate sections on (1) the evaluator's clinical findings and opinions of each matter referred for evaluation and (2) the sources of information and the factual basis for the clinical findings and opinions (p. 109). This occurrence is so consistent and widespread that it is not necessary to describe case law supporting this principle.

However, this does not mean that clinical characteristics are assessed without considering how they might be relevant to the forensic issues and, ultimately, to the legal question. Under Rule 401 of the *Federal Rules of Evidence*, "relevant evidence" is defined as "evidence having any tendency to make the existence of any fact that is of consequence to the determination of the action more probable or less probable than it would be without the evidence," reflecting the importance of the relationship between the clinical characteristics and the functional capacities. Further, under Rule 402, evidence that is not relevant under this definition is not admissible. The need to provide information about clinical characteristics is embedded in the statutes governing most forms of FMHA; the importance of making such clinical information *relevant* is apparent when considering evidence law.

EMPIRICAL

Empirical studies describing the approaches to collecting information on clinical functioning in FMHA generally fall into two kinds: studies that have obtained information directly from FMHA reports, and those using data reported by mental health professionals regarding their practice (in the form of a response to a survey, or a checklist completed following the evaluation, for example). Available studies of each kind will be discussed. In addition, the use of objective measures, and the issue of clinical versus actuarial prediction, will be discussed in this section.

Petrella and Poythress (1983) sampled 120 reports on the legal question of competence to stand trial (CST) and another 80 reports on criminal responsibility (CR). The reports of psychiatrists, psychologists, and social workers (on the issue of CST) and psychiatrists and psychologists (on CR) were examined. All reports contained information regarding the defendant's clinical functioning.

Heilbrun and Collins (1995) considered 277 Florida reports addressing CST (for 167 reports based on evaluations conducted in the hospital) and CST and/or sanity at the time of the offense (for 110 reports based on community evaluations). Virtually all reports noted that the evaluator had used an interview, with another 67% citing the use of a mental status exam and 20% describing psychological testing of some kind (when the evaluator was a psychologist). Also, 68% of reports cited the use of mental health records, relevant to the individual's clinical functioning. In a second sample of Virginia FMHA reports (Heilbrun et al., 1994), a total of 42% of evaluators reported on a postreport checklist that they had considered mental health records as part of their evaluation.

Several other studies involving surveys of mental health professionals also provide data relevant to the collection of clinical information in FMHA. A sample of 69 mental health professionals described their use of certain psychological tests in FMHA on a scale with 4 = always, 3 = frequently, and 2 = moderately, with the most frequently cited instruments the MMPI or the MMPI-2 (X = 3.33), the WAIS-R (X = 2.93) and the Rorschach (X = 2.14) (Lees-Haley, 1992). In a more recent survey of psychologists (N = 53) and psychiatrists (N = 43), about 80% of whom were board-certified, Borum and Grisso (1995) observed that "current mental status" was rated as "essential" by 91% of psychiatrists and 97% of psychologists for CST evaluations. It was also rated as "essential" by 88% of psychiatrists and 93% of psychologists for CR evaluation reports.

It is useful to consider this emerging picture on the pattern of usage (both actual and desirable) for various sources of information in FMHA in the context of the clinical versus statistical prediction discussion. Meehl's (1954) use of about 18 studies citing the statistical over clinical prediction advantage was addressed in greater detail by Sawyer (1966), who distinguished between (1) data collection (clinical versus objective) and (2) data combination (clinical versus actuarial). The number of relevant studies in this area had grown to about 100 by 1989, encompassing a range of tasks involving diagnosis and prediction in human behavior (Dawes et al., 1989). A noteworthy actuarial advantage was described for predictive tasks; in addition, this advantage "likely encompasses many of the unstudied judgment tasks" (Dawes et al., 1989). A more recent meta-analysis comparing actuarial versus clinical prediction incorporated a total of 136 studies. These studies yielded a total of 617 distinct comparisons between clinical and statistical prediction, with about half of these comparisons showing clear superiority of actuarial prediction and the other half showing no difference between clinical and actuarial judgment (Grove, Zald, Lebow, Snitz, & Nelson, 1996). While these results provide no evidence for the superiority of clinical over actuarial approaches for any predictive task, they also do not provide a compelling consistent advantage for actuarial approaches. Nonetheless, this study does underscore the advisability of using an actuarial approach when possible.

The Grove et al. (1996) meta-analytic results are consistent with the conclusion to be drawn from the literature in this area over the last five decades: Actuarial measures are preferable whenever they are available and appropriate (data collected with similar populations, outcomes measured systematically, predictors identified and weighted, and shrinkage assessed through cross-validation). In the present context, this would mean that instruments that are structured and well-validated, such as the Wechsler scales and the MMPI-2, are preferable for use in FMHA to those that are unstructured and not well-validated (e.g., most projective techniques, with the possible exception of the Exner-scored Rorschach). The use of structured diagnostic instruments and checklists would be preferred to unstructured clinical interview when considered according to these criteria (see Rogers, 1995, for a discussion of available instruments for structured and diagnostic interviewing).

However, there are also circumstances in FMHA in which the primary purpose is not diagnosis or prediction. Consider the example of violence risk assessment. There are some circumstances (e.g., capital sentencing) in which the forensic issue relevant to risk is primarily a question of the probability that a convicted offender will behave violently in the future. However, there are other circumstances (e.g., the conditional release of a Not Guilty by Reason of Insanity acquittee) in which the primary task is the reduction of risk, many of the contingencies relevant to risk are controlled by the decision-maker, and the "prediction" itself is contingent on the status of these factors (see Heilbrun, 1997). Under such circumstances, the use of a purely actuarial prediction tool, such as the Violence Risk Appraisal Guide (VRAG; Harris et al., 1993), would be less appropriate than the combination of such a tool with a measure sensitive to dynamic risk factors and relevant to risk reduction interventions.

Examples of such a combination are beginning to emerge in the literature. The VRAG has been combined with a measure of risk-relevant areas, most of which are sensitive to change,[18] in an approach known as the "Violence Prediction Scheme" (Webster et al., 1994). Another approach to violence risk which combines static and dynamic risk factors is the HCR-20[19] (Webster et al., 1995; Webster, Douglas, Eaves, & Hart, 1997). There are circumstances, therefore, in which the use of actuarial measures (yielding a prediction or classification) should be appropriately combined with clinical assessment approaches (using structured and semistructured interviewing to assess clinical functioning and intervention implications) (see Webster & Cox, in press, for a complete discussion of this point in the context of risk assessment).

STANDARD OF PRACTICE

One of the features of the respective Morse (1978a) and Grisso (1986a) models of FMHA is the demand for a description of clinical characteristics. The Morse model contains a specific section on clinical characteristics, noting that there is typically a "mental disease or defect" prong within statutory law on civil commitment and other legal decisions within mental health law. Grisso's model embeds the clinical characteristics within the causal component, and asks that the user address how functional characteristics are affected by clinical symptoms (and other influences). Within either model, it is important to describe clinical characteristics.

Viewing model forensic assessment reports is another way to weigh the importance of a description of clinical characteristics. In a chapter containing many "sample reports," on legal questions including CST, competence to plead and confess, mental state at the time of the offense, sentencing, civil commitment, workers' compensation, juvenile transfer, child custody, and evaluation under the Individuals with Disabilities Act,

---

[18]The "clinical factors" within the ASSESS-LIST scheme (Webster et al., 1994) include Antecedent history, Self presentation, Social and psychological adjustment, Expectation and plans, Symptoms, Supervision, Life factors, Institutional management, Sexual adjustment, and Treatment progress.
[19]HCR stands for Historical, Clinical, and Risk Management scales.

Melton et al. (1997) include reports that vary a good deal in their length, focus, and level of detail. One element common to virtually all reports, however, is a section on clinical functioning. For certain reports, this information may be embedded in another section (e.g., relating clinical symptoms to functional elements of trial competence), but most reports had a distinct section on clinical condition.

The early work on the issue of CST, involving the development of the Competency Assessment Instrument and the Competency Screening Test (McGarry et al., 1973), emphasized functional criteria largely to the exclusion of clinical characteristics. However, the pendulum has returned from that extreme to the incorporation of both clinical characteristics and functional criteria in instruments like the Interdisciplinary Fitness Interview (Golding et al., 1984). It would appear that most FMHA tools developed during the last decade have likewise included the explicit assessment of clinical characteristics among the domains being assessed.

However, the nature of "clinical characteristics" may be considered much more broadly in some kinds of FMHA cases. In child custody evaluation, for example, the emphasis is on making a decision in the best interest of the child, involving an evaluation of both parents' *fitness* to parent. While psychopathology may be relevant, it is likely that attributes such as parenting skills, consistency, and availability will be more important.

Likewise, in another kind of FMHA evaluation (juvenile transfer or decertification), the two areas most frequently cited in U.S. statutes (Heilbrun et al., 1997) are public safety/violence risk and treatment/rehabilitation needs and amenability. However, the latter includes symptoms of psychopathology as well as other characteristics (mental illness or mental retardation is another specific criterion that is included in only some jurisdictions). Among these symptoms and characteristics are many commonly observed in delinquent youth: anger and impulse control problems, school underachievement, family problems, peer group difficulties, substance abuse, limited job skills or prospects for developing them, and poorly structured leisure time (Grisso, 1998a; OJJDP, 1995). Forensic assessment of juvenile transfer involves a consideration of whether these (and other) areas are amenable to rehabilitation within the juvenile system, the availability of such interventions, and the relative risks to public safety that would be posed by treating the young offender in the juvenile system as contrasted with the adult criminal system.

DISCUSSION

The evaluation of clinical characteristics is one of the most basic parts of FMHA. To be optimally useful for legal decision-makers, however, the assessment of clinical characteristics must be relevant to the forensic issues and, ultimately, to the legal questions. It must also use reliable and valid measures whenever possible, and compensate for the potential loss in accuracy whenever reliable, valid measures are not available.

The importance of relevance is seen most clearly in law, where it is a basic component of evidence law. Relevance is also an explicit consideration apparent among sources of ethics authority, where it is recognized that a variety of procedures and instruments are available, but only some of these are indicated for a particular purpose.

Sources of ethics authority generally address the validity of the assessment of such clinical characteristics, although some differences are apparent between the disciplines. The importance of nomothetic empirical evidence to characterize such validity is more typical in psychology standards, while a more idiographic, hypothesis-testing approach is seen in psychiatric sources. The empirical literature offers evidence regarding the psychometric properties of various approaches to obtaining clinical information, with objective measures and actuarial data-combination showing a clear empirical superiority over clinical measures and judgment when the task is prediction. The importance of considering the legal context is apparent when we observe, however, that some FMHA tasks involve addressing questions that do not call for predictions so much as management and monitoring recommendations. In the latter kinds of cases, the empirical literature reflects the development of several tools featuring a helpful combination of actuarial and clinical approaches.

The importance of clinical characteristics in FMHA is pervasive within the structure of mental health law. An examination of the literature in the area of practice also yields no doubt about the importance of a relevant, reliable, valid appraisal of clinical functioning. This principle is clearly *established*.

ASSESS LEGALLY RELEVANT BEHAVIOR

This principle addresses gathering the information that is directly related to the forensic issues, and more generally relevant to the legal question that is being decided. A forensic assessment must obtain information that clearly describes capacities relevant to the forensic issue(s), and it should not obtain information that is not relevant to the forensic issue(s). This discussion will build on a previous principle in this chapter ["Use Relevance and Reliability (Validity) as Guides for Seeking Information and Selecting Data Sources"] by considering how such sources might be applied to the legally relevant behavior described in both the Morse and Grisso models discussed in the last chapter.

Information on the case's *context* is one important component of Grisso's (1986a) model of competencies. In his discussion of the tools used in evaluating different kinds of legal competencies, Grisso also summarized the major criticisms of forensic assessments in three categories: (1) *ignorance* and *irrelevance* (involving evaluation and testimony that does not reflect an awareness of the appropriate legal standard or included criteria, or presents information that is to some extent irrelevant; diagnostic evaluations are a frequently cited example), (2) *intrusion* into essentially legal matters (addressing the ultimate legal question directly, or attempting to use psychological or psychiatric concepts without attempting to adapt or modify them according to legal context), and (3) *insufficiency* and *incredibility* of information provided to the courts (information about the examinee may not be sufficient to reach certain conclusions credibly, or the interpretation of available data cannot be supported credibly by available research). The present principle will be described in the context of these observed deficits.

At a minimum, forensic assessments should reflect relevance to the forensic issues and legal questions, and a good awareness of the nature of these standards. The evaluator should know the differences between FMHA and legal decision-making goals, so that conclusions and testimony are not intrusive. Sufficient data should also be gathered in a way that promotes confidence in their accuracy, to allow conclusions that seem reasonable and well-supported. Elsewhere in this book, I address the importance of an awareness of the forensic issues and legal questions (in the principle "Identify Relevant Forensic Issues" in Chapter 2) and the need to avoid intrusiveness (in the principle "Do Not Answer the Ultimate Legal Question Directly" in Chapter 9). This principle is distinct from one discussed in Chapter 2 ("Identify Relevant Forensic Issues") in its focus on the active process of the assessment itself, as contrasted with certain important parameters that are relevant for such assessment. Clearly, however, these two principles share common material. Because of the detailed discussion of the earlier principle, this material will be presented in condensed form, and the reader can consult Chapter 2 for a more extended discussion of the "awareness" parameters. Discussion of the present principle will focus on relevance, sufficiency, and credibility, and their direct implications for assessment.

ETHICS

The *Ethical Principles of Psychologists and Code of Conduct* (APA, 1992) provides nothing that addresses this principle directly. In a less direct way, the importance of relevant behavior is noted by indicating that forensic assessments "are based on information and techniques … sufficient to provide appropriate substantiation for their findings" (p. 1610). To the extent that legally relevant behavior is necessary to assess forensic capacities, this principle is supported.

The *Specialty Guidelines for Forensic Psychologists* (1991) also provides little that is directly applicable to this principle. Since legally relevant behavior provides information necessary to "examin[e] the issue at hand from all reasonable perspectives, actively seeking information that will differentially test plausible rival hypotheses" (p. 661), this principle is supported indirectly.

The *Principles of Medical Ethics with Annotations* (American Psychiatric Association, 1998) offers nothing applicable. The *Guidelines for the Practice of Forensic Psychiatry* (AAPL, 1995) refers to the "clinical evaluation and the application of the data obtained to the legal criteria" (p. 3). The "data obtained" would hopefully include information about behavior that is relevant to the forensic issues being assessed.

LAW

Statutes requiring the assessment of a reconstructive, present-state, or future-capacity forensic issue typically begin with the need for accounts of current characteristics and clinical symptoms. Particularly for present-state issues (e.g., capacity to consult with one's attorney) and future-capacity issues (e.g., violence risk), the functional characteristics in the evaluation may also be assessed in large part through accounts of current behavior. Such present-state information is thus directly relevant to forensic capacities in some cases. In other instances, the relevance of present-state information is less direct, but such information still plays an important part in the assessment of reconstructive or future-capacity cases. As such, present-state information in FMHA appears to meet the standard for relevance in evidence law—it helps to "prove" something about forensic capacities (even past or future capacities).[20]

The *Criminal Justice Mental Health Standards* (ABA, 1989) stresses the necessity of gathering present state information through personal contact with the individual, rather than through other ways that the courts have recognized as sufficient to generate an expert opinion in the absence of a personal interview (hypothetical questions and courtroom observations).

---

[20]Evidence is relevant if it has "any tendency to make the existence of any fact that is of consequence to the determination of the action more probable or less probable than it would be without the evidence" (F.R.E. 401). See the discussion under Law in the principle "Identify Relevant Forensic Issues," Chapter 2, for a discussion of supporting case law.

Two examples of the importance of descriptions of legally relevant behavior may be seen in case law on the issue of the probability of future dangerous behavior. In *Levine v. Torvik* (1993), an insanity acquittee in Ohio filed a habeas petition in an attempt to avoid recommitment to a hospital. When evaluating staff were in agreement that the defendant's mental illness had been in remission for several years, the court held that a determination whether he met the criteria for continued hospitalization (a "substantial risk of physical harm to himself or others") must be made in the context of current or recent behavior as well as previous dangerous propensities. In this case, "legal relevance" was established through the violence of the behavior, whether current, recent, or remote. In another case involving the alleged negligent release of a Veterans' Administration patient who was released and subsequently killed his mother, the court stressed the importance of current violent or aggressive behavior in making predictions about the likelihood of future harm to others (*Soutear v. United States*, 1986).

Behavior and other indicators of functional capacities are, in many respects, more directly relevant to the forensic issue than are clinical characteristics (even when the latter are selected for their own relevance to the forensic issue). The question of whether an individual is able to think, feel, and act at a level sufficient to meet specified functional demands cannot be assessed meaningfully without information from sources (such as comparable behavior) that are directly relevant to those demands.

EMPIRICAL

Within the last decade, there has been significant growth in the number of tools that are both psychometrically respectable and legally relevant. Such relevance is clear for tools that directly assess forensic capacities and related issues such as response style, helping the evaluator to more accurately assess the nature and extent of deficits or aberrations in these areas. Examples of such measures include the MacArthur Research Network tools for the assessment of constructs relevant to CST (the MacSAC-CD; see Hoge, Bonnie, Poythress, Monahan, Eisenberg, & Feucht-Haviar, 1997; the MacCAT-CA; see Otto et al., 1998; Poythress, Monahan, Bonnie, & Hoge, 1999) and capacities to make treatment decisions (the MacCAT-T; Grisso et al., 1997). Other examples include the revision of existing instruments (the Interdisciplinary Fitness Interview, or IFI, to the IFI-R; see Golding, 1993; Golding et al., 1984) and the development of instruments to assess relevant constructs such as response style (the SIRS; see Rogers, 1992) and violence risk (the HCR-20 and the VRAG; see, respectively, Webster et al., 1997, and Harris et al., 1993) that have been introduced to measure constructs that are relevant to a variety of forensic issues. The growth in the number of such tools, and their focus on behavior and characteristics that are directly relevant to such forensic issues, support the importance of this principle.

The application of well-developed tools to FMHA whenever possible is important for reasons recently illustrated by a study on CST. Analyzing community examiners' reports ($N = 100$) on CST, Skeem, Golding, Cohn, and Berge (1998) rated evaluators' conceptualizations of CST and their reasoning in establishing a relationship between symptoms of psychopathology and CST functional impairments. Reports adequately documented clinical findings, but did not obtain legally relevant data regarding certain functional capacities (e.g., a defendant's decisional capacities).

STANDARD OF PRACTICE

With the increasing availability of such tools that are both psychometrically sophisticated and legally sensitive, it has become advisable to incorporate the use of such tools into the practice of FMHA. However, even before such tools were available, the importance of obtaining information that is directly relevant to the forensic issue was widely acknowledged. This has been discussed in detail by commentators who address the use of forensic assessment across a broad range of legal questions (Curran, McGarry, & Shah, 1986; Grisso, 1988; Melton et al., 1997; Rogers, 1986; Shapiro, 1984, 1991; Weiner & Hess, 1987).

DISCUSSION

The criterion of relevance is very important in considering this principle. Obtaining information that is directly relevant to the forensic issues, which in turn relate to the larger legal question, involves a form of face validity that is particularly important in legal contexts (Grisso, 1986a; Melton et al., 1997), and is also consistent with the standard for "relevance" in evidence law. Asking direct questions to assess forensic capacities can be somewhat problematic, considering that response style may render such information inaccurate. However, these problems can often be managed through detailed questioning, confrontation regarding previous behavior where the information was obtained from other sources, questioning over multiple sessions, and the like. Without such direct, relevant information, there is no opportunity to obtain self-reported symptoms and factual information, nor is there the chance to relate such information to the individual's thinking, feeling, and behavior at a certain time. Obtaining collateral information is likewise very important in this respect, as it allows both "checking" and "management" of information and problems, respectively. This will be discussed in more detail in Chapter 7 ("Assessing Response Style").

Sources of ethics authority emphasize the value of legally relevant behavior, albeit indirectly. Descriptions of relevant behavior, particularly those gathered directly, are valued by the law. The growth in the availability of instruments that obtain information about legally relevant behavior in a psychometrically sound fashion provides another source of support for the importance of such relevant behavior as an important part of forensic assessment. As the number of such instruments increases, sound practice will dictate their inclusion in FMHA. Such use will be important, as research suggests that some forensic clinicians do not communicate information about forensic issues in an accurate, detailed fashion in their reports, and may offer reasons for reaching conclusions on ultimate legal questions that are inconsistent with reasons offered by other forensic evaluators, even when the ultimate question is answered in the same direction. This principle appears to be *established*.

6

Administration

This chapter will focus on the stage in FMHA in which the forensic clinician, having conceptualized and prepared for the assessment, begins to meet with the individual(s) being evaluated. In certain respects, this phase is similar to that in any kind of mental health assessment; it is always important to ensure that administration conditions are reasonably good, and that the individual being assessed understands the purpose and parameters of the evaluation.

In other ways, however, these issues have unusual aspects in the forensic context. Individuals undergoing FMHA are evaluated in a wide variety of settings, ranging from jails and prisons to secure forensic hospitals, outpatient clinics, and private offices. There may be no appropriate facilities in some settings. If the individual is in secure custody, but the evaluation is scheduled for a nonsecure setting, then he or she may be accompanied by sheriff's deputies, who must ensure the security of that individual until returned to the facility. This creates some unique challenges for the evaluator, involving balancing security and evaluation priorities in a nonsecure setting. This will be discussed further in this chapter.

The consequences of FMHA can be very significant. Because the individual is involved in litigation, that individual has legal rights and must make decisions, which underscores the importance of appropriately notifying the individual about the purpose of the evaluation in a way that is clearly understood. In this chapter, we will consider administration conditions, notification of purpose, and the comprehension of such notification, and discuss the principles relevant to each area.

ENSURE THAT CONDITIONS FOR EVALUATION ARE QUIET, PRIVATE, AND DISTRACTION-FREE

This principle describes the degree of quiet, privacy, and freedom from distraction that are important in FMHA. The interviewing, testing, and other procedures that are part of forensic assessment must be conducted in a setting in which privacy is ensured and there are few visual or auditory distractions that might adversely affect the individual's ability to concentrate and to respond in a reasonable way over an extended period. This is so basic that it is almost a truism; relatively little attention is paid to this point in testing manuals and basic texts on mental health interviewing because it seems so evident. This is true as well for the literature on FMHA. While "privacy" is discussed in some detail by different authors, they usually address the "privacy" that pertains to the release of confidential information.

The issue of security in the forensic context is why this principle needs discussion, however. When FMHA is performed in criminal cases, the defendant is usually incarcerated or hospitalized in a secure setting. Forensic clinicians must be careful to respect security needs,[1] but must also be clear about the minimally acceptable conditions under which the evaluation can be considered meaningful. Some issues to be considered as part of this discussion involve the proximity of sheriff's deputies to the examining room when a defendant has been brought to a nonsecure setting for evaluation, the proximity of correctional officers or ward staff when a particularly high-risk or agitated individual is being evaluated in a secure setting, and the extent to which mechanical restraints (handcuffs, leg irons, or leather restraints) are removed during the evaluation.

Ethics

Neither the *Ethical Principles of Psychologists* (APA, 1992) nor the *Specialty Guidelines for Forensic Psychologists* (Committee on Ethical Guidelines

---

[1]My observation, based on working in secure forensic units and performing FMHA in jails, prisons, and juvenile detention facilities, is that one of the most pervasive conflicts can be between the need to maintain security (most prominently, preventing violence toward others, threats, escape, or other "disruptive" behavior that might escalate into a more serious problem or incite others in this direction) and the need to provide assessment/ classification and treatment/rehabilitation services. My related observation is that security is viewed as the primary goal by virtually all staff in such institutions. Security and assessment/rehabilitation goals need not be incompatible, but occasionally will conflict. At these times, it is prudent for the forensic clinician to respect the need for security while ensuring that adequate conditions for evaluation are provided. If this cannot be accomplished, then it may not be possible to conduct the evaluation at that time.

for Forensic Psychologists, 1991) provides commentary that is directly relevant to this principle. Relevant commentary is provided in *Standards for Educational and Psychological Testing* (APA, 1985), however, which is discussed in the Standard of Practice section on this principle.

The *Principles of Medical Ethics with Annotations* (APA, 1998) states: "A physician shall respect the rights of patients, of colleagues, and of other health professionals, and shall safeguard patient confidences within the constraints of the law" (p. 4). The obvious interpretation of this broad dictum would pertain to the communication of information between the physician and third parties. However, this would certainly encompass the importance of communication between patient and physician as well, which bears directly on the importance of privacy. Moreover, such communication is facilitated by a quiet, distraction-free setting; in a broad sense, respect for the rights of patients would include facilitation of communication through use of a setting in which such communication is easier.

The *Ethical Guidelines for the Practice of Forensic Psychiatry* (AAPL, 1995) notes that

> Respect for the individual's right of privacy and the maintenance of confidentiality are major concerns of the psychiatrist performing forensic evaluations. (p. 1)

Here the "right of privacy" is distinguished from the maintenance of confidentiality. Broadly interpreted, this supports having evaluation conditions that allow the individual being examined to communicate information that will not be overheard by others.

LAW

No sources of legal authority were located for this principle.

EMPIRICAL

Performance on psychological testing has received some research attention with regard to environmental influences; this is apparently the only available empirical research on this principle. Testing performance has been shown to be affected by variables seemingly as minor as the use of desks (chairs with desk arms) (Kelley, 1943; Traxler & Hilkert, 1942), the type of answer sheet (Bell, Hoff, & Hoyt, 1964), and the use of paper and pencil versus computer (see APA, 1986b; Hofer & Green, 1985, for approaches to understanding comparability of scores under these different types of administration). Whether the evaluator is familiar to the individual being examined may also make a significant difference (Sacks, 1952;

Tsudzuki, Hata, & Kuze, 1957). The implications of these findings have been summarized by Anastasi (1988), who recommends that those who administer psychological tests should (1) follow standardized procedures in detail, (2) record unusual testing conditions, however minor, and (3) take testing conditions into account when interpreting test results. The influence of such testing variables, some of which are relatively minor, is relevant to the present discussion because this principle describes influences that are potentially much greater. If relatively minor environmental factors affect performance, then more significant environmental influences have the potential for even greater impact.

STANDARD OF PRACTICE

The *Standards for Educational and Psychological Testing* (APA, 1985) provides important information regarding the conditions of evaluation applicable to psychological testing, which in many respects should be comparable to those needed for FMHA. In Standard 15.1, it is emphasized that particular instruments will offer a description of the conditions under which the instrument should be administered in the manual distributed by the test publisher:

> In typical applications, test administrators should follow carefully the standardized procedures for administration and scoring specified by the test publisher.... Exceptions should be made only on the basis of carefully considered professional judgment, primarily in clinical applications. (p. 83)

If there are significant deviations from specified conditions, it might become necessary to weight the test results less heavily, or even discount them altogether. Standard 15.2 provides more detail on the setting: "The testing environment should be one of reasonable comfort and with minimal distractions" (p. 83). Both standards are considered to be quite important, described as "primary" rather than "conditional."

Elaboration on important aspects of testing conditions (Anastasi, 1988) has specified that the room should be free from undue noise and distraction, and provide adequate lighting, ventilation, seating, and working space for test takers. Further, it is important to prevent interruption whenever possible.

Similar comments on the importance of evaluation conditions for clinical interviewing and mental status examination (Nurcombe & Gallagher, 1986) have emphasized the importance of (1) sufficient space for a desk, chairs, and necessary equipment without crowding, (2) an arrangement permitting free entry and egress for both clinician and client, (3) the avoidance of harsh lighting or other visual distractions, and (4) reasonably comfortable chairs. The importance of privacy is clearly implied, although it is not mentioned explicitly. These appear comparable to the recommendations made by others regarding clinical interviewing (Freedman, Kaplan, & Sadock, 1980; Nicholi, 1978).

DISCUSSION

In FMHA, privacy is often limited and distractions created. This can result from (1) security concerns (involved in the transportation of an individual in secure custody to a less secure setting), (2) the risk of harm to the evaluator or to the individual being evaluated, (3) the observation of the evaluation for training purposes, or (4) the recording (audio or video) of the evaluation for subsequent use in training, research, or other professional uses.

An individual being transported to an evaluation site in a nonsecure setting is typically accompanied by one or two sheriff's deputies (or other personnel from the agency responsible for the transportation). The first priority of such personnel is security and containment—preventing any kind of serious (e.g., escape, aggression) or disruptive incident from occurring. The issues to be negotiated between the evaluator and security personnel include the proximity of security personnel to the individual being evaluated during FMHA, and the continued use of any restraints that may have been used in the course of the transportation. In considering the former, it is important to balance security and privacy considerations. An additional issue, if the evaluation is being conducted in a clinic where other professional activities are occurring, concerns the policies and needs of the clinic. One acceptable compromise that I have negotiated involves having the deputies seated where they choose, even as close as immediately outside the evaluation room door, but with the door closed so that nothing in a conversational tone can be overheard. This compromise may be resisted by some deputies, particularly when they accompany an individual who is seen as volatile, unpredictable, or otherwise high risk. However, having a deputy actually present in the room would invalidate the evaluation. Two possible alternatives involve (1) leaving the leg restraints on throughout and removing the wrist restraints at times when the individual is asked to write or (2) having the officers observe from behind a one-way mirror, as long as another individual was also observing to ensure that no sound can be overheard.

The second issue involves the continued use of restraints. As noted, this may serve as a compromise, to permit privacy during the evaluation when officers would otherwise be very reluctant on this point. Restraints may be a distraction for some individuals. However, for many other individuals in secure custody, being in restraints will not impair the development of a working relationship with the evaluator. This may be explored with direct questioning of the individual on this point if the evaluator is in doubt, which can be part of a broader notification about the necessity for the safety and security of both the evaluator and the individual being evaluated.[2]

A related consideration arises when the conditions of the evaluation are not quiet or distraction-free, although they may be private. This can occur when FMHA is performed is a jail, a prison, or even a secure hospital in which there are inadequate facilities to conduct this kind of evaluation. It may not be realistic in some settings to achieve ideal quiet or freedom from any kind of distraction. However, if circumstances are not minimally adequate in these areas, the results of the evaluation cannot be considered representative of the individual. This "level" will vary according to considerations such as the requirements of the evaluation itself (e.g., responding to questions about one's experience versus performing on an IQ test), the amount of useful information that can be obtained from observing the individual's behavior, and the availability of relevant third-party information to supplement the information obtained directly from the individual being evaluated. The forensic clinician should describe the evaluation conditions carefully when documenting the results, particularly when the setting is likely to have affected the individual's performance significantly.

Sources of ethics authority consistently emphasize the importance of privacy and freedom from distraction. No legal authority was located on this principle. Empirical research relevant to psychological testing has described the impact of relatively minor environmental influences on performance; it seems likely that larger influences (such as significant auditory or visual distractions, or the presence of another individual not involved in conducting the evaluation) would have a comparable or greater impact on performance. Practice standards emphasize the importance of privacy and freedom from distraction, albeit sometimes indirectly: These are very basic components of standard approaches to interviewing and testing. This principle appears to be *established*.

---

[2]The following specific suggestions for evaluators assessing potentially violent clients have been made (Otto & Borum, 1997): (1) a sufficiently large room to permit comfortable space between the clinician and client, (2) an open area within visual (if not voice) contact with others, (3) two exits, so neither clinician nor client feels "trapped," (4) possible use of more than one evaluator, and (5) availability of a nonobvious signal of an emergency (e.g., "Please tell my next client, Elliott Ness, that I won't be able to meet with him"). In addition, it is important that the evaluating clinician not sit between the client and the door when working with clients who might respond aggressively if they feel "trapped." The room should be very carefully inspected, and items that could be easily used for weapons (e.g., scissors, heavy lamps, telephone cords, pens/pencils/letter openers, removable desk drawers, umbrellas) should be removed or made less accessible.

PROVIDE APPROPRIATE NOTIFICATION
OF PURPOSE AND/OR OBTAIN APPROPRIATE
AUTHORIZATION BEFORE BEGINNING

This principle concerns the information about the evaluation that must be communicated beforehand to the individual being assessed. The nature of the information so provided to the individual being evaluated will depend on whether the purpose of this communication is to obtain the individual's informed consent, or notify as to the evaluation's purpose and the associated limits on confidentiality. This distinction, which turns on the source of the authorization for the particular FMHA, should be very clear for the evaluator before the first contact with the individual being evaluated.

Some of the information provided to the client will be the same under both conditions. For example, the forensic clinician should always identify him- or herself, describe what the evaluation will involve, and make sure the individual is aware that the evaluation is not part of a treatment relationship. The information should be provided in clear, basic language, with limited use of technical terms and at a comprehension level (written or oral) no higher than that necessary to take a standardized objective test such as the MMPI-2. Indeed, in some cases it will be important to provide this information in even more basic terms, for individuals who have significant problems with verbal comprehension.

However, there will also be differences in this notification depending on the authorization and relationship. This information may differ on the following points: (1) the purpose of the evaluation, (2) who has asked/ordered the evaluator to perform it, (3) the purpose(s) for which it will be used, (4) the procedures involved, (5) the expected and possible limits on confidentiality, (6) whether any individual (such as the individual's attorney) can, in conjunction with the client, determine whether the evaluation will be used in legal proceedings, or whether a report will automatically be submitted, and (7) who will receive the products (e.g., verbal notification, report, possible testimony) of the evaluation. Specific examples of notifications will be discussed under this principle's Standard of Practice section.

ETHICS

The *Ethical Principles of Psychologists* (APA, 1992) addresses this principle as follows:

> When psychologists provide assessment, evaluation ... or other psychological services to an individual, a group, or an organization, they provide, *using language that is reasonably understandable* [italics added] to the recipient of those

services, appropriate information beforehand about the nature of such services
and appropriate information later about results and conclusions. (p. 1600)[3]

This language is relevant to both the present principle (regarding notification) and the next (concerning the determination of whether the individual
has understood this notification). The importance of this notification is
clear and unequivocal:

> Psychologists discuss with persons and organizations with whom they estab-
> lish a scientific or professional relationship (including, to the extent feasible,
> minors and their legal representatives) (1) the relevant limitations on confiden-
> tiality, including limitations where applicable in group, marital, and family
> therapy or in organization consulting, and (2) the foreseeable uses of the
> information generated through their services. (p. 1606)

This statement also offers more detail regarding the specifics of the notification. This can be particularly important in FMHA for circumstances
beyond the use of evaluative material for the original purpose for which it
was requested or ordered. At times, this material is collected in high-
profile cases, generating a great deal of media attention and public interest.
It is sometimes tempting for a forensic clinician to present some of the
FMHA results in such cases in a professional context, such as a workshop
or a conference, or to discuss the case in the media. A more extensive
discussion of the considerations regarding the desirability of such extraevaluative communication is provided in Chapter 10 in this book. What
this ethical principle clearly underscores, however, is the importance of
obtaining the individual's consent if any use of FMHA data beyond their
primary purpose is contemplated.

Unless it is not feasible or is contraindicated, the discussion of confidentiality occurs at

> the outset of the relationship and thereafter as new circumstances may war-
> rant.... Permission for electronic recording of interviews is secured from clients
> and patients. (APA, 1992, p. 1606)

Obtaining permission to use FMHA data for such extraevaluative purposes, moreover, should optimally occur at the time of the original notification.

---

[3]The ethical demand in therapeutic assessment for an explanation of results after completion
of the evaluation, as expressed in this standard, does not necessarily apply in forensic
assessment. See, e.g., Standard 2.09 (APA, 1992): Unless the nature of the relationship is
clearly explained to the person being assessed in advance and precludes provision of an
explanation of results (such as in some organizational consulting, reemployment or security
screenings, and forensic evaluations), psychologists ensure that an explanation of the results
is provided using language that is reasonably understandable to the person assessed or to
another legally authorized person on behalf of the client (p. 1604).

The *Specialty Guidelines for Forensic Psychologists* (Committee on Ethical Guidelines for Forensic Psychologists, 1991) provides elaboration on both the distinction between notification and informed consent, and the desirable procedure when the latter is needed but not obtained:

> Unless court ordered, forensic psychologists obtain the informed consent of the client or party, or their legal representative, before proceeding with such evaluations and procedures. If the client appears unwilling to proceed after receiving a thorough notification of the purposes, methods, and intended uses of the forensic evaluation, the evaluation should be postponed and the psychologist should take steps to place the client in contact with his/her attorney for the purpose of legal advice on the issue of participation. (p. 659)

The importance of informed consent *unless court ordered* (in which case notification of purpose is applicable) is described in this paragraph. When informed consent is not obtained, the forensic clinician is encouraged to facilitate a meeting between attorney and client to determine whether the client will provide consent after consultation with counsel.

The *Specialty Guidelines* also refers specifically to the importance of informing the individual of his or her relevant legal rights:

> Forensic psychologists have an obligation to ensure that prospective clients are informed of their legal rights with respect to the anticipated forensic service, of the purposes of any evaluation, of the nature of procedures to be employed, of the intended uses of any product of their services, and of the party who has employed the forensic psychologist. (p. 659)

This adds an additional dimension to the importance of the notification or consent portion of FMHA. Not only must the information provided to the client be factually accurate, but it must also be accurate with respect to that individual's legal circumstances. Clearly this is not the same as providing authoritative legal information, but it does require the forensic clinician to ensure that this information is consistent with applicable statutes, administrative code, and case law. Having such information reviewed by a legal professional for factual accuracy would be a desirable step.

It is also important that such information be provided in a way that can be understood:

> Forensic psychologists inform their clients of the limitations to the confidentiality of their services and their products by providing them with an *understandable statement* [italics added] of their rights, privileges, and the limitations of confidentiality. (p. 660)

This means that the information should be given using language that is no more complex than would be required for other aspects of the evaluation (e.g., a standard objective psychological test) if any portion is given in written form. If the entire notification is done orally, then the language should also be simple, and the evaluator should check to determine how much of the information has been understood. This will be discussed in greater detail in the next principle.

The *Principles of Medical Ethics with Annotations* (APA, 1998) indicates that

> Psychiatric services, like all medical services, are dispensed in the context of a contractual arrangement between the patient and the treating physician. The provisions of the contractual arrangement, which are binding on the physician as well as on the patient, should be *explicitly established* [italics added]. (p. 3)

> A physician shall respect the rights of patients, of colleagues, and of other health professionals, and shall safeguard patient confidences within the constraints of the law. (p. 4)

Although this language is less explicit than that in the *Specialty Guidelines*, there is an emphasis on two similar points. The first involves the understanding about the nature of the relationship, which is explicitly established, and the second involves a respect for confidentiality rights under the law. This is described even more explicitly, however, when the *Principles of Medical Ethics* addresses services that are closer to (or clearly contained within) FMHA:

> Psychiatrists are often asked to examine individuals for security purposes, to determine suitability for various jobs, and to determine legal competence. The psychiatrist must fully describe the nature and purpose and lack of confidentiality of the examination to the examinee at the beginning of the examination. (p. 4)

As do the other sources of ethics authority, the *Ethical Guidelines for the Practice of Forensic Psychiatry* (AAPL, 1995) emphasizes the importance of establishing the limitations on confidentiality at the beginning of the evaluation. They note that

> An evaluation of forensic purposes begins with notice to the evaluee of any limitations on confidentiality. Information or reports derived from the forensic evaluation are subject to the rules of confidentiality as apply to the evaluation and any disclosure is restricted accordingly. (p. 1)

The *Ethical Guidelines* alludes to the distinction between informed consent and notification of purposes in several places:

> The informed consent of the subject of a forensic evaluation is obtained when possible. Where consent is not required, notice is given to the evaluee of the nature of the evaluation. If the evaluee is not competent to give consent, substituted consent is obtained in accordance with the laws of the jurisdiction. (p. 2)

This addresses an important point: When informed consent is needed, but the individual being evaluated does not appear capable of providing it, then the forensic clinician must consider an alternative to obtaining such consent. The language in the previous paragraph is sufficiently broad to cover a variety of possibilities regarding who might provide such consent. Under the laws of different jurisdictions, and depending on the circumstances, these might include the individual's legal guardian, the individual's attorney, a family member, or a guardian ad litem appointed by the court.

The distinction between circumstances involving the need for informed consent, versus those requiring notification, is again made:

> It is important to appreciate that in particular situations, such as court ordered evaluations for competency to stand trial or involuntary commitment, consent is not required. In such a case, the psychiatrist should so inform the subject and explain that the evaluation is legally required and that if the subject refuses to participate in the evaluation, this fact will be included in any report or testimony. (p. 2)

In addition, the importance of emphasizing that the clinician is playing a forensic role, rather than providing treatment, is underscored:

> The forensic situation often presents significant problems in regard to confidentiality. The psychiatrist must be aware of and alert to those issues of privacy and confidentiality presented by the particular forensic situation. Notice should be given as to any limitations. For example, before beginning a forensic evaluation, the psychiatrist should inform the evaluee that although he is a psychiatrist, he is not the evaluee's "doctor." The psychiatrist should indicate for whom he is conducting the examination and what he will do with the information obtained as a result of the examination. (p. 2)

LAW

Legal authority relevant to informed consent and notification of purpose for FMHA may be contained in the statutes and administrative code of a given jurisdiction. Evaluators should consult these sources to help them with jurisdiction-specific questions in this area.

When the legal context is such that informed consent is indicated, it is useful to consider the legal standards for competence to consent to treatment (Melton et al., 1997; Roesch, Hart, & Zapf, 1996). Currently, the determination of whether consent to treatment is valid requires consideration of three elements: disclosure, competency, and voluntariness (Melton et al., 1997). The elements of disclosure and competency are most relevant to FMHA, as voluntariness as a construct less often applies in clinical-forensic evaluation.

The importance of disclosure as part of both notification of purpose and informed consent, in the context of FMHA, was highlighted in the case of *Estelle v. Smith* (1981). Following the finding of a court-appointed psychiatrist that the defendant appeared competent to stand trial, he was tried and convicted of a capital offense. At sentencing, the same psychiatrist provided testimony, based on material obtained in the competency evaluation, that the defendant would present an ongoing risk to society (one of the three "special issues" that must be answered affirmatively by a jury in Texas in order to impose a death sentence). The U.S. Supreme Court upheld the decisions of the lower district court and Fifth Circuit to vacate, holding that the defendant had not been notified that the competency evaluation interview could also be used at sentencing. This decision underscores the importance of informing a defendant of the purpose(s) of the FMHA and the associated limits on confidentiality, as well as the need for notifying defense counsel in advance regarding court-ordered evaluations.[4]

EMPIRICAL

No empirical research was located that is relevant to this principle.

STANDARD OF PRACTICE

The *Criminal Justice Mental Health Standards* (ABA, 1989) indicates that both the evaluating clinician and the defense attorney have independent obligations to provide a defendant with an explanation of (1) the purpose and nature of the evaluation, (2) the potential uses of any disclosures made during the evaluation, (3) the conditions under which the prosecutor will have access to information obtained and reports prepared, and (4) the consequences of the defendant's refusal to cooperate in the evaluation. There is a clear distinction drawn between informed consent and notifica-

---

[4]Mr. Smith would have received a notification of purpose rather than a request for informed consent for the competence to stand trial part of his evaluation; since the evaluation was court-ordered, he did not have a legal right to refuse. (Clearly an individual who refuses to speak with an evaluator may do so for a variety of reasons; the point here is that there is no legal justification for such a refusal under this circumstance. An evaluator may ask about other reasons for refusing and refer the individual to his attorney for further discussion.) However, he would have had a legal right to refuse to participate in a sentencing evaluation on the issue of future dangerousness, as the defense did not call any mental health experts at sentencing. The Court held that Fifth Amendment rights were present for the sentencing phase of a capital trial, so Mr. Smith would have needed to receive a *Miranda* warning and waive his Fifth Amendment right against compelled self-incrimination before mental health testimony about dangerousness at sentencing, absent defense testimony on the same topic, would be admissible. Under *U.S. v. Alvarez* (1975), the prosecution is barred from calling mental health experts to testify about a mental state issue unless the defense has raised that issue. For further discussion of this and related issues, see, e.g., Yates (1994).

tion of purpose (Melton et al., 1997) that is relevant to how this stage of FMHA is carried out.

The *Guidelines for Child Custody Evaluations in Divorce Proceedings* (APA, 1994) has two points relevant to informed consent and notification of purpose in child custody evaluation. First, it is recommended that informed consent be obtained from all adult participants and, as appropriate, child participants. The information provided includes (1) the purpose, nature, and method of the evaluation, (2) who has requested the evaluation, and (3) who is paying for it. Also, information is provided about the tests and techniques that will be employed, and how all of the data that are collected will be used. To the extent that children are able to understand this information, it is recommended that it be provided to them also. The second recommendation is that participants be informed about the limits of confidentiality and the disclosure of information. In particular, consent to the evaluation includes consent to the disclosure of this information in the context of the child custody litigation and other proceedings deemed necessary by the court (APA, 1994). These recommendations are generally consistent with the information that might be provided to an individual undergoing FMHA as part of personal injury litigation. In addition to informing the individual about the nature of the evaluation and describing the tools and procedures that will be used, Greenberg and Brodsky (in press) also recommend giving information about how the results will be communicated and characterizing the process as an independent, neutral, objective evaluation in which the "client" is the attorney, not the individual being evaluated.[5]

[5]Greenberg and Brodsky also recommend that the forensic clinician obtain informed consent prior to proceeding with FMHA focusing on personal injury. They acknowledge that in some cases such informed consent may be technically unnecessary (when the evaluation is court-ordered, for example); they also suggest that refusals to provide informed consent should be addressed by stopping the evaluation immediately, billing for the time reserved for the evaluation, and allowing the attorneys and the court to resolve the matter. In some respects, their recommendation is comparable to the approach advocated in this book: When an evaluation is requested by an attorney, then informed consent must be obtained from the individual being evaluated before the FMHA can proceed. However, when an evaluation is court-ordered, the differences between the Greenberg and Brodsky recommendation and that provided in this book center around the extent to which the forensic clinician stops the evaluation immediately (as Greenberg and Brodsky recommend) or discusses the refusal to participate with the individual, clarifies the basis for this refusal, and informs that person that a report may need to be written (although the evaluation will not be as accurate) since the FMHA has been ordered by the court. These differences may be a function of evaluation type and the nature of the individuals being evaluated in each context. In FMHA evaluations in criminal cases, on issues such as trial competence and sentencing, there may be a higher proportion of individuals who suffer from severe mental disorders and whose basis for refusing participation in motivated by unrealistic suspicions as opposed to realistic caution.

Purpose of Evaluation and Source of Authorization
Your lawyer [ask whether youth has talked with his or her lawyer; if so, use attorney's name] has asked me to come talk with you because you have some charges now that have been filed in adult court. Your lawyer wants to get those charges transferred back into juvenile court. Maybe you're wondering why a psychologist is talking to you about your charges. It's because the judge who will decide whether your case is decertified will consider your needs for treatment and rehabilitation and how you'll do in programs to help with these needs. The judge will also want to know about your risk to the public—whether you are likely to commit another crime or hurt someone else.

Procedures
I will talk with you today about how you are doing, and also ask you questions about family, school, friends, jobs, and medical or mental health problems that you may have had. We will also do some testing. Based on all of this information, plus what I've received from your lawyer's office, I will write a report.

Recipient(s) and Control of Report
This report will be sent to your lawyer. If he/she wants to use it in a decertification hearing, then a copy of the report will be sent to the district attorney and the judge. If he/she does not like the report—if he/she decides it would not be helpful to you—then the report stays in his/her office and nobody else sees it.

Uses of Evaluation
Our meeting today is not for counseling or therapy. It is only for court.

If this report is used in a decertification hearing, it is possible that I will be asked to testify about it.

[If additional potential uses of the evaluation have been agreed upon by attorney and clinician, these should be mentioned here. Such additional uses include, e.g., the use at sentencing if the youth is not decertified.]

Understanding
I need to make sure I said that right. Can you tell me what we're going to be doing today and how it's going to be used?

[If this request is administered orally, then the youth can be prompted with relevant questions on specific points. If the request is administered in writing, then the youth can see the written material, but the clinician needs to determine whether each main point is understood. It is helpful to have a checklist of the main points on which understanding is assessed, so the clinician can

FIGURE 6.1. Request for Assent: Defense-Requested Juvenile Decertification.

either check off "satisfactory" items or note difficulties with those for which understanding seems limited.]

If you do not understand any part of this, or do not agree for any reason to participate in this evaluation, please tell the evaluator, who will arrange for your attorney to contact you to discuss this.

If you understand this information and agree to participate in this evaluation, please sign below.

_____   _____

Name   Date

_____

Witness

FIGURE 6.1. (*Continued*).

Two examples of notification or informed consent request in FMHA are provided for discussion: assent[6] for participation in a juvenile decertification evaluation (see Figure 6.1) and notification of purpose for participation in an evaluation of competence to stand trial (Figure 6.2). A third example, informed consent for child custody evaluation, will also be discussed.

In the first example,[7] the information is provided verbally to the juvenile because of the limited reading skills of many youths who are evaluated for decertification ("transfer back") from criminal to juvenile court. However, the individual being evaluated is asked to paraphrase the main points of information provided, in order to assess the extent to which it was understood. If the individual does not appear to understand some important aspect of the information, the evaluator repeats it and may paraphrase it. This is not a task that should rely on verbal memory, and the

---

[6]This is termed *assent* rather than *consent* because most juveniles are under the age of 18 at the time they are evaluated, and under applicable law may thus be unable to provide independent consent. Additional authorization (e.g., defense attorney or court order) is typically needed to allow the evaluation to be conducted. Consent of the parent or guardian may not be needed, as it would be for treatment or research, if applicable law allows the juvenile's attorney to provide this authorization.

[7]I use this procedure in my own practice evaluating juveniles, primarily in Pennsylvania. Such evaluations are typically defense-requested and address the forensic issues of treatment/rehabilitation needs and amenability, and risk to the public, as part of the larger legal question of decertification under applicable state law.

Purpose
You have been referred by the Court/Your Attorney/[or Name] for an evaluation of your competence to stand trial. I will be assessing your understanding
of your legal situation, as well as your ability to assist your lawyer.

Procedures
You will be asked about the circumstances surrounding the alleged crime(s),
your understanding of the case against you, how legal proceedings work, and
your past and current psychological functioning. You may be given psychological tests or asked to complete forms that will assist us in learning more
about you. It may be necessary for us to talk with other professionals or family
members and to review prior records to obtain additional background information that may be important to the case.

Reporting
The information that is collected during the evaluation will be prepared for [the
referrer; if court referred, indicate if reports will also go to State/Defense
attorney] in the form of a report. I may be subpoenaed to Court and required to
testify at a pretrial competency hearing.

Other Limits on Confidentiality
Other than our report to [the person(s) who referred you] and the possible
testimony just noted, all information given by you is treated as confidential,
except under the following circumstances. The State requires that information related to known or suspected child abuse, or abuse of a person over 65
be reported to the state health department. Also, information may be released
if you present a risk to yourself or someone else.

Possible Outcomes
The findings may result in a recommendation for you to receive treatment
prior to proceeding with your case, or the evaluation may indicate that your
case should proceed at this time.

My signature below indicates that I have read this statement (or had it read to
me). I have had an opportunity to ask questions about the evaluation and to
have issues explained in terms that I understand. By my signature below, I
agree to the evaluation under the conditions stated herein.

Signature of Participant   Date

[*Note*. Language may need to be simplified, depending on client.]

FIGURE 6.2. Notification of Purpose: Competence to Stand Trial (from Melton et al., 1997, p. 89).

evaluator is free to use whatever other prompts (verbal or written) may be necessary to ensure a basic understanding of the main points of information. If these do appear to be understood, the evaluator "checks off" each point and obtains the individual's consent. If the individual does not agree to participate, or wishes to discuss the question with counsel, then contact between the juvenile and his attorney is arranged before proceeding.[8] This consent approach provides somewhat less detailed information than either of the other two examples that will be discussed, reflecting my emphasis on the importance of the juvenile's understanding the main points of the information. It also has the advantage of being developed specifically for a given legal question and associated set of forensic issues, but could not be used for another kind of FMHA without modification.

The second example involves a notification of purpose for a court-ordered evaluation of competence to stand trial (see Figure 6.2). It contains information specific to this legal question, but provided in similar areas (e.g., purpose, procedures, reporting, other limits on confidentiality, and possible outcomes). It is clearly labeled "Notification" rather than "Consent," although it may appear confusing because the defendant is asked at the end of the notification to (1) indicate that the information has been provided and understood and (2) agree to participate under the conditions described therein. While this is advantageous in terms of documenting an essential step in the FMHA process, it may confuse the defendant unless the forensic clinician is very clear about the steps to be taken if the defendant does not agree to participate. These include questioning the individual about his or her reasons for refusing, advising that there is no legal right to refuse participation in this situation, offering to facilitate the defendant's contact with his or her attorney to clarify this, and advising that a report may need to be written even if the defendant does not participate, although the observations and conclusions in the report will necessarily be more limited than they would had the defendant participated (Melton et al., 1997).

A third example involves the informed consent, or notification of purpose, that would be obtained as part of a child custody evaluation. If the parties were participating in this evaluation at the request of one of the attorneys, or an agreement between the parents and their respective attor-

---

[8]In my experience, such initial refusals are very rare in defense-requested evaluations of juveniles. However, what occurs somewhat more often is a "partial agreement" to proceed: A youth may agree to be interviewed and tested on relevant aspects of history and functioning, but defer discussing the circumstances of his or her alleged offense until specifically advised to do so by counsel. In such cases, a second visit is necessary to complete the evaluation, assuming the individual agrees to participate after discussing the matter with the attorney.

neys, then the forensic clinician would obtain informed consent. In contrast, if the evaluation had been ordered by the court, with the stipulation that both sides receive the resulting report, then notification of purpose would appear to be indicated. In either circumstance, information in several areas should be provided to all parties. Such information would include the nature of the evaluation (forensic, not therapeutic; contact will be limited to that necessary for the evaluation; an appropriate description of the limitations on confidentiality and the ways in which the information obtained could be used; and the general areas in which information would be collected, and how), the expectations of the parents (the importance of cooperation with the evaluation process, the provision of necessary material and information), and the communication of results (the circumstances under which a report will be written; to whom the report will be provided; the possibility of the forensic clinician's testimony in a hearing or deposition; and whether an additional feedback will be provided regarding the results of the evaluation). In addition, it is important to inform the parties about the nature of the appointment (court-ordered versus requested by one of the parties), in part to clarify whether informed consent will be needed. Following the recommendation from APA (1994), informed consent should be obtained from adult participants or their legally authorized representatives, and children should be informed about the contours of the evaluation to the extent feasible and in a way that is developmentally appropriate.

In the context of psychological testing that is a part of FMHA, the *Standards for Educational and Psychological Testing* (Standard 16.1) reflects the following role of informed consent:

> Informed consent should be obtained from test takers or their legal representatives before testing is done except (a) when testing without consent is mandated by law or governmental regulation ... (b) when testing is conducted as a regular part of school activities, or (c) when consent is clearly implied (e.g., application for employment or educational admissions). When consent is not required, test takers should be informed concerning the testing process. (APA, 1985, p. 85)

DISCUSSION

The need to either provide notification of purpose or obtain informed consent prior to beginning FMHA is very clear from ethics authorities. There is an important distinction between these two, particularly in the implications for action if the information is not understood, which will be discussed in more detail under the next principle. This distinction is made more clearly by the ethical guidelines that are more specialized in their application to FMHA.

There is a noteworthy absence of empirical evidence on the role and impact of notification/informed consent in FMHA in the criminal context. It is helpful to consider how the empirical work done on civil constructs, such as competence to consent to treatment (see, e.g., Grisso & Appelbaum, 1998a,b), may have implications for defendants' capacities to understand and agree to the contours of criminal FMHA.

The legal authority for providing the appropriate notification or obtaining consent (even extending to the provision of *Miranda* warnings in some capital contexts) is given in *Estelle v. Smith* (1981). It is also likely that jurisdiction-specific legal authority is available within many states, whether from statute, administrative code, or case law relevant to FMHA.

Examples of notification of purpose or informed consent request were used to discuss the implications for standard of practice of this principle. It is important to "tailor" this information to the specific legal context and included forensic issues that form the basis for the evaluation, as it is impossible for a generic "FMHA Information" form to provide the appropriate level of specific, accurate detail. However, there is some question about the level of detail that ought to be provided with any consent request or information notification. When the notification has covered the essential points in understandable form, there may be little to be gained from providing additional information.

This principle appears to be *established*. As much as any principle discussed in this book, it represents a condensation of a number of important points about FMHA. To provide the appropriate notification or obtain indicated consent, the forensic clinician must be aware of the implications of the legal context of the particular FMHA. This provision should represent the initial contact between evaluator and evaluee(s), and is important in establishing the shared purpose behind the evaluation itself. One of the important distinctions between therapeutic assessment and FMHA is the purpose and conditions established by the notification. Moreover, specific courses of action are indicated by (1) the failure to understand the important information presented in the notification or request for consent or (2) unwillingness to provide consent when needed. These will be discussed as part of the next principle.

DETERMINE WHETHER THE INDIVIDUAL UNDERSTANDS THE PURPOSE OF THE EVALUATION AND ASSOCIATED LIMITS ON CONFIDENTIALITY

This principle describes the importance of assessing such understanding when providing notification of purpose or obtaining informed consent in FMHA. The forensic clinician must have an accurate awareness of the nature, purposes, limits on confidentiality, possible uses, and authority for the evaluation if this information is to be provided with accuracy to the individual(s) being evaluated.

In the discussion of this principle, two related issues will be covered: how to assess understanding of the relevant information, and how to proceed if the individual being evaluated does not understand the initial information.

ETHICS

The *Ethical Principles of Psychologists and Code of Conduct* (APA, 1992) addresses this principle directly:

> When psychologists provide assessment ... or other psychological services to an individual, a group, or an organization, they provide, using language that is reasonably understandable to the recipient of those services, appropriate information beforehand about the nature of such services. (p. 1600)

"Reasonably understandable" suggests that such language would be simple. Even when it is, however, there must be some way of determining whether it is understood by a given individual being evaluated.

In the *Specialty Guidelines for Forensic Psychologists* (Committee on Ethical Guidelines for Forensic Psychologists, 1991), it is noted:

> In situations where the client or party may not have the capacity to provide informed consent to services or the evaluation is pursuant to court order, the forensic psychologist provides reasonable notice to the clients' legal representative of the nature of the anticipated forensic service before proceeding. If the client's legal representative objects to the evaluation, the forensic psychologist notifies the court issuing the order and responds as directed. (p. 659)

In order to determine whether a client or party has the capacity to provide informed consent to participating in FMHA, it is necessary to assess whether the initial request for informed consent was understood. The *Specialty Guidelines*, like the *Ethical Principles*, cite the need to provide an "understandable statement" of rights, privileges, and limitations of confidentiality applicable to FMHA (p. 660). This was discussed under the previous principle.

The *Principles of Medical Ethics with Annotations* (APA, 1998) does not address the need for understandable notification quite so directly. However, there is an implication that it is important to determine whether the "explicitly established" provisions of the contractual relationship are understood (p. 3).

In the *Ethical Guidelines for the Practice of Forensic Psychiatry* (AAPL,

1995), there is a somewhat different approach to determining whether the initial notification or request for consent was understood:

> There is a continuing obligation to be sensitive to the fact that although a warning has been given, there may be slippage and a treatment relationship may develop in the mind of the examinee. (p. 2)

This describes the importance of assessing understanding throughout the assessment, to prevent "slippage" in the examinee's awareness of the distinction between the forensic and treatment roles. In some cases, it may be insufficient to assess only the basic intellectual awareness of relevant information in the beginning of the assessment. This notification may need to be repeated, and perhaps even discussed further, at additional times during the evaluation.

LAW

There are three broad elements that are contained in the legal doctrine of informed consent: disclosure, competency, and voluntariness (Melton et al., 1997). The first and second of these are relevant to this principle, although the case law to be discussed was developed in the context of informed consent regarding treatment decisions rather than participation in FMHA. Under *Nathanson v. Kline* (1960), the questions of whether information was disclosed and could be understood are addressed from the perspective of the "reasonable clinician"—whether such a clinician would disclose such information under comparable circumstances. A second line of case law considers the disclosure and understanding of relevant information from the patient's perspective, considering whether the information disclosed was sufficient to make a reasonable decision (*Canterbury v. Spence*, 1972). The majority of U.S. jurisdictions apply the former ("reasonable clinician") test (Reisner, Slobogin, & Rai, 1999).

No case law has been located on how such legal precedents might apply to informed consent in FMHA. With some kinds of FMHA, at least, there is the obvious problem that the basis for the individual's incompetence to provide informed consent (e.g., being impaired in capacities for communication, understanding, and/or reasoning; see Grisso & Appelbaum, 1998a) might very well be the basis for the referral (e.g., in questions of competence to stand trial or sanity at the time of the offense). Moreover, in those instances requiring informed consent, the source of the referral is typically the defense attorney, who is, in some respects, the primary "consumer" of FMHA. Nonetheless, the forensic clinician is well advised to obtain informed consent (when needed) that is specific to the particular evaluation and understandable to the client. Further, when the forensic clinician observes deficits that might suggest incompetence to consent to the FMHA, this should be communicated to the defense attorney, who can advise the clinician on how to proceed.

A series of studies on competence to consent to treatment, performed by the MacArthur Research Network on Mental Health and Law, provide relevant conceptual and empirical information on the particular legal question of competence to consent to treatment. They also have implications for other kinds of FMHA.

In several studies on the capacities of patients to provide consent to treatment, it was first observed that there have been four commonly applied legal standards that have served as the basis for competence to consent to treatment. These include the abilities to (1) communicate a choice, (2) understand relevant information, (3) appreciate the nature of the situation and the likely consequences, and (4) rationally manipulate information (Appelbaum & Grisso, 1995).

A second article (Grisso et al., 1995) described the development and psychometric properties of three standardized, objectively scored measures that are relevant to these constructs. These MacArthur Treatment Competence Research Instruments include Understanding Treatment Disclosures, Perceptions of Disorder, and Thinking Rationally About Treatment. Very good interscorer reliability was described with three samples of hospitalized patients: (1) individuals with schizophrenia, (2) those with major depression, and (3) individuals with ischemic heart disease.

In a third article (Grisso & Appelbaum, 1995), the authors described a validation study that included patient groups with schizophrenia, major depression, and ischemic heart disease as well as community control groups of nonill individuals matched for age, gender, race, and socioeconomic status. Statistically significant differences between experimental and control groups were observed in understanding (for those with schizophrenia versus controls for all subtests of the UTD and for those with depression for two of three UTD subtests) and reasoning (for both those with schizophrenia and those with depression versus controls) in the direction of poorer performance by those with mental disorder. There were no differences on either measure between those with ischemic heart disease and the community control group. However, it should be noted that only a minority (less than 30%) of any group performed in the "impaired" range on these measures.

These measures of understanding relevant information, reasoning about potential risks and benefits of choices, appreciating the nature of their situation and the consequences of their choices, and expressing a choice have now been combined into a single tool appropriate for clinical use. The MacArthur Competence Assessment Tool–Treatment (MacCAT-T; see Grisso & Appelbaum, 1998a,b) is described as distinguishing between 40 individuals hospitalized with schizophrenia or schizoaffective disorder and 40 matched community control subjects without mental disorder, although many subjects in the hospitalized group performed as well as community controls (Grisso et al., 1997).

An assessment process to address the question of "competence to consent to a competence assessment" has been described in the civil context, developed at the "Competency Clinic" at the Baycrest Center for Geriatric Care in Toronto (Pepper-Smith et al., 1992). This clinic is a multi-disciplinary facility whose primary mission is the development of criteria and procedures for the assessment of specific competencies. This is a rare (published) example of a formal procedure developed to determine whether an individual has the necessary capacity to understand the nature of a certain kind of FMHA, and thereby provide meaningful consent for participation. For individuals who do not appear to be competent to consent to participate in the full evaluation, specialized interventions are provided designed to improve the individuals' relevant understanding and allow them to participate in the formal evaluation.

When a more standard form is used in FMHA for obtaining informed consent, it may facilitate individuals' understanding to make it shorter and less detailed. In a study of undergraduates' comprehension of two consent forms for research participation, Mann (1994) found that longer consent forms, which attempted to describe the procedure fully, are not understood as well. It is also noteworthy that the act of signing the form apparently caused subjects to believe that they had lost the right to sue the investigator. While subjects in this study (Stanford undergraduates) may have lacked the experience and maturity of some individuals undergoing FMHA, there is no doubt that their cognitive and conceptual skills were significantly better than many others who are assessed in a forensic context.

It is also important to provide relevant information more than once, when indicated. In a recent study involving individuals with schizophrenia ($N = 49$), informed consent forms were read and explained to all individuals participating in clinical treatment research trials. Investigators repeated this information until all participants had responded correctly to 100% of the questions, requiring a second trial for 53% of participants and a third trial (or more) for 37% of participants (Wirshing, Wirshing, Marder, Liberman, & Mintz, 1998). These results underscore an important consideration in providing relevant information regarding FMHA to participants, particularly those with severe mental disorder: Repetition and careful questioning increases the probability that the information is actually understood. Moreover, it is also important to repeat the notification and questioning, perhaps more than once, on each separate occasion that the individual is seen for evaluation. Forensic clinicians can draw on the research conducted involving other approaches to helping individuals understand the process of a research study (such as videotapes, computer programs, or family involvement; see, e.g., Pincus, Lieberman, & Ferris, 1998; Silva & Sorrell, 1988; Tymchuk, 1997). Making such information comprehensible to individuals with severe mental disorders is not impossible, but typically more difficult (Appelbaum, 1998).

STANDARD OF PRACTICE

The importance of determining whether a notification of purpose or request for informed consent has been understood is also emphasized in the *Criminal Justice Mental Health Standards* (ABA, 1989). As indicated with the previous principle, the nature of this notification should include an explanation of (1) the purpose and nature of the evaluation, (2) the potential uses of any disclosures made during the evaluation, (3) the conditions under which the prosecutor will have access to information obtained and reports prepared, and (4) the consequences of the defendant's refusal to cooperate in the evaluation.

Although there has been little research on the very specific issue of individuals' understanding of the request for informed consent or the notification of purpose in FMHA, there has been a great deal of work done in the area of understanding and communication of information (see, e.g., Flynn, 1987; Lezak, 1995; Prifitera & Saklofske, 1998; Wechsler, 1981, 1992). In addition, recent research on closely related topics such as competence to consent to treatment (Grisso & Appelbaum, 1998a) allows extrapolation from such work to FMHA in order to describe reasonable and legally sensitive approaches.

First, after information relevant to informed consent or a notification of purpose[9] is provided, the evaluee should be questioned about his or her understanding of this information. The complexity of the language in the notification and subsequent questions should be appropriate to the age and cognitive capacity of the individual. In the *Standards for Educational and Psychological Testing* (APA, 1985), it is observed that

[9]As should be clear from the examples of each discussed in this chapter, the request for informed consent and the notification of purpose are similar in much of the information that is provided—and in the assumption that this information is understood.

Young test takers should receive an explanation of the reasons for testing. Even a child as young as two or three and many mentally retarded test takers can understand a simple explanation as to why they are being tested. For example, an explanation such as "I'm going to ask you to try to do some things so that I can see what you know how to do and what things you could use some more help with" would be understandable to such test takers. (p. 85)

Likewise, even when the source of the difficulty in understanding is related to mental disorder or cognitive limitation, the evaluator should attempt to determine whether the concepts can be grasped on a more basic level when they have been simplified.

Second, the individual should be asked to paraphrase the information in the form of a concept. Particularly when individuals are responding to written material or verbal cues, there is the risk that they are simply repeating the words without understanding their meaning. Short inquiries, sometimes asking for different language (e.g., "what does that mean?"), sometimes for applicability (e.g., "so how would that work in your case?"), and at other times using brief hypothetical vignettes (e.g., "if Joe is getting an evaluation like this and he doesn't want to, what can he do?"), can yield useful information in a relatively brief time about the individual's understanding.

The third recommendation concerns the consequences if the evaluator determines that the individual has (1) limited understanding of the relevant information or (2) no meaningful understanding of the information. In such cases, the question of legal context is particularly important, because the consequences for impaired understanding of a request for informed consent differ from the consequences when a notification of purpose is not understood. When informed consent is needed, the evaluator must judge "how much is enough" understanding. At a minimum, the individual should be able to understand major points (even if continued prompting or brief explanation is needed). Significant doubts regarding the meaningfulness of consent because of the failure to understand relevant information should be resolved by notifying the individual's attorney, and obtaining "substituted consent" in accordance with the laws of the jurisdiction.

However, when the legal context requires notification of purpose but not informed consent, the "next step" for the evaluator is somewhat different when the individual shows problems in understanding important aspects of the notification. While it is essential that the evaluator respect the individual's legal rights, this is best accomplished by ensuring that the individual's attorney is aware that the evaluation has been ordered and is about to be conducted. It may be, however, that the deficits interfering with the individual's understanding of the notification also interfere with the capacities to perform tasks related to relevant forensic issues. Hence, it seems best to carefully observe and document any apparent problems with understanding, and to describe in the report the apparent basis for this difficulty. Particularly when cognitive limitations or symptoms of mental illness grossly impair the abilities to understand and reason, it can be most helpful to the court to indicate that "for reasons to be described more fully later in this report, it is unlikely that Mr. A. understood several important aspects of this notification"—and then to explain *why* this is so, and describe the impact on other legally relevant capacities.

DISCUSSION

In evaluating this principle, there are two major points that are particularly important. The first involves how an individual's understanding of information about the FMHA should be assessed; the second involves the indicated procedure when such understanding is impaired, or when (in cases in which informed consent is needed) the individual is unwilling to provide consent. Sources of ethics authority emphasize that language should be "understandable," and also offer guidance regarding the need to notify and consult with the individual's attorney in the event of limited understanding. Another important point concerns the need for ongoing assessment of understanding *throughout* the FMHA, lest there be "slippage" in the individual's awareness that the evaluation is for forensic rather than treatment purposes.

Legal authority in the related area of competence to consent to treatment has provided guidance for the development of measures in the areas of understanding, communication, appreciation of the situation and its consequences, and the capacity to rationally manipulate information. The emphasis on "understanding" is consistently observed in ethical standards, but the other three standards for competence to consent to treatment may also provide conceptual guidance for notification of purpose or capacity to provide informed consent for FMHA.

Suggestions for assessing an individual's understanding of the information in a notification or request for informed consent include asking particular questions, presenting hypothetical situations, and asking that the individual paraphrase the information. When understanding appears somewhat limited, it is always advisable to consult with the individual's attorney to apprise her of this difficulty. In cases in which informed consent is needed, the attorney may need to provide the forensic clinician with guidance, as valid consent cannot be given unless the individual has at least a basic understanding of the important points. Consultation with counsel is also indicated in cases in which there appears to be a limited understanding of the notification of purpose, but the response would be different. Instead of seeking some kind of substituted judgment in accordance with the laws of the jurisdiction, as would be needed for informed consent, it seems advisable under court-ordered/notification circumstances to document the difficulties in understanding carefully but proceed with the evaluation and report, as some of the same deficits potentially relevant to the forensic issues and legal question may be interfering with the individual's understanding of the notification information.

This principle appears to be *established*, but much clarification is needed. Establishing a consistent procedure for notification of purpose and informed consent in FMHA would not be helpful, unless it could accommodate the variety of information and circumstances across different legal contexts in which forensic assessments are performed. However, the clarification of broader standards, within which specific procedures could be developed for particular kinds of FMHA, would represent an important advance in this area.

IV

Data Interpretation

7

Assessing Response Style

One of the more important distinctions between FMHA and therapeutic assessment concerns the presumed accuracy of the self-report of the individual being evaluated. There are some circumstances under which a patient might want to distort the accuracy of information provided to a therapist. However, there is always the assumption in FMHA that such self-reported information may be inaccurate. An important consideration concerns the individual's incentives to exaggerate or minimize certain kinds of experiences. It has long been recognized that the accuracy of therapeutic communication may be limited by influences such as resistance, limited trust or rapport, or embarrassment about the nature of the information. However, there is an additional incentive in FMHA to distort information—the nature of the legal circumstances—and such an incentive should always be considered in terms of potential impact on the accuracy of self-report.

Response style has been defined to include four particular styles: (1) *reliable/honest* (a genuine attempt is made to be accurate; factual inaccuracies result from poor understanding or misperception), (2) *malingering* (conscious fabrication or gross exaggeration of psychological and/or physical symptoms, understandable in light of the individual's circumstances and not attributable merely to the desire to assume the patient role, as in factitious disorder), (3) *defensive* (conscious denial or gross minimization of psychological and/or physical symptoms, as distinguished from ego defenses, which involve intrapsychic processes that distort perception), and (4) *irrelevant* (failure to become engaged in the evaluation; responses are not necessarily relevant to questions and may be random) (Rogers, 1984, 1997b). It is useful to broaden the fourth response style to include instances in which the individual refuses to respond, or responds minimally, and call this *uncooperative* rather than *irrelevant*.

The assessment of response style is a very important step in FMHA, because of special incentives in forensic contexts and the role of the perception of the decision-maker regarding whether the self-reported information *is* consistently accurate. This kind of perception of accuracy, comparable to "face validity," is among the most important forms of validity in legal decision-making contexts (Grisso, 1986a).

Beyond the issue of whether the results of FMHA *appear* accurate is the question of whether they *are*. The accuracy of clinical judgment in detecting dissimulation is not impressive (Melton et al., 1997; Rogers, 1997a,b), nor have disciplines including mental health, legal, and law enforcement displayed above-chance levels of detecting lying (Ekman & O'Sullivan, 1991). The explicit assessment of response style and the corroboration of relevant information through multiple sources are two steps that can help compensate for this problem. There has also been an effort to move from research using the "global-signs-of-lying" model (which is based on the assumptions that such signs are universal, independent of context or content, have a strong psychophysiological undercurrent, and cannot be inhibited very well by individuals who are lying, even if they know about them) to research that uses *accuracy of knowledge* about a given condition (reflected by both self-report and behavior) and *attempts to personally influence* the examiner (Lanyon, 1997). Research using the "global-signs-of-lying" model has yielded discouraging results in the accuracy of identifying simulators, while research on "accuracy of knowledge" has been somewhat more encouraging.

Such research will be discussed in this chapter, which will focus on the assessment of response style. Important advances in this kind of assessment have been made during the last decade, improving the opportunities for a more rigorous and reliable assessment. However, there are still empirical gaps in the theoretical assumption that patterns of response style will vary consistently between FMHA and therapeutic assessment, and across different kinds of FMHA.

Important implications follow from the conclusion about response style in a given case. When the examinee's response style appears to be reliable, then the self-reported information concerning relevant thoughts, feelings, and behavior can be weighed along with other sources of information. However, there must be less emphasis on the role of self-report when the individual's response style does not appear to be reliable. Moreover, explicit assessment and communication regarding response style not only allows the forensic clinician to determine how self-reported information will be used, but can also enhance the credibility of the entire evaluation by addressing an issue that the legal decision-maker is likely to regard as of considerable importance.

USE THIRD-PARTY INFORMATION
IN ASSESSING RESPONSE STYLE

This principle describes the importance of third-party information in assessing response style, and the ways in which this can be done. Using third-party information to assess response style is part of a multitrait, multimethod approach to FMHA. In this approach, third-party information is used not only to assess response style, but also to provide valuable information discussed in other principles in this book: identifying the relevant legal issue, obtaining history, and learning about the context in which the relevant legal behavior occurred. Instruments that are proving particularly useful in FMHA, such as the Psychopathy Checklist-Revised (Hare, 1991), require that the evaluating clinician consider third-party information as part of the assessment. Given the limited accuracy with which clinicians (and others) can detect deception from personal observation in an interview (see, e.g., Ekman & O'Sullivan, 1991), the use of corroborative data from collateral sources is particularly important.[1]

Third-party information can also increase the face validity of FMHA and enhance communication with judges and attorneys regarding such assessment. The commonsense notion that individuals may selectively exaggerate or minimize certain kinds of information about themselves to avoid trouble may be accurate in some cases, but it is difficult to refute effectively (when it does not apply) without third-party information. Finally, the use of third-party information may help the forensic clinician to distinguish between deliberate distortion and genuine memory loss, by providing prompts or cues that can facilitate recall in cases of genuine amnesia (Schacter, 1986).

ETHICS

The *Ethical Principles of Psychologists and Code of Conduct* (APA, 1992) provides the following caution regarding considerations that may reduce the accuracy of assessment:

[1]It would not be accurate to conclude from this research that the interview is not useful in detecting deception of various kinds. Ekman and O'Sullivan showed brief video vignettes of subjects, some of whom had been instructed to lie about their feelings and others of whom were told to convey their feelings accurately. When these video vignettes were observed, raters had to use cues like facial expression and tone of voice in making their judgments. These were unlike typical FMHA circumstances, where the forensic clinician can conduct a lengthy personal interview, can consider the substance as well as the style of responding, and has the benefit of access to other information about the person against which the accuracy of their responses can be considered. It would be more accurate to say that legal, mental health, and law enforcement professionals generally are no better than chance at recognizing deception from a brief exposure to a subject, using only facial and vocal cues for guidance.

When interpreting assessment results, including automated interpretations, psychologists take into account the various test factors and characteristics of the person being assessed that might affect psychologists' judgments or reduce the accuracy of their interpretations. They indicate any significant reservations they have about the accuracy or limitations of their interpretations. (p. 1603)

Certainly among the "characteristics of the person being assessed" are relevant behavioral histories best obtained through multiple third-party sources in addition to self-report. The review of information coming from third-party sources can enhance accuracy, and limit the need to describe "significant reservations" about the accuracy of the observations and the resulting conclusions.

The *Specialty Guidelines for Forensic Psychologists* (1991) describes the role of third-party information (and other sources of information) in FMHA when it is observed that the forensic clinician conducting an evaluation actively seeks information "that will differentially test plausible rival hypotheses" (p. 661). Common "rival hypotheses" relevant to response style in FMHA involve the possibilities that an individual (1) experiences a genuine mental disorder and presents these symptoms accurately, (2) experiences a genuine mental disorder but exaggerates or otherwise distorts the experience of symptoms, or (3) presents but does not actually experience the symptoms of a mental disorder.

The *Principles of Medical Ethics with Annotations Especially Applicable to Psychiatry* (APA, 1998) contains nothing directly relevant to this principle. The *Ethical Guidelines for the Practice of Forensic Psychiatry* (AAPL, 1995) also considers the potential contribution of third-party information to both enhancing the accuracy of observations and facilitating the reasoning about their meaning:

Forensic psychiatrists ... adhere to the principles of honesty and they strive for objectivity. Their clinical evaluation and the application of the data obtained to the legal criteria are performed in the spirit of such honesty and efforts to attain objectivity. Their opinions reflect this honesty and efforts to attain objectivity.... Practicing forensic psychiatrists enhance the honesty and objectivity of their work by basing their forensic opinions, forensic reports and forensic testimony on all the data available to them. They communicate the honesty of their work and efforts to attain objectivity, and the soundness of their clinical opinion by distinguishing, to the extent possible, between verified and unverified information as well as between clinical "facts," "inferences," and "impressions." (p. 3)

LAW

There are competing considerations that can be identified from sources of legal authority on the use of third-party information in FMHA, particularly on the question of response style. On one side is the importance of increasing the relevance and reliability of FMHA information provided to the decision-maker. To the extent that third-party information relevant to response style does this, and enhances the accuracy of decision-making, then its use in FMHA is desirable.[2]

There may be some limiting considerations in the use of third-party information on the issue of response style as part of FMHA. Sources of third-party information described in this chapter (see Standard of Practice under this principle) may be challenged as inadmissible hearsay, on the grounds that they constitute out-of-court statements being presented to prove the truth of the in-court statement. Under Rule 703, facts or underlying data need not be admissible if they are of a type "reasonably relied on by experts ... in forming opinions or inferences upon the subject." Some states have evidentiary rules similar to Rule 703, while others require that expert testimony be based on sources of information that would be independently admissible (e.g., *Mayer v. Baiser*, 1986). In such a jurisdiction, it is possible that certain kinds of third-party information or their specific content could be held inadmissible, in turn possibly rendering the entire FMHA inadmissible if it relied significantly on the use of such third-party information in supporting its conclusions.[3] For a detailed discussion of the legal considerations in the admissibility of third-party information, see Melton et al. (1997).

However, it seems likely that this would occur only rarely. First, as Melton et al. (1997) point out, the court may not consider the admissibility of each source of information cited in FMHA independently, but rather rule on the admissibility of the FMHA more broadly unless there is a specific reason to do otherwise. Indeed, to do otherwise in practice would be extraordinarily cumbersome. A recent review of appellate cases citing *Daubert* (1993) in the context of FMHA would suggest that specific sources of information included in FMHA are rarely singled out for admissibility scrutiny. Not one of the 276 appellate cases that had been decided as of March 1996 cited *Daubert* as a justification for admitting or excluding document review, third-party interviews, or third-party observations[4] (Heilbrun, 1996).

---

[2]For an example of a deposition arguing for the use of third-party information in a single case, see Greenberg and Brodsky (in press).

[3]It may be that the court's perception of the credibility of the third-party information will be relevant to the ruling on the admissibility of this evidence. It seems likely that no court would exclude an official criminal history as a source of third-party information relevant to judging the credibility of a defendant's account that he had never previously been arrested. However, it is possible that the court would exclude the report of a close relative who was asked about the defendant's criminal history.

[4]Anecdotally, I would observe that I have performed or supervised approximately 2000 forensic mental health assessments in the last 15 years, and testified about 200 times. I have never had a court exclude third-party information from my testimony, nor have I ever learned that such information has been excluded from my reports when they have been used during a negotiation, hearing, or trial.

EMPIRICAL

There is empirical support from several sources for using third-party information to assess response style in FMHA. In a review of the research on clinicians' detection of deception, Faust (1995) concluded that clinicians should not let subjective confidence guide them regarding the accuracy of self-report. Rather, it was suggested that obtaining and incorporating collateral information, as well as interview and data from other sources, would provide more accuracy in determining self-report accuracy. A similar conclusion was reached following a review of the literature on the detection of malingering and assessment instruments used by clinical neuropsychologists; there is no clear evidence for the effectiveness of specific measures for detecting neuropsychological malingering and dissimulation, suggesting that collateral information should be incorporated on this issue (Frazen, 1990; McCann, 1998; Rogers, 1997b).

Several studies published within recent years provide some empirical basis for judging the normative use of third-party information in FMHA. Possibly one of the reasons evaluators would use such information would be to help them assess the response style of the individual being evaluated, although no empirical evidence was located to support this possibility.

Heilbrun and Collins (1995) described a total of 277 reports on competence to stand trial and/or mental state at the time of the offense, based on evaluations performed either in a Florida forensic hospital ($N = 167$) or in various communities in Florida ($N = 110$). A great majority of hospital reports (81%) but a minority of community-based reports (30%) cited the use of third-party information as part of the evaluation. Third-party information of two kinds was cited most frequently in hospital evaluations: (1) *interview* with other hospital staff (70% of reports, 38% of evaluators always used it) and (2) *arrest report* (95% of reports, 62% of evaluators always used it). Community evaluations cited the use of the arrest report (48% of reports, 23% of evaluators always used it), other third-party information (33% of reports, 15% of evaluators always used it), and interview with jail staff (17% of reports, 7% of evaluators always used it) most often as sources of third-party information.

A second study (Heilbrun et al., 1994) expanded on the Florida research by comparing the use of third-party information by forensic clinicians in Florida (a total of 277 evaluations on the issues of CST and sanity at the time of the offense) with that in Virginia (316 evaluations addressing the same legal issues). Evaluations in each state were performed in either a community or a hospital setting. Third party information was composed of (1) basic information about the offense, (2) records of prior mental health evaluation or treatment, and (3) specific statements by victims or witnesses. Across states and settings, most of the evaluations incorporated this information. There was less consistency in the use of mental health records and victim/witness statements, with significant differences observed across settings and states.

In a survey of the beliefs of forensic psychologists and forensic psychiatrists regarding appropriate content for reports on CST (N = 102) and criminal responsibility (CR) (N = 96), Borum and Grisso (1996) asked participants to rate various report components as "essential," "recommended," "optional," or "contraindicated." For CST reports, the two elements of third-party information were mental health records and police information. The importance of mental health records was rated as quite high (93% of psychologists and 82% of psychiatrists rated it as either essential or recommended), while the value of police information was more moderate (57% of psychiatrists and 44% of psychologists described it as essential or recommended). Third-party information was valued even more highly for CR reports. Mental health records (100% of psychologists and 98% of psychiatrists called them essential or recommended) and police information (98% of psychiatrists and 94% of psychologists considered it essential or recommended) were considered extremely valuable, as was a collateral description of the circumstances of the alleged offense (96% of psychologists and 93% of psychiatrists rated this as essential or recommended).

Another recent study focused on reports addressing CST (50 from a New Jersey forensic hospital and 16 from a Nebraska public defender's office) (Robbins, Waters, & Herbert, 1997). They noted that "third-party information" (not specified further) from "one source" was cited in 39% of the reports, and from "more than one source" in another 38% of reports.

One of the logistical problems with obtaining third-party information involves the difficulty in obtaining face-to-face contact for interviews with collateral informants. Recent evidence suggests that telephone interviews, which can be obtained much more easily, are comparable to direct interviews in the quality of the information obtained from the client concerning Axis I and Axis II disorders, suggesting that the quality of the information obtained from third parties about the individual being evaluated might also be as good as in face-to-face interviews. In this particular study (Rohde, Lewinsohn, & Seeley, 1997), 60 young adults from the community were interviewed face-to-face and over the telephone regarding Axis I disorders, and another 60 young adults were interviewed twice regarding Axis II disorders. Subjects with a history of disorder were oversampled, and the order of interviews was counterbalanced. Agreement between telephone and face-to-face interviews was contrasted with interrater values, which were obtained by having a second interviewer rate a recording of the original interview. The kappa value was used as a measure of agreement between interviews of different kinds, and was good for anxiety disorders (.84), substance use disorders (.73), alcohol use disorders (.70), and major depressive disorder (.67). It was more problematic for adjustment disorder with depressed mood (.31), but this concern did not appear sufficient to override the economic and logistic advantages of telephone interviewing using structured interviews for these kinds of disorders.

There is other evidence regarding the value of collateral information, beyond that obtained in records and self-report, in detecting aggression. In the MacArthur Risk Study (Steadman et al., 1998), a total of 1136 male and female patients with mental disorders between the ages of 18 and 40 were monitored for violence toward others every 10 weeks during the first year following discharge from psychiatric hospitalization, and these results were compared with violence toward others by a comparison group ($N = 519$) randomly sampled from the same census tracts as the discharged patient group. Outcome behavior was divided into two categories of seriousness: *violence* (battery resulting in physical injury, sexual assaults, and threats with a weapon) and *other aggressive acts* (battery that did not result in a physical injury). Information sources included self-report (every 10 weeks), collateral report (obtained every 10 weeks from a person nominated by the subject at the beginning of the study), and agency records (arrest and hospitalization). The addition of collateral report to self-report and records resulted in an increase in the recorded frequency of violence from a cumulative percentage of 23.7% of subjects over the course of the yearlong outcome period to a total of 27.5%. The collateral report increased the overall recorded frequency of other acts of violence over the same period from 47.7% to 56.1% beyond that provided by self-report and records. It is important to note that this collateral information was also obtained from a structured interview, based on indicated acts of very specific kinds. Both of these studies suggest that collateral data can add valuable information to the results obtained in FMHA, particularly when it is obtained in a structured interview format and is in response to very specific questions about observable behavior.

STANDARD OF PRACTICE

Support for the use of third-party information in FMHA is consistent and broad. When the evaluator does not assume that self-reports of symptoms and experience will necessarily be accurate, this is part of a broader "role shift" that is necessary for mental health professionals who perform FMHA. This has been described as assuming the role of a "forensicist" (P.S. Appelbaum, 1990), similar in some important respects to that of an investigative journalist (Levine, 1980).

Some commentators, in discussing the usefulness of collateral information, offer reasons that are specific to response style. Using the example of personal injury litigation, it has been observed that

> one of the most useful means of detecting malingering is third-party information. Indeed, obtaining information contradicting the client's version of events is probably the most accurate means of detecting fabrication and may be the only viable one with clients who sabotage interview and testing efforts. (Melton et al., 1997, pp. 57–58)

However, these comments about the value of third-party information are not limited to personal injury litigation. The authors also note that forensic clinicians can appropriately use evidence from a variety of sources, including third-party information, to confront clients when there is suspicion that symptoms or experience are not being reported accurately. It is observed that the clinician loses little if there is no admission of feigning, but gains a great deal if there is (Melton et al., 1997). A similar view is advanced by Shapiro (1984, 1991), who cautions that "disastrous results" can ensue if a psychologist does not do the investigative work necessary in a forensic case. A clinical interview is never sufficient, it is noted; a careful review of records, history, and interviews with family, friends, or employees must be integrated into FMHA, partly to assess response style.

The value of third-party information in enhancing the accuracy of information about response style and other FMHA issues has been made as well by a variety of commentators on clinical and legal questions including child custody (Otto, 1996), juvenile CST, transfer, and sentencing (Grisso, 1998a), trauma in personal injury and workman's compensation litigation (Resnick, 1995), dissociative disorders in both civil and criminal litigation (Coons, 1989), and employment discrimination (Goodman & Foote, 1995). It also appears important when it is necessary to discriminate between genuine and simulated memory problems (Schacter, 1986).

A variety of sources of third-party information relevant to response style (and other forensic issues) have been described (Heilbrun & Warren, 1999) (see Table 7.1). Both individuals and documents may serve as sources of such information. While the list of sources in Table 7.1 is not exhaustive, it does provide a reasonable overview of many third-party sources that might be used in FMHA.

The accuracy of information provided by third parties is important, if such information is to increase the overall accuracy of FMHA. Some discussion of the influences that could potentially diminish such accuracy, as well as how to handle such influences, has been provided (Heilbrun & Warren, 1996). Problems for the accuracy of information obtained from third parties include

TABLE 7.1. SOURCES OF THIRD-PARTY INFORMATION IN FORENSIC ASSESSMENT

Individuals	Documents
Spouses or partners	Statements
Roommates	Transcripts of previous hearings,
Family members	depositions
Employers, supervisors, and fellow workers	Previous FMHA reports
Police	Police reports
Jail staff	Crime scene evidence
Nurses	Autopsy reports
Officers	Mental health records
Social workers	Medical records
Consultants	Criminal juvenile history
Community case managers	School records
Hospital or correctional facility line staff	Employment records
Neighbors	Military records
Medical and mental health professionals who have	Department of Social Service
previously been involved in assessing or treating	records
the individual being evaluated	Letters, journals, diaries

1. *Bias.* Just as the defendant may have reason to distort information provided to the clinician, so may the third-party source. Bias of one kind may be seen when the sources are family, friends, or defense attorneys, or of a different sort when the sources are correctional officers or crime victims.

2. *Expertise.* Often the sources of third-party information will be without training or experience in psychopathology, and will not pick up on the more subtle indicators of mental disturbance, such as a formal thought disorder manifested through a mild speech disturbance.

3. *Suggestibility.* Sources of third-party information may be prone to influence from leading questions, particularly when the questioner is an individual with some status and authority, such as a mental health professional.

4. *Memory loss.* Individuals who observed the defendant only one time, such as witnesses, or who routinely make arrests, such as police officers, may have difficulty remembering relevant details.

Problems in these areas may be handled as follows:

1. *Bias.* Potential bias should be considered from the beginning. It may be assessed near the end of the interview with some question such as, "What do you think should happen with [the individual

being evaluated]?" Third-party information should be obtained from multiple sources whenever possible, particularly when bias is suspected, and conclusions developed from trends rather than single-source observations.

2. *Expertise.* Examiners should preselect particularly relevant symptoms on which to focus, rather than leave this selection to untrained observers. Initial questions should elicit observations (What did the defendant say? do? act like?), not conclusions (Did he act bizarre? confused? crazy?).

3. *Suggestibility.* To avoid "leading" the source, the interview should begin with very general questions (see #2, above) and gradually proceed to more specific areas. This allows some comparison between the uncontaminated description (namely, that given with little guidance from the interviewer) with the more specific but possibly less objective version given when asked about specific relevant areas.

4. *Memory loss.* This can be assessed in generally the same way as suggestibility. By beginning with general questions and gradually moving to more specific areas, and providing the source with some details supplied by the defendant or other observer, the examiner can get some idea of the source's general familiarity as well as specific recollections (Heilbrun & Warren, 1996).

DISCUSSION

Using third-party information for assessing response style is a very important part of FMHA. It is consistent with other justifications for using third-party information, increases the face validity of the evaluation, and helps to overcome the limited accuracy in detecting deception that has been demonstrated to characterize interviewers.

Sources of ethics authority vary in specificity with which they support this principle. While the APA's *Ethics Code* reflects the general importance of accuracy, and is indirectly consistent with using third-party information to assess response style because it reduces sources of inaccuracy, both forensically specialized ethics codes in psychology and psychiatry stress the need for hypothesis testing and distinguishing between facts and inferences. In this regard, they directly support the need to assess response style in order to help gauge the accuracy of self-reported symptoms and experience.

Reviews of empirical research also justify using third-party information, integrated with other sources of FMHA data, to assess response style and increase the overall accuracy of the assessment. Recent studies on the use of third-party information in FMHA suggest that at least some kind of collateral information is frequently included in such assessments. A survey among mental health professionals, many of whom were forensically specialized, indicates that third-party information is highly valued. Two empirical studies suggest that collateral information obtained from third-party informants in a structured interview fashion (1) provides data that are as reliable as those obtained in face-to-face interviews when they are obtained from telephone contact and (2) adds to the detection of the occurrence of specific kinds of behavior during an outcome period, beyond that obtained from self-report and records.

It is clear, however, that the empirical evidence about third-party information has not kept pace with the recommendations for its use. Concern about the accuracy of the information provided by third parties was discussed under this principle. Although four potential sources of unreliability (bias, suggestibility, expertise, and memory loss) were identified, and recommendations made for minimizing their influence, these recommendations need to be tested empirically. This principle appears to be *established*, but there remain ongoing research needs that are apparent in considering its current status within FMHA.[5]

USE TESTING WHEN INDICATED
IN ASSESSING RESPONSE STYLE

This principle describes the value in using psychological and specialized testing to assess response style in FMHA. Response style can be assessed through such testing, broadly considered to include structured interviews and instruments specifically developed to assess response style as well as traditional psychological tests.[6] However, it is noteworthy that relatively few traditional psychological tests have any built-in measure of response style. For this principle, the analysis will emphasize the distinction between tests for which there is theoretical or empirical evidence that they can measure response style, and those for which there is no such evidence. There will also be discussion of the particular tests that *are* sensitive to response style. One of the distinctions that has been made

---

[5]One of the first studies involving the way in which certain third party observers—ward staff on an inpatient forensic unit—make judgments about response style (Philipson, 1998) has recently been conducted.

[6]There is also some literature on assessing dissimulation through the use of procedures that are specialized but would not be considered psychological tests even under a broad definition. Such procedures include drug-assisted interviews, polygraphy, and hypnosis. For a detailed discussion of each, see Rogers (1997b).

regarding the ways in which an individual can feign deficits has involved the exaggeration or fabrication of psychopathology versus the failure to respond accurately that is associated with feigning of cognitive deficits (Melton et al., 1997; Rogers, Harrell, & Liff, 1993). This distinction will be reflected in the discussion under this principle.

ETHICS

The *Ethical Principles of Psychologists and Code of Conduct* (APA, 1992) indicates that

> Psychologists who develop, administer, score, interpret, or use psychological assessment techniques, interviews, tests, or instruments do so in a manner and for purposes that are appropriate in light of the research on or evidence of the usefulness and proper application of the techniques. (p. 1603)

Since the overwhelming majority of psychological tests have been developed without explicit attention to the issue of response style, and have no way of assessing this formally, they are not applicable to the specific question of whether the individual is reporting symptoms and experiences reliably, is exaggerating or fabricating some such material, is underreporting or denying relevant information, or is responding uncooperatively. The latter may be readily discerned from overtly antagonistic behavior or very minimal involvement on the part of the examinee, but the other three response styles cannot be described as accurately unless by the relatively few tests that either contain validity indices or have been developed specifically to assess response style.

The *Specialty Guidelines for Forensic Psychologists* (Committee on Ethical Guidelines for Forensic Psychologists, 1991) contains nothing specifically about this principle. Neither the *Principles of Medical Ethics with Annotations Especially Applicable to Psychiatry* (APA, 1998) nor the *Ethical Guidelines for the Practice of Forensic Psychiatry* (AAPL, 1995) contains anything specific about the use of testing to assess response style. Under the *Ethical Guidelines*, it is important to distinguish "to the extent possible, between verified and unverified information as well as between clinical 'facts,' 'inferences' and 'impressions'" (p. 3). To accomplish this meaningfully, it is important to determine the accuracy of self-reported symptoms and experiences.

LAW

No specific legal authority on the use of testing in response style was located. However, there are two sources that will be discussed in this section that provide a framework for considering the application of testing or other sources of evidence to response style. They will be discussed under this principle because of the association between forensic psychology and formal testing and measurement.

In a discussion of the admissibility of expert evidence on malingering and deception, Ogloff (1990) provided a useful framework for considering how courts might make this decision.[7] Using the *Federal Rules of Evidence* as underlying structure for his discussion, he observed that the Rules contain three general criteria for the admissibility of expert evidence: (1) relevance (under F.R.E. 401, evidence is admissible when it makes a determination "more probable or less probable" than without the evidence), (2) more probative than prejudicial (under F.R.E. 403, evidence may be excluded if its "probative value is outweighed by the danger of unfair prejudice"), and (3) satisfies other admissibility criteria set forth in *Frye* (1923). Since the *Daubert* (1993) decision, the latter criterion would need to be expanded to read "meets admissibility criteria of the given jurisdiction," since the federal and some state jurisdictions are now guided by *Daubert* and others have retained *Frye*. Using these three, Ogloff offered a broader decision model that might be employed by courts in determining whether to admit (and, if so, how heavily to weigh) expert evidence on malingering and deception. First, the testimony must be relevant. Second, the witness must be qualified as an expert. Third, the testimony must be necessary to assist the trier of fact in making a determination. Fourth, the probative value of such testimony must not be outweighed by its prejudicial value. Finally, it meets the *Frye* test in other respects (or, currently, meets *Daubert* criteria if those apply in the given jurisdiction). If the testimony were to be given in a *Daubert* jurisdiction, it is possible that the court could further inquire about whether the evidence regarding malingering or deception could be tested, in a scientific sense, about whether it had been tested, and the "error rates" reflected by such empirical scrutiny. This is a potentially useful decision framework, although it would be relatively rare for malingering or deception to be targeted as the primary forensic issue. More often, it would be among the "included" forensic issues addressed as part of FMHA relevant to a given legal question. It may be that courts will not scrutinize these "included" forensic issues separately, but will evaluate a forensic clinician's expertise at the level of the legal question or the most prominent forensic issues.

---

[7]Ogloff's discussion is relevant to both third-party information and psychological testing in assessing malingering and deception. It would also appear to apply to courts' consideration of expert evidence on a number of other forensic issues as well. In this sense, he has provided a framework that is helpful in understanding the legal admissibility of a range of issues that are part of FMHA.

While the admission of FMHA evidence on malingering and deception may be fairly common, the admissibility of evidence on litigants' credibility (on issues that go beyond self-report of relevant symptoms and characteristics to reflect truthfulness more broadly) appears far more problematic. In discussing the issue of credibility assessment, Melton et al. (1997) observed that the *Federal Rules of Civil Procedure* 35 only allow mental examination of parties to the litigation and only when there is good cause for such an evaluation (and do not even mention nonparties), and about half the states have rules that cannot compel even parties to undergo such evaluation. Likewise, they noted that the *Federal Rules of Criminal Procedure* 16(a)(1)(D) and 16(b)(1)(B) allow for disclosure of results of evaluation only of defendants on issues of trial competency and sanity, and do not mention nondefendants. While it is conceivable that courts could hold that such an evaluation be ordered to produce a just result, with "relevance" being the determining criterion for whether the Sixth Amendment guarantee to right of compulsory process and to confront accusers is sufficient, they suggest that this will occur only rarely, if at all. Given the discussion in this chapter of the present scientific evidence on credibility assessment, as contrasted with the current evidence on response style evaluation, it is likely that a credibility assessment performed as a part of FMHA could be challenged on scientific grounds under *Daubert*.

EMPIRICAL

One study on the frequency of different kinds of response styles in forensic inpatients (Heilbrun, Bennett, White, & Kelly, 1990) used a sample of 159 forensic inpatients and an MMPI-based approach to classifying response style, and found the following distribution of response styles on admission: Reliable (22%), Malingering (9%), Defensive (21%), and Irrelevant (16%) (the remainder could not be classified). A sufficient number of studies like this would allow a better estimate of such base rates. However, the accuracy of such an estimate would also depend on the validity of the predictor and outcome measures. These will be discussed further in this section.

There is some recent evidence that one forensic assessment tool, the Georgia Court Competency Test (GCCT; Wildman et al., 1980), can be interpreted in light of data regarding its dissimulation. While offenders appear to be able to simulate incompetency, and tended to score lower on the GCCT than genuinely incompetent individuals, several strategies have been developed empirically to detect possible dissimulation. Such strategies include the consideration of an Atypical Presentation scale, the failure of very simple items (a floor effect), and variable success on items of increasing difficulty (a performance curve), with optimal cutting scores recommended for screening for feigned incompetence (Gothard, Rogers, & Sewell, 1995).

In a chapter in a recent book (Rogers, 1997a) devoted to assessing malingering and deception, Greene (1997) discussed the assessment of malingering and defensiveness by multiscale personality inventories. His primary focus was the MMPI-2 (Butcher, Dahlstrom, Graham, Tellegen, & Kaemmer, 1989), but the chapter also includes discussion of the California Psychological Inventory (2nd edition) (CPI; Gough, 1987), the Millon Clinical Multiaxial Inventory-III (MCMI-III; Millon, 1994), the Personality Assessment Inventory (PAI; Morey, 1991), and the 16 PF (Karson & O'Dell, 1976), and their respective roles in assessing malingering and defensiveness. Evidence on the consistency of item response and the accuracy of responding (encompassing underreporting versus overreporting) is addressed. Response consistency on the MMPI-2 is assessed either through visual inspection for obvious patterns (e.g., TFTF, TTFTTF) or the elevation of the F Scale (Carlin & Hewitt, 1990; Sewell & Rogers, 1994). MMPI-2 response inconsistency is also detectable through scales VRIN and TRIN. Additional research is needed to provide information on the optimal cutting score for VRIN, with various such scores ranging from 10 to 14 having been suggested (cf. Berry, Baer, & Harris, 1991; Butcher et al., 1989; Greene, 1991). It is likely that the "optimal" cutting score will vary according to population and circumstances, but a conservative strategy of using a lower cutting score and subsequently investigating the meaning of the inconsistent responding using other sources would be indicated. There is also some recent support for the use of MMPI-2 scales Mp (Positive Malingering) and Wsd (Wiggins Social Desirability) in child custody and personal injury litigation in detecting defensiveness (Posthuma & Harper, 1998).

Response consistency can also be estimated through the examinations of particular scales on multiscale inventories. As Greene observed, the CPI has a "Communality Scale" measuring the number of responses in a "nonpositive" direction (Gough, 1987; Megargee, 1972). The MCMI-III has a three-item Validity Index, containing nonbizarre items endorsed by fewer than 0.01% of individuals from clinical populations, with one such item endorsed indicating that interpretive caution should be exercised, and two items indicating an invalid profile (Millon, 1994). The PAI has both an Infrequency scale (8 items rarely endorsed and unrelated to psychopathology) and an Inconsistency scale (10 highly correlated items); respective T scores of 73 and 75 render the profile invalid (Morey, 1991). Finally, the Random scale on the 16 PF contains 31 items, with a score ≥ 5 reflecting an invalid profile (Karson & O'Dell, 1976). Each of these respective inventories has the potential for detecting inconsistent responding, although there is limited research on their forensic applications. On the issue of the accuracy of item endorsement, the MMPI-2 contains a variety of scales that are relevant to the underendorsement and over-endorsement of psychopathology. Although a number of studies have demonstrated that such scales can distinguish clinical patients or correctional/forensic patients from those given global instructions to malinger, this kind of research has been criticized for its poor external validity (Sivec, Lynn, & Garske, 1994; Wetter, Baer, Berry, & Reynolds, 1994). Further studies, in which participants were provided with more detailed information on the nature of the psychopathology to be faked, have demonstrated that (1) MMPI-2 validity scales are fairly effective in distinguishing genuine mental disorders characterized by severe pathology, such as schizophrenia (Rogers, Bagby, & Chakraborty, 1993), but (2) those instructed to malinger a less severe, more circumscribed disorder are able to do so readily and are hard to detect (Lamb, Berry, Wetter, & Baer, 1994; Wetter, Baer, Berry, Robinson, & Sumpter, 1993). Finally, it appears that the more information about validity scales that one provides to those who dissimulate, the more effective they are in avoiding detection (Lamb et al., 1994; Rogers, Bagby, & Chakraborty, 1993).

The CPI-R, MCMI-III, PAI, and 16 PF also each have some form of validity scale, although they are again less well-researched in the forensic context. The Well-Being scale on the CPI-R uses a very low score as a criterion for malingering, although there is apparently little research on its effectiveness. The MCMI-III Debasement scale (Scale Z) has been shown to identify college students instructed to malinger on the MCMI-II (Bagby, Gillis, Toner, & Goldberg, 1991). The PAI Negative Impression (NIM) scale contains nine items with very unusual psychopathology. In what has been considered the best forensic study to date on the PAI, a total of 182 naive and coached simulators feigning specific disorders were compared with 221 patients with these genuine disorders (Rogers, Sewell, Morey, & Ustad, 1995). The NIM was somewhat effective with naive simulators (but not coached), and overall less effective than statistical discrimination.

In another chapter in Rogers (1997b), Schretlen (1997) reviews the research on the use of the Rorschach and other projective tests in detecting malingering and deception. After reviewing studies done between Stermac's (1988) review and his, he concluded (as did Stermac) that available research findings still preclude the development of a decision model using the Rorschach to accurately detect malingering. Further, Schretlen notes that the available research does not support the conclusion that the Rorschach adds any incremental validity to the detection of malingering.

In an additional chapter on structured interviews in his edited book,

Rogers (1997a) discussed the use of the Schedule for Affective Disorders and Schizophrenia (SADS; Spitzer & Endicott, 1978) and the Structured Interview of Reported Symptoms (SIRS) (Rogers, 1992) in assessing malingering and defensiveness. Three samples using the SADS for this purpose were described: (1) forensic patients (N = 104) from two university-based clinics evaluating a broad range of patients (Rogers, 1988), (2) patients with schizophrenia (N = 90) involved in a partial hospitalization program (Duncan, 1995), and (3) metropolitan jail inmates referred for psychiatric evaluation, divided into those for whom there was no indication of feigning (N = 50) and suspected malingerers (N = 22) (Ustad, 1996). Using a strategy previously described by Rogers (1988), the following criteria were used to identify relevant SADS symptoms: rare symptoms, contradictory symptoms, symptom combinations, symptom severity, and indiscriminant symptom endorsement. A "threshold model" for malingering classification was then derived for contradictory symptoms (cutting score ≥1 yielded 68% malingering), symptom combinations (cutting score ≥2 detected 82% malingering), symptom severity (cutting score ≥16 found 32% malingering), and indiscriminant symptom endorsement (≥47 revealed 55% malingering).

The SIRS (Rogers, 1992) is a 172-item structured interview that was developed specifically for the evaluation of feigning psychopathology. There are eight primary scales, originally selected from the empirical literature (Rogers, 1984): (1) rarely endorsed symptoms, (2) unusual symptom combinations, (3) very atypical symptoms, (4) blatant symptoms, (5) symptoms likely to be seen as everyday problems, (6) proportion of symptoms, (7) severity of symptoms, and (8) discrepancy between self-reported and other-observed behavior. Each of these scales reportedly has a weighted mean interrater reliability coefficient greater than .90, and internal consistency (alpha) rates between .77 and .92. Effect size estimates (using Cohen's d) were calculated to describe the differences between clinical versus malingering subjects (using a known-groups design) and between clinical versus simulating subjects (using a simulation design), with a resulting mean effect size for both given as 1.74 (Rogers et al., 1992). Other research (see Rogers, 1997b, for a full description) has also provided evidence for the effectiveness of the SIRS in discriminating between feigners and genuine patients. Two significant caveats are noteworthy, however. First, the SIRS is somewhat dependent on the "more is better" strategy employed by many individuals who malinger, and hence will not detect the malingerer who falsely reports a single symptom (e.g., hearing voices) combined with a failure to respond meaningfully (e.g., "I don't know") to a number of questions. Second, the SIRS and its validation research focuses on distinguishing malingering from genuine subjects, and can provide less information concerning the "partial malingerer"— the individual who experiences genuine symptoms, but who also selectively reports, exaggerates, or fabricates some symptoms depending on the circumstances. For these reasons, Rogers and others recommend a multistep strategy for assessing response style, which will be discussed in the next section.

In a third chapter in Rogers (1997b), Pankratz and Binder (1997) discuss malingering on intellectual and neuropsychological measures. They note that research in this area must address the same "outcome problem" applicable to research on the malingering of psychopathology: There are problems with both the "known groups" and the "simulator" research designs; researchers and scholars in this area tend to rely on studies that use each, and look for consistent findings across designs. There is mixed evidence on the accuracy of neuropsychologists' detection of malingered deficits. As Pankratz and Binder note, the studies by Heaton, Smith, Lehman, and Vogt (1978) and Faust, Hart, and Guilmette (1988) suggest that malingering detection is at no greater than chance levels when neuropsychologists do not explicitly consider the possibility of malingering. In contrast, in a study in which they are forewarned that some vignettes will reflect malingered material, the rates of accurate detection of malingering are much higher (Trueblood & Binder, 1995). This should strongly reinforce the notion, discussed elsewhere in this book, that response style should always be explicitly considered in FMHA.

The development of "forced-choice testing" represented an important step in the detection of malingered cognitive deficits. This approach involves (1) assessing a specific ability with a large number of items presented in multiple-choice format and (2) comparing the performance on these items to the likelihood of success based on chance alone (that is, assuming no ability). Scores significantly below chance suggest that the information has been understood, but the pattern of responding has been deliberately toward the incorrect option. Several standardized forced-choice tests of cognitive ability include those developed by Hiscock and Hiscock (1989), which reflected apparent increased levels of item difficulty, and a further modification of this procedure into the Portland Digit Recognition Test (PDRT; Binder, 1990). In a further series of studies on the PDRT, there was performance comparison between groups with genuine cognitive deficits (e.g., brain-injured individuals) but no financial incentive to exaggerate or fake symptoms, and other groups with incentive to feign or who had been instructed to simulate cognitive deficit (Binder & Kelly, 1996; Binder & Willis, 1991). These comparisons, replicated across sites, reflected the more "impaired" performance of both the simulators and the groups with financial incentive to feign deficits. These studies have allowed the calculation of cutting scores on the PDRT, so that sensitivity and specificity can now be calculated against more than the "chance alone" decision standard. Cutting scores are apparently not yet available on the Hiscock procedure, but should become so with further research. The Hiscock procedure is also available in computerized version (the Multi Digit Memory Test).

The Validity Indicator Profile (VIP; Frederick, 1997), designed to distinguish between genuine and feigned cognitive deficits, also uses forced-choice methodology. It has both verbal and nonverbal subtests. Criterion and comparison groups described in the manual include honest normals ($N = 100$), brain injury patients ($N = 61$), coached normals ($N = 52$), suspected malingerers ($N = 49$), random responders ($N = 50$), and persons with mental retardation ($N = 40$). Sensitivity rates reported for the nonverbal subtest (.74) and verbal subtest (.67) are both reasonably good, as are specificity rates (.86 and .83, respectively), with overall classification accuracy reported between .75 and .80. Clearly the VIP is a promising tool for the assessment of response style relevant to cognitive deficit, and may become even more impressive as continued research adds to its empirical base.

One of the important considerations in assessing response style in FMHA concerns the base rates of individuals in a given population who respond in a way that is reliable, defensive, malingering, or uncooperative. Such estimates would be best if they were obtained through a series of studies across sites and jurisdictions, but within a population.

STANDARD OF PRACTICE

There are two issues regarding standard of practice relevant to the use of psychological testing to assess response style. The first question involves whether it is desirable to use such testing; the second concerns how testing should be applied when it is used. Both will be discussed.

Considering tests in eight categories (Rorschach, "other projectives," MMPI/MMPI-2, PAI, CPI-CPI-R, MCMI-II/MCMI-III, intelligence, and neuropsychological batteries), Rogers (1997a) offered several conclusions about their usefulness in assessing response style. First, he observed that all tests in these categories are susceptible to being influenced by response style, and that relatively little progress has been made in adjusting the interpretation of results to accommodate different response styles. The MMPI/MMPI-2 and the PAI were described as particularly appropriate for detecting both malingering and defensiveness, and the MCMI-II/MCMI-III was described as indicated for malingering but not defensiveness. He added, however, that only the MMPI/MMPI-2 and the PAI have even partial support for their respective capacities to detect "coached" deception (when research subjects are provided with relevant information about the disorder, or when forensic clients prepare, typically by observing those with genuine disorders). When specialized inventories are considered as well, there is support for the use of the SIRS for detecting malingering (both coached and uncoached), as well as some capacity for compensation in interpretation. There is also support for the use of the SADS in the assessment of both malingering and defensiveness, although less so when the detecting is coached.

In a separate study of the effectiveness of MMPI-2 validity indicators in detecting defensive responding, both a clinical group (patients diagnosed with schizophrenia, $N = 38$) and a nonclinical sample (college undergraduates, $N = 49$) were instructed to take the test and conceal any symptoms (Bagby et al., 1997). Both groups were able to produce profiles that were significantly less pathological when given these instructions. The Other-Deception and Superlative Scales were best able to distinguish honest from fake-good profiles within the nonclinical sample, while the Edwards Social Desirability Scale and the L scale were most effective in discriminating honest from fake-good profiles in the patient sample.

Several commentators have addressed the question of how it is desirable to use psychological testing in FMHA. In discussing malingering and deception in adolescents, McCann (1998) concluded that "the MMPI-A and SIRS are the only two instruments whose utility in assessing adolescent malingering has been the object of any significant degree of research" (p. 148). He also noted that the Millon Adolescent Clinical Inventory (MACI; Millon, 1993) enjoys a number of advantages over the MMPI-A, including brevity, applicability to a broader age range, lower required reading level, and superior internal consistency, suggesting that research on malingering using the MACI may result in its applicability toward this end.

Two additional analyses of the use of psychological tests in legal settings also address the desirability question regarding psychological testing in forensic contexts. Heilbrun (1992) offered guidelines that included the explicit assessment of response style, and the suggestion that tests such as the MMPI/MMPI-2 and the SIRS, with empirical support toward this end, be used.[8] Marlowe (1995) described a framework for determining whether the use of a given test is appropriate in a forensic context. Among the criteria in this framework are (1) support by a suffi-

[8]This short list might be expanded to include the PAI and the MCMI-II, which both have some empirical support for the assessment of response style in adults (see McCann & Dyer, 1996; Rogers, 1997b).

cient body of literature, (2) having items with adequate range that represent all relevant content domains, (3) yielding sound data (integrity can be assured for this specific case because standard administration was used and justified norms were applied), and (4) yielding valid expert reasoning linking data to conclusions.

It is possible to examine the empirical literature and reach some conclusions regarding how psychological tests might be used to assess response style. In each of the chapters reviewed in Rogers (1997b), there is discussion about the criteria that would create a suspicion of malingering or deception on the instrument reviewed. For the MMPI-2, there are three levels of decision to be made, concerning item omission, item consistency, and item accuracy (Greene, 1997). It is recommended that forensic clinicians using the MMPI-2 first verify that the first two levels are satisfied; it is difficult to draw conclusions about malingering or defensiveness if they are not. If they are satisfied, however, then scales such as F, K, and L, and indices such as F-K can be considered to help draw the conclusion regarding whether the profile's response style is reliable, exaggerated/malingered, or defensive.

Likewise, Pankratz and Binder (1997) present seven considerations in a "threshold model" for malingered neuropsychological impairment: (1) lying to health care providers, (2) marked inconsistency between present diagnosis and neuropsychological findings, (3) marked inconsistency between reported and observed symptoms, (4) resistance, avoidance, or bizarre responses on standard tests, (5) failure on any specific measure of neuropsychological faking, (6) functional findings on orthopedic or neurological exams, and (7) late onset of cognitive complaints following an accident. To this would be added a score at or above cutoff threshold on any of several instruments described in the last section under the discussion of malingered cognitive deficits.

Finally, Rogers (1997a) presents both a "threshold model" (associated with a conclusion of "suspected malingering") and a clinical decision model (consistent with the conclusion of malingering). Under the threshold model, he listed any of the following: (1) four or fewer SIRS scales in the honest range, (2) two SIRS scales in the probably feigning range, and (3) a total SIRS score above 66. For the clinical decision model, he indicated the importance of any of the following: (1) any SIRS scale in the definite feigning range, (2) three or more SIRS scales in the probably feigning range, and (3) a total SIRS score above 76. It is important to note, however, that he also listed a second criterion necessary to establish the conclusion that an individual has malingered: corroborative data from self-reporting, collateral interviews, or psychometric measures.

A consistent theme cited by researchers describing measures relevant to response style is the importance of using multiple measures in a given case. In this sense, the use of a relevant psychological test, specialized inventory, or structured interview is complemented by the need for collateral information. Likewise, even when third-party information has been collected in some detail, it appears helpful to administer a relevant instrument of the kind described under this principle. Ogloff (1990) observed that expert testimony regarding malingering and deception might not be legally admissible if not corroborated through collateral sources. While it is unclear how often a court might actually rule such testimony inadmissible, there is no question that desirable practice in assessing response style involves both corroboration and, when indicated, assessment using a specific test or tool like those discussed in this section.

Finally, there are interview strategies that can help to clarify the question of response style as well. Asking specific, detailed questions about symptoms, recording the responses, and asking again at a later time can help assess consistency. Being alert to descriptions of atypical history, onset, or nature of symptoms, particularly when they are reported at sensitive times (that is, circumstances under which there seems to be strong external incentive to either appear ill or suffer deficits). The confrontation of a suspected malingerer after most of the information has been collected, particularly if it is done in a way that allows the individual to acknowledge responding inaccurately without feeling coerced into doing so, can occasionally result in such an acknowledgment (Melton et al., 1997; Resnick, 1997). In assessing the prospect of possible malingered amnesia, it is helpful to incorporate the useful review of the (few) known sources of genuine amnesia in the criminal context, and use Schacter's (1986) suggestion that the evaluator incorporate one of the few factors that, experimentally, seem to distinguish genuine from simulated loss of memory—the "feeling of knowing" (e.g., "do you think it would help if I gave you some hints?") question that is more likely to be answered "no" by simulators.

DISCUSSION

The principle involving using psychological testing when indicated in assessing response style has mixed support. There are a few psychological tests that meet fairly stringent criteria for reliability and validity, for the assessment of both symptoms and response style. This number may grow, as further research allows the development and validation of additional tests that are relevant in FMHA. At present, however, this principle appears to be *emerging*.

There is a particularly important conclusion to be drawn from considering the two principles in this chapter. If the response style does not appear reliable, then it is important to weigh it less heavily than information obtained from other sources. In some instances, it may be necessary to disregard self-reported information to a great extent, and rely instead on behavioral observations and collateral reports, including the observations by others and the history that can be reconstructed through interviews with third parties. While corroboration is always an important component of FMHA, and collateral sources should consistently be obtained for that reason, they can serve the purposes of both primary description and corroborating sources in cases in which the evaluation of response style indicates that it appears to provide inaccurate information regarding symptoms and experience.

8

Incorporating Scientific Reasoning and Data

Scientific evidence is important to FMHA. One of the most important goals in research and practice of FMHA is the application of empirical evidence to better inform legal decision-making (Heilbrun, 1997). However, empirical evidence is not the only potentially valuable aspect of science in FMHA. Rather, both scientific data *and* reasoning can offer important contributions. In this chapter, three relevant principles will be discussed. The first, addressing the use of case-specific information in FMHA, will involve the application of scientific procedures and reasoning in the context of a single case, comparable to what appears in other mental health specialty areas as single case studies. The second principle will address the integration of behavioral scientific evidence and the FMHA case. The third principle focuses on the role of scientific reasoning, as distinguished from data, and identifies the contours of the appropriate role for such reasoning in FMHA.

There are a number of epistemological differences between clinical sciences and the law. In a broader discussion of psychology and law, Haney (1980) described two of the more important as (1) nomothetic versus idiographic research and reasoning and (2) the way in which certainty is communicated. Most research in the medical and behavioral sciences is nomothetic, involving a comparison of group differences. Legal decision-making is typically done in a context in which the specific behavior of an identified individual in a particular circumstance is at issue; it is this information, rather than group data, that is most immediately applicable. Also, legal decision-making is often dichotomous, and there is more emphasis on categorical communication (e.g., the litigant "is" or "is not" able to meet a certain test) than continuous probability communication (e.g., the litigant is "70% likely" to be able to meet a certain test). Nevertheless, there is a role for both idiographic and nomothetic data, as well as scientific reasoning, in FMHA. The respective roles for each are discussed in this chapter.

USE CASE-SPECIFIC (IDIOGRAPHIC) EVIDENCE IN ASSESSING CAUSAL CONNECTION BETWEEN CLINICAL CONDITION AND FUNCTIONAL ABILITIES

This principle emphasizes the importance of gathering information specific to the case and the individual when assessing the relevant domains in FMHA. This involves information about the particular circumstances that are relevant to the forensic issues being assessed. It also involves information about the individual that is immediately relevant to the forensic issues.

There are two important reasons to begin with the use of case-specific data. The first is accuracy. FMHA and therapeutic assessment both use data from a variety of sources (including behavioral science research, psychological testing, interviewing, and third-party information) to create hypotheses. An important difference, however, is the extent to which the evaluator seeks to verify such hypotheses *as part of the evaluation* (in FMHA), as contrasted with during the ongoing process of therapeutic intervention. Idiographic (case specific) information is used as part of both the hypothesis-forming and the verification steps, and plays a critical role in both. Without such case specific information, the data and resulting conclusions usually cannot be as accurate.

Nor would they *appear* as accurate, or as relevant, to the individual case. It has been observed that face validity, the weakest form of validity in behavioral scientific terms, is actually the strongest in legal contexts (Grisso, 1986a). When evidence is not perceived as reliable and relevant, it may not even be admitted; if it is, the emphasis placed on such evidence by the decision-maker is likely to be diminished. It is simply easier to see the relevance and reliability of expert evidence that is obtained directly from, and about, an individual in a specific case. For both of these reasons, the discussion of the application of scientific contributions to FMHA will begin with the idiographic.

ETHICS

The *Ethical Principles of Psychologists and Code of Conduct* (APA, 1992) notes the importance of using information and techniques that are sufficient to substantiate findings, typically including personal contact with the individual. This is cited both in the broader section, and the section of the *Principles* focusing specifically on Forensic Activities:

> Psychologists' assessments, recommendations, reports, and psychological diagnostic or evaluative statements are based on information and techniques (including personal interviews of the individual when appropriate) sufficient to provide appropriate substantiation for their findings. (pp. 1603, 1610)

The *Principles* further indicates that

> Except as noted ... below, psychologists provide written or oral forensic reports or testimony of the psychological characteristics of an individual only after they have conducted an examination of the individual adequate to support their statements or conclusions. When, despite reasonable efforts, such an examination is not feasible, psychologists clarify the impact of their limited information on the reliability and validity of their reports and testimony, and they appropriately limit the nature and extent of their conclusions or recommendations. (p. 1610)

The *Specialty Guidelines for Forensic Psychologists* (1991) first outlines the importance of testing "plausible rival hypotheses" using information that may come from a variety of sources:

> In providing forensic psychological services, forensic psychologists take special care to avoid undue influence upon their methods, procedures, and products, such as might emanate from the party to a legal proceeding by financial compensation or other gains. As an expert conducting an evaluation, treatment, consultation, or scholarly/empirical investigation, the forensic psychologist maintains professional integrity by examining the issue at hand from all reasonable perspectives, actively seeking information that will differentially test plausible rival hypotheses. (p. 661)

A more specific example of the importance of corroborating FMHA data is provided in the context of hearsay evidence:

> While many forms of data used by forensic psychologists are hearsay, forensic psychologists attempt to corroborate critical data that form the basis for their professional product. When using hearsay data that have not been corroborated, but are nevertheless utilized, forensic psychologists have an affirmative responsibility to acknowledge the uncorroborated status of those data and the reasons for relying upon such data. (p. 662)

Such corroboration may be obtained, in part, from an interview with the individual. Hence, it *is* indicated that

> Forensic psychologists avoid giving written or oral evidence about the psychological characteristics of particular individuals when they have not had an opportunity to conduct an examination of the individual adequate to the scope of the statements, opinions, or conclusions to be issued. Forensic psychologists make every reasonable effort to conduct such examinations. When it is not possible or feasible to do so, they make clear the impact of such limitations on

the reliability and validity of their professional products, evidence, or testimony. (p. 663)

The *Principles of Medical Ethics with Annotations Especially Applicable to Psychiatry* (APA, 1998) does not provide any specific reference to this principle. The *Ethical Guidelines for the Practice of Forensic Psychiatry* (AAPL, 1995) alludes to it by indicating that

> Practicing forensic psychiatrists enhance the honesty and objectivity of their work by basing their forensic opinions, forensic reports and forensic testimony on all the data available to them. They communicate the honesty of their work, efforts to attain objectivity, and the soundness of their clinical opinion by distinguishing, to the extent possible, between verified and unverified information as well as between clinical "facts," "inferences" and "impressions." (p. 3)

LAW

Under the *Federal Rules of Evidence*, expert evidence must be both relevant and reliable in order to be admissible. Most of the discussion of the relationship between the *Federal Rules* and scientific aspects of evidence has been under the "reliable" portion of this evidentiary requirement, which was elaborated by the U.S. Supreme Court in their decision affirming the applicability of the *Federal Rules* to scientific testimony in *Daubert v. Merrell Dow Pharmaceuticals* (1993). However, it should be noted that FMHA expert evidence may become more "relevant" to the immediate case when this principle is applied. When findings suggested by interview, testing, and third-party information are treated as hypotheses and subsequently verified through comparable information from different sources, then it becomes much clearer how each of the findings is relevant to the specific case (particularly when some of the test findings are based on actuarial approaches that involve comparison of the individual to others on whom the test was validated). At least one court (*U.S. v. Downing*, 1985) has commented that one aspect of relevancy under Rule 702 is "whether the expert testimony proffered in the case is sufficiently tied to the facts of the case that it will aid the jury in resolving a factual dispute" (p. 1242).

The test for the reliability of scientific evidence set forth in *Daubert* (1993) is particularly important for this FMHA principle in jurisdictions in which *Daubert* and the *Federal Rules of Evidence* or their comparable state equivalents apply. Rather than focusing primarily on the results of a scientific study or the acceptance of the method within the scientific community, the court (in dicta in which seven of the nine justices joined) suggested a number of criteria that might be applied by the court toward evaluating whether the "reasoning or methodology underlying the testimony is scientifically valid" (p. 592) and could be applied to the immediate case. These criteria include whether the basis for the opinion is testable, whether it has been tested, the known error rate, and other criteria such as level of general acceptance and indices of peer review. Two observations are particularly relevant. First, the focus on reasoning as well as testing methodology suggests the court is considering "scientific" evidence broadly to include reasoning, case-specific evidence, and nomothetic data (to be discussed further under the other two principles in this chapter). Second, the court's emphasis on relevance to the facts at issue would indicate that approaches to providing more case-specific evidence would not be excluded under *Daubert* so long as the methodology is acceptable. As Shuman (1997) has observed, "*Daubert* struggles to articulate a method of analysis, beyond mere popularity, to assess being right" (p. 556). To the extent that case-specific evidence contributes to this goal, it should be admissible under *Daubert*.

EMPIRICAL

Studies that provide normative information about the idiographic use of science in FMHA have not been located. However, there are published examples of the idiographic use of research in contexts that are comparable to FMHA. The U.S. Secret Service, for example, has a primary mission to protect the President, the Vice President, and their families:

> Essentially, the Secret Service must conduct a very specialized assessment of dangerousness—that is, dangerousness toward the President or other protectee—based on consideration of a range of risk factors that often include significant clinical data. Recognizing the need for professional expertise related to a thorough understanding of mental illness in general, and familiarity with clinical and forensic practice standards for risk assessment in particular, the Secret Service turned to the behavioral sciences as a resource to assist with investigative decision-making and inform policy. (Coggins, Pynchon, & Dvoskin, 1998, p. 59)

However, relatively little useful empirical data are available to help agents assigned to the task of investigating and evaluating individuals who may pose a risk to Secret Service protectees. There are two ways in which data might be helpful: (1) in the nomothetic sense, to allow the *prediction* of a specific kind of violence (toward a protectee) or the *classification* of risk level, and (2) in a more idiographic sense, to determine whether dynamic risk factors for a given individual have changed over time and whether Secret Service *risk reduction* strategies have been sufficient to lower an individual's dynamic risk factors over time (Heilbrun, 1997).

There has apparently been no empirical research that would identify objective, quantifiable risk factors that would allow application of research in the first way. Two studies by Dietz and colleagues (Dietz, Matthews, Martell, & Stewart, 1991; Dietz, Matthews, Van Dayne, et al., 1991) provide data that can be applied in the second way, allowing agents to confirm or disconfirm assumptions about dynamic risk factors that are used in their work (Coggins et al., 1998). This has been done in a more organized fashion through the Secret Service Exceptional Case Study Project (Fein & Vosse-kuil, 1998), allowing observations regarding assassination in the United States through cases such as a near-lethal approacher and an attacker.

There is also a study that addresses the perceived desirability of using this principle in FMHA. Borum and Grisso (1996) found several elements cited by forensic psychiatrists and psychologists as important to FMHA that are also relevant to this principle. These include (1) "mental illness rationale" (76% of responding psychiatrists rated this as "essential" or "recommended" in evaluations of CR and CST, while 81% of responding psychologists considered it essential or recommended), (2) rationale for the relation of mental illness and CST abilities (93% of responding psychiatrists and 95% of responding psychologists described this as essential or recommended), and (3) rationale for the relation of mental illness to CR (88% of responding psychiatrists and 87% of responding psychologists rated this as essential or recommended in evaluations of CR).

STANDARD OF PRACTICE

Both the need for accuracy and the scrutiny in FMHA have been cited as justifications for obtaining case-specific information in the form of records and interviews of third parties (Melton et al., 1997). This has been discussed as well in a case report (Heilbrun, 1990), in which the need for extensive third-party information in the form of staff observations was essential in a high-profile case in which the defendant, although hospitalized as incompetent to stand trial, was entirely uncooperative with attempts at interview and testing as part of the evaluation.

Greenberg and Brodsky (in press) offer several guidelines for forensic clinicians in the context of civil FMHA that are particularly relevant to this principle. Although their review of the literature and analysis of relevant procedures is intended for application to FMHA in personal injury litigation, it can be generalized reasonably well to FMHA performed to address other legal questions and forensic issues. They first describe the importance of "hypothesis testing" as a forensic assessment strategy:

> Test results will be considered as hypotheses only, to be confirmed or disconfirmed by additional data.

a. reasonable attempts will be made to corroborate critical test data which may form the basis of the examiner's opinions, reports, or testimony.

b. the examiner will consider both directly assessed data from the examinee and collateral data from multiple other sources when attempting to arrive at corroborated valid conclusions regarding the interpreted meaning of psychological tests.

c. when using test data and hypotheses that have not been corroborated, the examiner will acknowledge the uncorroborated status of such data and the reasons for relying, or not relying, upon that data.

I. major test hypotheses that are not corroborated by other data will be discussed in the report along with hypotheses that are corroborated by evidence from the current examination. (in press)

These steps include the process of attempting to confirm (or disconfirm) hypotheses by using other case-specific data obtained in the course of the evaluation. Next is the importance of the use of multiple sources in testing such hypotheses, with the goal of "integrated, convergent" data:

> If significant negative or positive impression results from any single aspect of the examination, there will be further assessment to confirm that the impression is representative and not aberrant. The goal is to generate integrated convergent data. (in press)

Finally, they comment on the importance of thoroughness, and the necessity of avoiding opinions that are preliminary or based on incomplete information:

> Examiners will not offer opinions until they have considered sufficient data ... adequate to form that opinion and have also considered sufficient data that might refute that opinion. Opinions and recommendations will (be) based on an integration of ... data. (in press)

The importance of confirming or disconfirming possible explanations for relevant capacities and behavior is a recurring theme that can be seen in other major works on forensic assessment (e.g., Grisso, 1986a, 1998a; Melton et al., 1997; Shapiro, 1991). It is one of the important links that connects the sources of information and the raw data that they yield with the conclusions regarding relevant forensic capacities. More specifically, this principle is consistent with one particular aspect of using a model in FMHA: the need to address the causal relationship between clinical symptoms and legally relevant deficits (see the discussion in Chapter 4).

DISCUSSION

It is important to use idiographic scientific approaches in FMHA for two reasons: accuracy, and the perception of increased accuracy and relevance. Sources of ethics authority in psychology emphasize that the assessment should be based on information and techniques that are sufficient to substantiate findings. These include direct contact with the individual being evaluated, and allowing the evaluator to obtain case-specific information for hypothesis formation and testing. More specific reference to such hypothesis testing is seen in the forensic ethical standards for psychology and psychiatry, which refer to "hypothesis testing" and "verification of information," respectively.

Relevance also appears to be an important legal justification for using idiographic approaches in FMHA, addressing one of the two major evidentiary criteria for the admissibility of expert evidence. Reliability, at least as construed under *Daubert*, is judged with an emphasis on the method and considered broadly enough to include idiographic as well as nomothetic approaches, as well as scientific reasoning.

There is apparently no empirical research on the effectiveness of using idiographic approaches in FMHA. This represents a clear need for the field, given the support that is apparent for this principle in ethical, legal, and standard of practice areas. One of the areas in which this need is most apparent is FMHA involving risk assessment, with individualized intervention-planning based on dynamic risk factors. This is a current theoretical trend, but it has not been tested sufficiently empirically. There are some limited data on the extent to which forensic psychiatrists and psychologists favorably perceive the need for an explicit "rationale" between clinical condition and functional abilities, but even these data need replication and expansion.

The support for this principle in the standard of practice literature is very clear, however. A number of influential sources cite the importance of hypothesis testing, the generation of integrated and convergent data, and the value of idiographic approaches for both accuracy and perceived accuracy. Idiographic approaches in FMHA are also consistent with the use of a model, with the emphasis on the causal connection between clinical and functional areas. While this principle clearly needs further empirical investigation, it is reasonably well supported in other areas, and will be considered to be *established*.

USE NOMOTHETIC EVIDENCE IN ASSESSING CAUSAL CONNECTION BETWEEN CLINICAL CONDITION AND FUNCTIONAL ABILITIES

This principle describes the value of applying scientific data gathered with groups to assess the relevant domains in FMHA. A conventionally accepted contribution of science to a forensic assessment is the application of scientific research data that have been gathered for various purposes.

Several of these purposes are particularly noteworthy in their applicability to FMHA. One is validation. Research can provide data on the reliability and validity of various tools (e.g., psychological tests, structured interviews, specialized inventories) and their relation to outcomes of interest in FMHA (e.g., response style, functioning in certain diagnostic categories, behavior in functional legal areas). A second purpose is prediction. Research can provide important information on base rates, and provide relatively sophisticated ways of constructing actuarial approaches and gauging the accuracy of these (and other approaches to decision-making) with measures such as sensitivity and specificity. This aspect of science is an indispensable part of the development of tools, the measurement of accuracy, and the determination of outcomes that are so important in FMHA. In this section, the support for the nomothetic applications of science to FMHA will be discussed.

ETHICS

The *Ethical Principles of Psychologists and Code of Conduct* (APA, 1992) provides a number of sections that are relevant to this principle. First, the value of scientifically derived knowledge is emphasized:

> Psychologists rely on scientifically and professionally derived knowledge when making scientific or professional judgments or when engaging in scholarly or professional endeavors. (p. 1600)

A number of sections relate directly to various phases of psychological assessment (including FMHA). The importance of research on the usefulness and applications of various tests or instruments is cited:

> Psychologists who develop, administer, score, interpret, or use psychological assessment techniques, interviews, tests, or instruments do so in a manner and for purposes that are appropriate in light of the research on or evidence of the usefulness and proper applications of the techniques. (p. 1603)

The interpretation of assessment results should be guided by research on the reliability and validity of the procedures used in the assessment:

> Psychologists who perform interventions or administer, score, interpret, or use assessment techniques are familiar with the reliability, validation, and related standardization or outcome studies of, and proper applications and uses of, the techniques they use. (p. 1603)

A number of considerations can affect such interpretation. With the use of automated scoring and interpretation services increasingly common in psychological assessment, there is an important question about the factors that affect the applicability of such assessment in an individual case:

> When interpreting assessment results, including automated interpretations, psychologists take into account the various test factors and characteristics of the person being assessed that might affect psychologists' judgments or reduce the accuracy of their interpretations. They indicate any significant reservations they have about the accuracy or limitations of their interpretations. (p. 1603)

However, there is no question that scoring and interpretation services are subject to the same ethical demand for scientific validation that applies to all psychological assessment:

> Psychologists select scoring and interpretation services (including automated services) on the basis of evidence of the validity of the programs and procedures as well as on the other appropriate considerations. (p. 1604)

As a result of these considerations, the interpretation of psychological assessment results must be qualified and communicated to indicate the limits on certainty:

> Psychologists recognize limits to the certainty with which diagnoses, judgments, or predictions can be made about individuals. (p. 1603)

The *Specialty Guidelines for Forensic Psychologists* (1991) addresses this principle in a more limited way. Both the awareness of current scientific information and the application of such information to the selection of data collection methods and procedures in FMHA are cited:

> Because of their special status as persons qualified as experts to the court, forensic psychologists have an obligation to maintain current knowledge of scientific, professional and legal developments within their area of claimed competence. They are obligated also to use that knowledge, consistent with accepted clinical and scientific standards, in selecting data collection methods and procedures for an evaluation, treatment, consultation or scholarly/empirical investigation. (p. 661)

Neither the *Principles of Medical Ethics with Annotations Especially Applicable to Psychiatry* nor the *Ethical Guidelines for the Practice of Forensic Psychiatry* addresses this principle directly.

LAW

The issue of whether FMHA will be construed by the courts as a "scientific" or "other technical" procedure is discussed elsewhere in this book. It is more straightforward to discuss the law's support for science in FMHA if we assume that FMHA will be treated as scientific evidence, at least by some courts. Legal support for the use of science as part of FMHA would be quite clear for this principle, since it encompasses that aspect of science that is most commonly associated with the scientific enterprise: group data that are gathered, analyzed, and interpreted according to accepted scientific procedures.

Under the *Frye* (1923) standard, scientific evidence must be "sufficiently established to have gained general acceptance in the particular field to which it belongs." This standard tends to focus a court's attention on the status of the evidence within the field; to the extent that the FMHA "field" values instruments and tools that are reliable and valid for the purpose of measuring constructs relevant to the legal question, then *Frye* is consistent with the importance of empirical research findings to FMHA. However, this could be argued in the other direction as well. To the extent that *Frye* has rarely been used to exclude any kind of clinical testimony from legal proceedings, it has been observed that the *Frye* standard has not been effectively used by courts to distinguish between clinical testimony that is research-based and that which is not.[1]

Under *Daubert*, it seems clearer that a court inclined to consider FMHA as scientific evidence has a stronger basis for excluding components of the assessment if they are not properly validated. It is unclear how often trial courts will apply *Daubert* to FMHA evidence. Some (e.g., Rotgers & Barrett, 1996) have argued that clinical psychology, for example, has been increasingly based on science and, having "adopted the mantle of science," should be held to the requirements of *Daubert*. Others (e.g., Zonana, 1994) have suggested that at least some forensic applications of psychiatry will also be relevant to screening under this case. There is also a slowly emerging body of case law reflecting instances in which *Daubert* has been applied to FMHA. To date, courts have used *Daubert* criteria to consider the admissibility of evidence from tools or techniques in cases involving alleged sexual offending (e.g., victim and perpetrator "profiling," including testimony about Posttraumatic Stress Disorder, Rape Trauma Syndrome, Child Sexual Abuse Accommodation Syndrome, the accuracy of "recovered memories") and violence and victims more generally (e.g., risk assessment, victimology, partner abuse, and Battered Spouse Syndrome). The techniques most often considered are psychological tests, interview approaches, and conclusions regarding syndromes and profiles; no appellate courts have cited *Daubert* in ruling favorably on the admis-

---

[1]Melton et al. (1997) make precisely this observation, noting that some courts would apply *Frye* to the physical sciences but not the behavioral sciences, and others apparently conclude that if a technique, procedure, or diagnosis is sufficiently well accepted to be a part of clinical practice, that it is sufficiently well accepted to satisfy *Frye*.

sibility of FMHA procedures such as documents review, third-party interviews, or other third-party observations (Heilbrun, 1996; Bersoff, Glass, Dodds, Eckl, & Peters, 1999).[2]

It may be that whether courts regard FMHA as "scientific" or "technical," or even "other specialized knowledge," is not always crucial to the role that empirical scientific data will play in the admissibility of such evidence. Under Rule 702 of the *Federal Rules of Evidence*, it is noted that an

---

[2]It is useful to consider the ground(s) cited by appellate courts in cases in which *Daubert* has been cited as a basis for admitting or excluding FMHA evidence. Under *Daubert*, there are several possible grounds: testability, known or potential error rate, peer review and publication, and general acceptance. In the area of sexual offending, expert evidence regarding the following has been admitted: (1) credibility and suggestibility of child witnesses (*U.S. v. Reynolds*, 1996, *Daubert* grounds not specified), (2) Repressed Memory Syndrome (*Hoult v. Hoult*, 1995, *Daubert* grounds not specified; *Shahzade v. Gregory*, 1996, on grounds of testability, error rate, peer review, and general acceptance; *Isley v. Capuchin Province*, 1995, on grounds of error rate, peer review, and general acceptance), (3) Posttraumatic Stress Disorder (*State v. Alberico*, 1993, admitted in part on grounds of testability and general acceptance; *State v. Martens*, 1993, admitted on ground of general acceptance), and (4) symptomatology of sexual abuse based on clinical experience and experience with the plaintiff (*Frohne v. State*, 1997, *Daubert* grounds not specified). Courts have also excluded expert evidence in the area of sexual offending under *Daubert*: (1) credibility of child witnesses (*U.S. v. Rouse*, 1997, rejected on peer review and general acceptance grounds), (2) interviewing techniques (*U.S. v. Reynolds*, 1996, rejected but *Daubert* grounds not specified; *Gier v. Educational Service Unit No. 16*, 1994, rejected on grounds of testability and peer review), (3) the psychological phenomenon of recantation (*Newkirk v. Commonwealth*, 1996, rejected on testability and error rate grounds), (4) profiling of sexual offenders (*S.V. v. R.V.*, 1996, rejected on grounds of testability and general acceptance; *Tungate v. Commonwealth*, 1995, *Daubert* grounds not specified; *State v. Cavaliere*, 1995, rejected on grounds of testability and error rate; *State v. Parkinson*, 1996, rejected on grounds of error rate and general acceptance), and (5) profiling of sexual abuse victims (*State v. Alberico*, 1993, rejected on grounds of testability and general acceptance; *State v. Foret*, 1993, rejected on grounds of testability, error rate, and peer review; *Steward v. State*, 1995, rejected on grounds of testability and error rate; *S.V. v. R.V.*, 1996, rejected on grounds of testability and error rate). Courts have also applied *Daubert* to scrutinizing FMHA evidence on violence and victims of violence more generally. Such expert evidence has been held admissible on (1) future dangerousness (*U.S. v. Evanoff*, 1993, *Daubert* grounds not specified), (2) victimology (*U.S. v. Alzanki*, 1995, *Daubert* grounds not specified), (3) Posttraumatic Stress Disorder (*Chester v. State*, 1996, *Daubert* grounds not specified), (4) Battered Spouse Syndrome (*U.S. v. Brown*, 1995, *Daubert* grounds not specified), (5) Battered Person Syndrome (*Chester v. State*, 1996, *Daubert* grounds not specified), and (6) "cycle of abuse" (*State v. Maelega*, 1995, on grounds of testability and general acceptance). Expert evidence of several kinds within the areas of violence and victimology has also been excluded using *Daubert*: (1) victimology (*Karabian v. Columbia University*, 1996, *Daubert* grounds not specified), (2) future dangerousness (*Rodriguez Cirilo v. Garcia*, 1995, *Daubert* grounds not specified), (3) Battering Parent Syndrome (*State v. Picklesimer*, 1996, for inappropriate use of character evidence), and (4) Steroid Rage Syndrome (*Pennington v. State*, 1995, rejected on ground of general acceptance). For a further discussion of courts' use of *Daubert* to evaluate both FMHA and social science evidence, see Bersoff et al. (1999).

expert in any of these three areas, if qualified by knowledge, skill, experience, training, or education, may testify in the form of an opinion or otherwise to assist the trier of fact in understanding such evidence. As Melton et al. (1997) observe, a court in a *Daubert* jurisdiction might be more likely to scrutinize FMHA and the scientific support for its components if it considers FMHA to be "scientific." It might be less inclined to consider a research base to be essential for decisions in which FMHA was considered "technical" or "other specialized knowledge," and therefore scrutinize applicable research only in the cases in which it existed.

The U.S. Supreme Court has written one decision stressing the importance of establishing the underlying scientific validity of the scientific expert's testimony (*Daubert*), and another in which there was little apparent concern with the underlying scientific validity of testimony in the sentencing phase of a capital case. In the latter instance, in *Barefoot v. Estelle* (1983), the Court supported the admissibility of expert testimony on future dangerousness that was based on the clinician's experience, made no reference to research, and described the probability of future criminal acts of violence (a "one hundred percent and absolute chance"; see p. 919) in a way that could not be supported by either available research results or research-based thinking (see Shuman, 1997, for a fuller discussion). Courts using *Daubert* as a basis for evaluating the admissibility of FMHA evidence will clearly be inclined to consider the basis for the opinion beyond "clinical judgment and experience," while courts applying the *Barefoot* precedent may not.

The U.S. Supreme Court has now decided a case that should provide some guidance concerning the applicability of *Daubert* to FMHA evidence. In *Kumho Tire Company, Ltd. v. Carmichael* (1999), the Court held that the Eleventh Circuit (in *Carmichael v. Samyang Tire, Inc.*, 1997) had incorrectly reversed a trial court decision to apply *Daubert* to the testimony of an expert on tire failure. This expert was prepared to testify, based on his experience (but, according to the plaintiffs, not based on his scientific expertise or the application of scientific principles), that a tire manufactured by the defendant was defective and the proximate cause of an automobile accident in which the plaintiffs were involved. The Eleventh Circuit Court of Appeals described the distinction between scientific and nonscientific expert testimony by quoting a Sixth Circuit decision in *Berry v. City of Detroit* (1994):

> The distinction between scientific and non-scientific expert testimony is a critical one. By way of illustration, if one wanted to explain to a jury how a bumblebee is able to fly, an aeronautical engineer might be a helpful witness. Since flight principles have some universality, the expert could apply general principles to the case of the bumblebee. Conceivably, even if he had never seen

a bumblebee, he still would be qualified to testify, as long as he was familiar with its component parts. On the other hand, if one wanted to prove that bumblebees always take off into the wind, a beekeeper with no scientific training at all would be an acceptable witness if a proper foundation were laid for his conclusions. The foundation would not relate to his formal training, but to his firsthand observations. In other words, the beekeeper does not know any more about flight principles than the jurors, but he has seen a lot more bumblebees than they have. (pp. 1349–1350).

The Eleventh Circuit decision went on to reason that *Daubert* should be applied to experts who are scientific (e.g., aeronautical engineers), but not experts who base their opinion on observations and experience (e.g., beekeepers). The U.S. Supreme Court, however, rejected this distinction, and held that *Daubert* may be applied to evaluating experts who testify on the basis of *either* scientific *or* technical or other specialized knowledge regarding a matter before the court. However FMHA is classified, therefore, it would appear after *Kumho* that it may be scrutinized under *Daubert*.

EMPIRICAL

Relatively little empirical information is available on the normative ways in which scientific data have been applied in FMHA. However, there are examples of how such empirical data can be integrated into FMHA. A volume of *Behavioral Sciences and the Law* (Winter 1998) was devoted to the integration of research and practice in forensic psychology and psychiatry. Several articles in this issue are particularly applicable to this principle. Kuehnle (1998) discusses the scientist-practitioner model as it applies to child sexual abuse evaluations, focusing the conclusions on the empirically established associations between empirical data and relevant behavior that are validated by research. Child sexual abuse is treated as a "life event" rather than a clinical syndrome, allowing better incorporation of base rates of this behavior into evaluation of the distinctions between sexually abused children and those who have not been sexually abused. Also considered are the predictive characteristics, such as sensitivity and specificity, of instruments used in such evaluations. Although she presents a good discussion of the importance of incorporating scientific data and focusing on decision-making models, it is unclear whether she recommends that an ultimate opinion (whether the child being evaluated "was" versus "was not" abused) in such cases be avoided, in favor of the data and reasoning relevant to each.

Dammeyer (1998) also focused on issues of child sexual abuse, and discussed the empirical considerations relevant to the sources of information in child sexual abuse evaluations. "Commonly used indicators" of child sexual abuse were discussed. These included (1) physical indicators (sexually transmitted diseases, pregnancy, tears in the skin, enlargements, or other medical problems), (2) age-inappropriate sexual knowledge, (3) consistency over time of the child's report of abuse, (4) the idiosyncratic nature of the child's abuse account, and (5) a statement by the child relating a progression of sexual activity. Also discussed were procedures such as anatomically detailed dolls, free drawings, anatomically correct drawings, puppets, and psychological tests (see Conte, Sorenson, Fogarty, & Rosa, 1991, for details of a survey of professionals at child protection agencies and rape crisis centers, as well as other knowledgeable professionals, about the use of such sources). He reviews the empirical evidence in each of the following areas: (1) medical examinations, (2) the child's report, (3) assessment procedures using anatomical dolls, drawings, puppets, and dollhouses, (4) sexualized behavior, and (5) psychological testing. The best support appears to be for factors such as the results of medical examinations, the child's report, and sexualized behavior, although cautions are given regarding the possible inaccuracies of each; assessment procedures using dolls, puppets, dollhouses, and the like, and psychological tests, receive very mixed support and are frequently nonspecific in their results. Hence, they have a very limited capacity to discriminate between abused and nonabused children.

Cruise and Rogers (1998) reviewed the efficacy of specialized forensic assessment instruments for CST, including the Competency to Stand Trial Assessment Instrument (McGarry et al., 1973), the Competency Screening Test (Lipsitt, Lelos, & McGarry, 1971), the Georgia Court Competency Test–Mississippi Version Revised (Johnson & Mullet, 1987), and the recently developed MacArthur Structured Assessment of the Competencies of Criminal Defendants (MacSAC-CD; Hoge, Bonnie, et al., 1997). In reviewing the research relevant to the psychometric properties and validation of each of these instruments, Cruise and Rogers emphasized the importance of research that measures constructs that are related to trial competence. These include, for example, the clinical symptoms that are relevant to the capacities for factual understanding, communication, and decision-making, as well as the related issue of response style.[3]

Additional information on recent research in the area of CST has been summarized for the years 1991–1995 in seven areas: (1) the systemic context of CST, (2) conceptual definitions of CST, (3) research on CST assessment

---

[3]The approach to applying empirical research to a legal question taken by Cruise and Rogers (1998) is consistent with that used by other scholars in FMHA most recently—rather than focusing on the legal question as an outcome variable, the primary variables of interest are the forensic issues that are included within, and relevant to, the legal question.

methods, (4) characteristics of incompetent defendants, (5) interpretation and communication of CST evaluation data, (6) issues in CST assessment of special populations (juveniles, persons with mental retardation), and (7) treatment to restore competence (Cooper & Grisso, 1997). Several of these areas are particularly important in the use of nomothetic data in FMHA. Research on the characteristics of incompetent defendants can inform an evaluator's judgment about whether certain kinds of psycho-pathology or functional deficits have been sufficient for an adjudication of incompetence across a large number of cases. Likewise, research on the interpretation and communication of CST evaluation data can allow the forensic clinician to compare her practices with those of other evaluators. Finally, a recommendation that a given defendant appears incompetent to stand trial may trigger the need for a further judgment regarding whether the individual can be restored to competence, and possibly the anticipated length of time for such restoration (*Jackson v. Indiana*, 1972). Such a judg-ment is essentially a prediction about whether the individual's response to treatment, usually in a secure hospital, will be sufficiently favorable to diminish the functional deficits interfering with the individual's compe-tence to stand trial to a manageable level. As such, research on treatment response among incompetent defendants is clearly relevant, as it provides information about base rates and particular kinds of deficits that may be applicable to the immediate case.

STANDARD OF PRACTICE

Given the demands for both accuracy and perceived accuracy in FMHA, it is important to be able to describe the degree of empirical scientific support that has been demonstrated for a particular FMHA procedure. It is also important to select and use procedures that have such an empirical base. This has been strongly advocated for psychological tests that are used in FMHA, with some of the guidelines described (by Heilbrun, 1992) relevant to this principle: (1) the test is commercially available and has a manual documenting its psychometric properties, (2) tests with a reliability coefficient of less than .80 would require explicit justification explaining why they are used, (3) the test's relevance to the legal issue or an underlying psychological construct should be supported by validation research, and (4) objective tests and actuarial data combina-tion are preferable when there are appropriate outcome data and a "for-mula" exists.

Although these guidelines were written with psychological tests in mind, they can be applied to other procedures (e.g., interviewing) that are also important in FMHA. This would be consistent with the position espoused by others (e.g., Blau, 1984b; Grisso, 1986; Melton et al., 1997) regarding the importance of empirical support for procedures used in FMHA. Guidelines that are more broadly applicable have recently been proposed (by Greenberg & Brodsky, in press), who note that instruments used in FMHA should be reliable and valid to an extent adequate to the scope of statements, opinions, and conclusions. They further propose that instruments without adequate levels of reliability and validity should be considered only as a source of self-report, and identified as such.

DISCUSSION

Nomothetic data can be used in two important ways in FMHA. The first is validation; the collection of such data allows the establishment of reliability and validity for tools that are used in forensic assessment. The second is prediction and management, with the establishment of base rates and the measurement of the accuracy with which legally relevant constructs and behavior can be either predicted or changed through planned interventions.

Sources of ethics authority for this principle are drawn entirely from psychology. Heavy and detailed support is seen from the APA's *Ethics Code*, with primary emphasis on the reliability and validity of psychological assessment procedures, the application of automated scoring and interpretation, and the recognition of the limits of certainty that can be clarified through empirical data. Less detailed support is seen in the *Specialty Guidelines for Forensic Psychologists*; however, there is emphasis on the importance of scientific knowledge as it contributes to competent practice, and is applied to the selection of procedures for FMHA.

The legal support for this principle no longer depends on whether FMHA is considered by courts to be scientific, technical, or "other specialized knowledge," since the *Kumho* decision in which the U.S. Supreme Court held that expert evidence may be evaluated under *Daubert* regardless of whether the nature of the expertise is scientific, technical, or other specialized knowledge. The *Frye* standard would help to gauge whether scientific research helps establish an FMHA procedure's general acceptance in the field, but it has rarely been used to exclude such procedures from admission into legal proceedings. The *Daubert* decision is somewhat more likely to be applied toward considering the empirical scientific base for FMHA, and there is an emerging body of case law involving the use of *Daubert* criteria in evaluating the admissibility of FMHA procedures, particularly in cases involving sexual abuse and other kinds of violence, and their impact on victims.

The empirical trend seen particularly within the last 10 years has been toward measuring the forensic issues relevant to the larger legal questions that courts use FMHA to address. This trend should help the discipline to mature, allowing the measurement of such constructs to facilitate better comparisons with relevant groups, and more accurate prediction. As this empirical research has been applied with more sophistication toward describing the functioning of relevant forensic constructs, the standard of practice literature has become increasingly specific. At present, the literature generally emphasizes the importance of reliable and valid psychological tests that are relevant to such forensic constructs. With better research support for an increased number of these constructs, it should be possible for forensic clinicians to apply the research toward a better-supported description of an individual being evaluated, when compared with others in a similar population being evaluated for comparable reasons.

Strong support for nomothetic research is apparent among ethical standards in psychology, and there is flexibility within some present legal standards for the evaluation of FMHA in the context of such empirical support. Although the trend within the last decade has clearly been toward allowing empirical scientific research to measure relevant forensic constructs, the development of this research base is not sufficient to conclude that the standard of practice in FMHA must involve the consistent selection of tools that are well validated. This principle appears to be *established*, but the research base must continue to develop.

USE SCIENTIFIC REASONING IN ASSESSING CAUSAL CONNECTION BETWEEN CLINICAL CONDITION AND FUNCTIONAL ABILITIES

This principle describes the value of using scientific reasoning to reach conclusions in FMHA using data gathered in a particular case. There are several aspects of scientific reasoning that are particularly relevant to this principle. They include the operationalization of variables, hypothesis formulation and testing, falsifiability, parsimony in interpretation, and the awareness of limitations on accuracy and the applicability of nomothetic research to the immediate case. Within the constructs that are being evaluated as part of FMHA, there are usually a number of explanations that could account for the existing clinical symptoms or relevant personality characteristics, the degree of deficit in the relevant legal capacities, and the causal relationship between the two. Such explanations might be considered as hypotheses, with one of the goals of FMHA being the "testing" of various hypotheses in order to determine which is best supported. In order to make such "testing" meaningful, however, the hypothesis must be evaluated using constructs that have been operationalized, and formulated in a way that allows it to be rejected when it is not supported. In Popper's (1968) language, the hypothesis is then "falsifiable." Parsimonious interpretation involves determining which explanation is "best," in the sense that it is the least complex while accounting for the most data.[4] In the following discussion, the role of scientific reasoning, as reflected in hypothesis formulation and testing, will be considered.

ETHICS

The *Ethical Principles of Psychologists and Code of Conduct* (APA, 1992) has a number of sections relevant to this principle. The selection of instruments and other procedures for use in FMHA is relevant to the way in which constructs are operationalized. To some extent, appropriate operationalization depends on selecting a procedure developed for a purpose that is comparable to that in the present evaluation:

> Psychologists who develop, administer, score, interpret, or use psychological assessment techniques, interviews, tests, or instruments do so in a manner and for purposes that are appropriate in light of the research on or evidence of the usefulness and proper application of the techniques. (p. 1603)

Also, how the procedure has been applied previously should be comparable to how it is being used presently:

> Psychologists who perform interventions or administer, score, interpret, or use assessment techniques are familiar with the reliability, validation and related standardization or outcome studies of, and proper applications and uses of, the techniques they use. (p. 1603)

Error in the selection of procedures can have adverse consequences for the successful operationalization of variables. Also, such error would limit both the overall accuracy of findings and the extent to which nomothetic results are applicable:

> Psychologists refrain from misuse of assessment techniques, interventions, results, and interpretations.... Psychologists do not base their assessment or

---

[4]There is an inherent conservatism in science and the interpretation of scientific findings that is a function of the value placed on accumulated knowledge. Such conservatism also characterizes FMHA, which draws its strength from existing relevant scientific knowledge. It may be that the *Daubert* decision, with its emphasis on method as well as general acceptance, will diminish such conservatism. This may be true occasionally in FMHA. However, forensic clinicians are still well advised to consider their clinical formulations and causal explanations of functional behavior in light of existing scientific evidence. When there is no scientific evidence (that is, the proposition is *untested* rather than *unsupported by relevant research*), then explanations should be made with more caution, and their lack of nomothetically based support readily acknowledged.

intervention decisions or recommendations on data or test results that are outmoded for the current purpose.... Similarly, psychologists do not base such decisions or recommendations on tests and measures that are obsolete and not useful for the current purpose. (p. 1603)

Next, the *Ethics Code* addresses the importance of personal contact with the individual being evaluated. In the context of the present principle, such personal contact is important because it facilitates hypothesis formation and testing:

> Except as noted ..., psychologists provide written or oral forensic reports or testimony of the psychological characteristics of an individual only after they have conducted an examination of the individual adequate to support their statements or conclusions. (p. 1610)

When such contact is not possible, then it becomes more difficult to test hypotheses, because the reaction of the individual to specific questions or procedures cannot be observed:

> When, despite reasonable efforts, such an examination is not feasible, psychologists clarify the impact of their limited information on the reliability and validity of their reports and testimony, and they appropriately limit the nature and extent of their conclusions or recommendations. (p. 1610)

Finally, there are two sections in the *Ethics Code* that are relevant to the interpretation of FMHA results. The applicability of validation research for a test or procedure used with the individual is addressed:

> Psychologists attempt to identify situations in which particular interventions or assessment techniques may not be applicable or may require adjustment in administration or interpretation because of such factors as individuals' gender, age, race, ethnicity, national origin, religion, sexual orientation, disability, language, or socioeconomic status. (p. 1603)

Parsimonious interpretation requires the consideration of various sources of uncertainty, including error that may have been introduced in selection, administration, scoring, and interpretation—or from the absence of relevant, validated procedures. In some cases, for some questions, the parsimonious conclusion is "I don't know":

> Psychologists recognize limits to the certainty with which diagnoses, judgments, or predictions can be made about individuals.... When interpreting assessment results ... psychologists take into account the various test factors and characteristics of the person being assessed that might affect psychologists' judgments or reduce the accuracy of their interpretations. (p. 1603)

The *Specialty Guidelines for Forensic Psychologists* (1991) offers one particularly relevant section, which emphasizes the value of hypothesis testing:

> In providing forensic psychological services, forensic psychologists take special care to avoid undue influence upon their methods, procedures, and products, such as might emanate from the party to a legal proceeding by financial compensation or other gains. As an expert conducting an evaluation, treatment, consultation, or scholarly/empirical investigation, the forensic psychologist maintains professional integrity by examining the issue at hand from all reasonable perspectives, actively seeking information that will differentially test plausible rival hypotheses. (p. 661)

This is consistent with the *Ethical Guidelines for the Practice of Forensic Psychiatry*, which (less directly) supports hypothesis testing by stressing the distinction between "verified" and "unverified" information. However, the *Principles of Medical Ethics with Annotations* does not address this principle directly.

LAW

The U.S. Supreme Court's holding in *Daubert* (1993) may have implications for the role of reasoning as part of the "method" of science that the trial judge must consider to determine the admissibility of expert evidence. In dicta outlining criteria that might be used to determine the scientific validity of the evidence, the Court used the phrase "reasoning or methodology." Further, examining the criteria described in the Court's dicta (whether the basis for the opinion is testable, whether it has been tested, and the known error rate, as well as other criteria such as level of general acceptance and indices of peer review) would suggest that the *Daubert* Court takes a broad view of the nature of "science," and that both reasoning and case-specific evidence (as well as nomothetic data) are components to be considered.

Under Rule 703 of the *Federal Rules of Evidence*, it is noted that "[t]he facts or data in the particular case upon which an expert bases an opinion *or inference* [italics added] may be those perceived by or made known to the expert at or before the hearing," explicitly suggesting some role for reasoning in FMHA. The nature of such reasoning may be considered in more detail by examining Rule 702:

> If scientific, technical, or other specialized knowledge will assist the trier of fact to understand the evidence or determine a fact in issue, a witness qualified as an expert by knowledge, skill, experience, training, or education, may testify thereto in the form of an opinion or otherwise.

Melton et al. (1997) have observed that at least seven levels of inference are possible as part of such an opinion. Ranging from requirement for the lowest to the highest level of inference, and increasingly approaching the legal questions, they include (1) perception of behavior, (2) perception of general mental state, (3) formulation of perception of mental state into theoretical or research-supported constructs , (4) diagnosis, (5) relationship of formulation or diagnosis to legally relevant behavior, (6) elements of the ultimate legal issue, and (7) ultimate legal issue. Some significant degree of reasoning is required for levels three and higher; the authors suggest that common judicial practice is to expect at least level six.

EMPIRICAL

Relatively little empirical evidence is available on the role of scientific reasoning in FMHA. However, in a recent survey of forensic psychologists and psychiatrists, Borum and Grisso (1996) obtained information regarding the desirability of descriptions in reports for evaluations of CST and CR. Some of these elements are clearly relevant to reasoning. Rating the value of providing a "mental illness rationale" describing how the examiner reached an opinion about the presence and degree, or absence, of mental illness, the majority of responding psychiatrists ($N = 45$) rated this rationale as either essential (24.4%) or recommended (51.1%), while the responding psychologists ($N = 57$) also saw it most often as either essential (36.8%) or recommended (43.9%). The language of this element ("presence" and "degree" versus "absence" of mental illness) is quite consistent with a reasoning process that is explicitly hypothesis testing. Other relevant elements were also strongly endorsed, with more than 75% of responding psychiatrists and psychologists rating each as either essential or recommended. These elements included an explanation for (1) how the examiner reached an opinion about relevant trial competence abilities, (2) the relation between observed symptoms of mental illness and observed deficits in CST abilities, (3) alternative ways (other than mental illness) of explaining the deficits in CST abilities, (4) the relation between symptoms of mental illness that existed at the time of the offense and the concurrent capacities relevant to the legal definition of CR, and (5) how the examiner reached an opinion regarding the relationship between mental illness and capacities relevant to CR. Although questions in the survey were limited to evaluations of CST and CR, the elements described in the last sentence would apply as well to FMHA involving other legal questions and forensic issues. It is unclear, however, whether the values assigned to them by other forensic clinicians, when applied to other kinds of FMHA, would be comparable.

STANDARD OF PRACTICE

The process of FMHA has been analogized by Heilbrun (1992) to Meehl's description of "quasi-experiments in real-life settings" (Meehl,

1989, p. 521). Sources of information that might assist in formulating and testing hypotheses include history, psychological testing, medical testing, interview data, and third-party observations. Heilbrun further observed:

> Following the formulation of falsifiable hypotheses, the verification process can proceed much as it would in a scientific experiment. Does the defendant exhibit behavior consistent with the presence of the hypothesized psychological characteristic? (A researcher might call this construct validity.) Does the defendant show the absence of behaviors that are not consistent with the presence of the hypothesized construct? (We could analogize this to discriminant validity.) The remaining task is then to offer conclusions in terms that reflect the consistency of support for the hypothesis that was framed in psychological rather than legal terms (e.g., psychosis, cognitive awareness, and volition rather than insanity). (p. 269)

The importance of reasoning, particularly in the context of hypothesis formation and testing as well as interpretation, is strongly advocated in this particular article.

Greenberg and Brodsky (in press) discuss the following aspirational guidelines for civil FMHA that are relevant to this principle:

> Reports and testimony will consider both the strengths and the limitations of psychological tests, of using such tests in forensic contexts, and of the individual examinee's functioning.
> a. An explanatory statement as to the meaning, weight, applicability, and limitations of psychological tests and interpretations in a forensic context will be included in each forensic report and expressed before providing testimony that might otherwise be misleading.
> b. Ambiguous test results, when relevant and significant to the matter, will be so identified and fair consideration will be given to additional testing in those instances.
>   i. Alternative explanations for such ambiguity will be offered in the report and testimony.
> c. Examiners will remember, and not misrepresent in their reports or testimony, that much of what is predicted in personality test interpretations is that a particular quality or trait is more likely to be present in this test taker than its base rate likelihood for the population. This is not to say, and it should not be implied in reports or testimony, that the particular quality or trait has a greater than 50% chance of being present in this individual unless adequate research support exists for such a prediction.

They also address the importance of fairly considering alternative explanations:

> Reports will contain at least a substantial paragraph making the fairest and best reasonable argument possible supporting the position of the party against whom the overall recommendation falls, so that person's best legitimate position and perspective may be fully considered by the court. This will be accompanied by a full explanation as to why this position is flawed or is outweighed by the examiner's ultimate opinion.

Discussion

The components of scientific reasoning that are particularly relevant to FMHA include the operationalization of variables, hypothesis formulation and testing, falsifiability, parsimony in interpretation, awareness of the limits on accuracy, and the applicability of nomothetic research to the immediate case. Like idiographic evidence, scientific reasoning is an element of the larger scientific process that is less frequently identified but quite important to FMHA.

Sources of general ethics authority in psychology provide direct support for the applications of scientific reasoning of several kinds in FMHA. These include hypothesis testing, the applicability of psychological assessment procedures, avoiding their misapplication, and parsimonious interpretation of results. Sources of ethical guidance in the more specialized forensic areas of both psychology and psychiatry provide further support for reasoning as demonstrated through hypothesis testing in FMHA.

With the change in the legal standard for the admission of expert scientific evidence that is now apparent in jurisdictions in which *Daubert* (rather than *Frye*) is now applicable, the role of scientific reasoning in FMHA is more explicit. Both *Daubert* and the *Federal Rules of Evidence* cite the importance of reasoning, as well as data, in constituting scientific evidence.

There is relatively little available research on how scientific reasoning is used in FMHA. One study has addressed how it is *valued* by those involved in forensic practice; the great majority of psychiatrists and psychologists who were surveyed in this study rated elements of reasoning in FMHA as either essential or recommended.

There have been several attempts by those writing in the area of FMHA standard of practice to describe how scientific reasoning *should* be applied in forensic assessment. These descriptions have focused on hypothesis testing, the applicability of validated procedures to the individual case, and the interpretation of results.

This principle appears *established*. However, a better explanation of how reasoning might be used in FMHA should be developed. Empirical study of how reasoning is used, and how it is valued, are also needed.

Making Assertions and Clarifying Limits

When relevant data are collected in a thorough manner and weighed through the input of multiple sources, this provides important information on the forensic issues being evaluated. However, various considerations can affect the strength of the assertions that are made in a given case. One consideration is the absence of data in the specific case. A second limitation can result from the unavailability of empirical research relevant to the tools or other important steps used in the assessment. Yet a third limitation is imposed by the structure and procedures of the law under which the FMHA is performed. In particular, the question of how the "ultimate legal issue"—in the terms of this book, the legal question that the court must answer—is to be addressed by the evaluating clinician has been discussed and debated by a number in the field for years (Bonnie & Slobogin, 1980; Grisso, 1986a; Melton et al., 1997; Morse, 1978a,b, 1982b; Poythress, 1982; Rogers & Ewing, 1989; Slobogin, 1989). In this chapter, the ultimate legal question will be discussed in the context of this debate and its implications for communicating FMHA results. This chapter will also discuss two other principles involving making assertions and describing limits in the course of FMHA communication.

DO NOT ANSWER THE ULTIMATE LEGAL QUESTION DIRECTLY

This principle describes the importance of refraining from answering the legal question directly, and focusing on the description of capacities that are part of the "forensic issues" included within, and relevant to, the legal question. The debate about whether the forensic clinician should directly answer the ultimate legal question has encompassed a number of positions. As part of his larger analysis of the relationship between mental health law and FMHA, Morse (1978a,b, 1982a,b) has argued that any attempt to answer the ultimate legal issue directly will inevitably confound relevant clinical and scientific evidence with values that are political, moral, and societal. However, in a practical sense, the attempt to limit one's communication in a report or testimony by avoiding a direct conclusion regarding the ultimate legal issue may result in the entire evaluation being excluded in some jurisdictions, or the weight of the evidence considerably reduced. A vivid example of some of the problems that can result in a hearing or trial when the expert attempts to limit her communication in an unexpected way has been described by Poythress (1982), who once attempted to define "reasonable medical/psychological certainty" for the court and encountered surprise and confusion, with the court eventually going onto a separate record outside the presence of the jury. Clearly, the attempt to describe cautions or limit one's communication can encounter significant practical problems. Others (e.g., Rogers & Ewing, 1989) have argued that the issue is less important than some have described it in the debate, that any ban on addressing the ultimate issue is not presently supported by empirical evidence, and that such evidence should be obtained if the debate is to be settled properly.

Communication relevant to the ultimate legal issue will be analyzed in light of the literature in this area. In this analysis, the balance between asserting findings and describing the limits of those findings will be considered throughout.

ETHICS

The *Ethical Principles of Psychologists and Code of Conduct* (APA, 1992) provides no explicit guidance on the issue of addressing the ultimate legal issue as part of FMHA. The *Specialty Guidelines for Forensic Psychologists* (1991) alludes to this issue by contrasting mental health and scientific material with legal facts, opinions, and conclusions. In providing this explanation, the *Guidelines* makes it clear that the forensic clinician should be prepared to explain the distinction between the two areas:

> Forensic psychologists are aware that their essential role as expert to the court is to assist the trier of fact to understand the evidence or to determine a fact in issue. In offering expert evidence, they are aware that their own professional observations, inferences, and conclusions must be distinguished from legal facts, opinions, and conclusions. Forensic psychologists are prepared to explain the relationship between their expert testimony and the legal issues and facts of an instant case. (p. 665)

Neither the *Principles of Medical Ethics with Annotations Especially Applicable to Psychiatry* (APA, 1998) nor the *Ethical Guidelines for the Practice of Forensic Psychiatry* (AAPL, 1995) addresses this principle.

LAW

Under common law, evaluators were generally barred from giving conclusions about the ultimate legal question because it invaded the legal decision-making province of the judge or jury (Melton et al., 1997). Analyzing this justification further, it is useful to consider that a decision on an ultimate legal question is affected by relevant statutory and evidentiary standards, established legal precedent, and the moral and "community standards" values brought to the interpretation of these standards by the decision-maker. In contrast, the findings on a relevant forensic issue should be affected primarily by the results of scientifically supported clinical procedures.

This is related to another legal principle. It is well established that it is for the judge, not for witnesses, to instruct the jury regarding applicable principles of law (*Marx & Co. v. Diners' Club, Inc.*, 1977; *United States v. Newman*, 1995). A number of circuit courts have held that the *Federal Rules of Evidence* prohibits testimony in which a witness provides such instruction or interpretation. One such example is *Burkhart v. Washington Metro. Area Transit Auth.*, (D.C.Cir. 1997), in which the court found reversible error in allowing an expert in police practices to offer an opinion on whether police officers' efforts in communicating with a deaf plaintiff were enough to satisfy federal disability statutes. In a Sixth Circuit case (*Berry v. City of Detroit*, 1994), the court held inadmissible the testimony of an expert in police practices with respect to defining the legal term *deliberate indifference* in a civil rights case. This inadmissibility of testimony can be seen even in cases in which the witness's expertise would arguably include matters of law. In one such case in the Tenth Circuit, it was deemed reversible error to allow an expert witness who was an attorney to give his opinion on the requirements for effective consent to a search (*Specht v. Jensen*, 1988). In a Second Circuit case, the court held that a securities lawyer called as an expert could not testify to the legal obligations created under a contract (*Marx & Co. v. Diners' Club, Inc.*, 1977).

Currently under the *Federal Rules of Evidence*, there are two parts to the language relevant to ultimate issue opinions. Under F.R.E. 704 (a):

> Except as provided in subdivision (b), testimony in the form of an opinion or inference otherwise admissible is not objectionable because it embraces an ultimate issue to be decided by the trier of fact.

However, under F.R.E. 704(b):

> No expert witness testifying with respect to the mental state or condition of a defendant in a criminal case may state an opinion or inference as to whether the defendant did or did not have the mental state or condition constituting an element of the crime charged or of a defense thereto. Such ultimate issues are matters for the trier of fact alone.

Ultimate issue testimony is thus explicitly barred in mental state at the time of offense evaluations in the federal jurisdiction, and in state jurisdictions that have adopted the equivalent of F.R.E. 704(b). It is not *per se* inadmissible in criminal cases involving other kinds of legal questions. However, one court has cautioned that the abolition of the "bar on 'ultimate issue' opinions ... is not a carte blanche for experts" (*Dinco v. Dylex, Ltd.*, 1997, p. 973), reasoning that an expert's conclusion about the ultimate legal issue, even when offered, should be viewed in light of the rule against expert opinion on questions of law. Under such reasoning, it should be made clear by both the expert and the judge that such an opinion may be advisory to the jury, but should not substitute for the jury's consideration of questions of law within the instructions provided by the court.

Other courts have gone further in reasoning about certain disadvantages of ultimate issue testimony. When a deaf bus passenger sued the city transit authority for alleged violations of the Americans with Disabilities Act (ADA) and the Rehabilitation Act of 1973, the district court allowed an expert witness to give ultimate opinions regarding whether the transit authority had violated these statutes. These opinions concerned whether the means of communication employed by a transit officer with the passenger were as effective as the means of communication with others, whether the ADA required the transit authority to grant a passenger's request for a translator, and whether the transit authority was proficient in the requirements of the ADA and the Rehabilitation Act. The appellate court held that the admission of such testimony was in error, reasoning that testimony that consists of legal conclusions cannot properly assist the trier of fact in either understanding the evidence or determining the fact in issue, and therefore is not "otherwise admissible" (*Burkhart v. Washington Metro. Area Transit Auth.*, 1997).

Another case providing a good example of how ultimate opinion testimony under some circumstances (but perhaps not others) is problematic involved the expert's use of the term *deliberately indifferent* to describe conduct of defendant prison officials in a 1983 suit arising from the murder of an inmate (*Woods v. Lecureux*, 1997). Such testimony, which was excluded at the trial court level, would not have been helpful because of its apparently conclusory nature—the expert was not providing the fact finder with a full description of the data and reasoning which led to the conclusions that there had been "deliberate indifference." The court also commented that the use of a term such as *deliberate indifference* that has a very specific legal meaning may result in the exclusion of the opinion. In this case, since the expert apparently failed to fully describe the basis for the opinion, it would have been difficult to determine whether the meaning of *deliberate indifference* as used by the expert was comparable to that within the law.

EMPIRICAL

Relatively little empirical information is available on the frequency with which ultimate opinions are expressed, either in reports or in testimony, or the forms in which opinions are expressed and the impact of different kinds of communication. Each of these issues merits study, a point made strongly by Rogers and Ewing (1989), in order to better gauge the importance of the way in which opinions are presented as part of FMHA. In this section, the limited empirical data that *are* available will be reviewed.

A study described but not published (Poythress, 1981, cited in Melton et al., 1997) provides some evidence about the attitudes of Michigan judges regarding various relevant communications that could be provided in testimony or a report as part of FMHA. Although the study was done almost 20 years ago and had a fairly small number of judges responding (N = 30), it does offer an example of how such investigation might be pursued. In this study, the judges surveyed were asked to rank-order various aspects of testimony in terms of probative value using a nine-point scale, with 7–9 reflecting "essential," 4–6 "desirable," and 1–3 "undesirable." In order of ranking, the aspects of testimony were as follows: (1) *descriptive testimony* (median rating: 7.83), (2) *ultimate legal issue* (7.60), (3) *interpreting the legal standard for mental disorder* (6.83), (4) *theoretical accounts or explanations for legally relevant behavior* (6.00), (5) *diagnosis* (5.83), (6) *weighing of different motives or explanations for legally relevant behavior* (5.50), (7) *statistical/actuarial data on diagnosis or clinical observations* (5.25), and (8) *statistical/actuarial data on the relationship between clinical and legally relevant behavior* (3.20). When researchers rated each of the items on the extent to which they "stayed close to data" (which was rated in the direction of being more appropriate) versus addressed broader, legal considerations (less appropriate), the correlation between judges' rankings and the appropriateness values was −.55. This suggested that, for the most part, the judges viewed as probative and valuable testimony that directly addressed legal elements, including ultimate legal issues.

Two studies conducted by Rogers and colleagues (Rogers, Bagby, Crouch, & Cutler, 1990; Rogers, Bagby, & Chow, 1992) considered the impact of having the ultimate legal question answered directly. In the first (Rogers et al., 1990), the investigators examined the influence of "ultimate opinions" in the context of an abbreviated transcript of a trial in which an insanity defense was asserted. Subjects were 274 adults (18+ years old) who read a transcript that included direct and cross-examination of a psychiatrist's testimony both when an ultimate legal opinion was delivered and when such an opinion was not given. There were no significant differences in subjects' ratings of outcome (voting for a verdict of not guilty by reason of insanity versus a verdict of guilty) between these two conditions, suggesting minimal impact of answering the ultimate legal question. In the second study (Rogers et al., 1992), a total of 460 undergraduates and adults received a packet of materials that included an abbreviated transcript, a judge's instructions, and a rating form. While subjects appeared to be influenced in their vote for an insanity acquittal versus a guilty verdict by the defendant's account ("crazy" versus "argument") and the expert testimony ("psychotic" versus "alcoholic"), their verdicts were not affected by whether an ultimate opinion was given. In neither of these studies, therefore, did an expert's rendering of an ultimate legal opinion make a significant difference in subjects' verdicts.

The limited available normative evidence suggests that the ultimate legal question is frequently answered directly in forensic practice, however. In a study of FMHA reports on the issues of trial competence and sanity at the time of the offense performed by hospital and community evaluators in Florida, Heilbrun and Collins (1995) reported that the ultimate legal question was answered directly in virtually all reports on trial competence (95% of community evaluations and 99% of hospital evaluations). In reports on the issue of sanity (which were all done in the community; this study could not sample from hospital FMHA reports on sanity, since they were rarely done in this hospital), the ultimate legal question was answered directly in 47% of reports. Excluding reports in which the evaluator declined to reach a conclusion due to insufficient information, the proportion of reports addressing the sanity issue directly increased to 66%.

In another survey (Borum & Grisso, 1996) of forensic psychologists and forensic psychiatrists on CST ($N = 102$) and CR ($N = 96$), a majority of respondents indicated that it was either "essential" or "recommended" to include an ultimate issue opinion as part of an evaluation on these issues. Some differences were observed on ratings of CST and CR. On the issue of CST, a total of 78% of psychiatrists and 74% of psychologists rated the ultimate issue conclusion as either essential or recommended. For CR, by comparison, a total of 71% of psychiatrists and 56% of psychologists indicated that the ultimate issue opinion was essential or recommended. One conclusion to be drawn from the findings of these two studies (Borum & Grisso, 1996; Heilbrun & Collins, 1995) is that ultimate issue conclusions on FMHAs involving CST or sanity are both valued (rated as essential or recommended) and given (at the conclusion of reports) by a majority of forensic clinicians. This must be tempered with the observation that a very limited amount of research is available on the normative aspects of FMHA, and that these two studies may not generalize well to other legal issues or to the larger domain from which they sample.

STANDARD OF PRACTICE

There are a number of ways in which FMHA conclusions can be communicated. Seven levels, ranging from the least to the most direct in terms of addressing the ultimate legal issue, have been described (Melton et al., 1997): (1) *the application of meaning (perception) to a behavioral image* (e.g., "he was wringing his hands"), (2) *perception of general mental state* (e.g., "he appeared anxious"), (3) *"formulation" of the perception of general mental state to fit into theoretical constructs or the research literature and/or to synthesize observations* (e.g., "his anxiety during the interview was consistent with a general obsession with pleasing others"), (4) *diagnosis* (e.g., "his behavior during the interview and his reported history are consistent with a generalized anxiety disorder"), (5) *relationship of formulation or diagnosis to legally relevant behavior* (e.g., "at the time of the offense, his anxiety was so overwhelming that he failed to consider the consequences of his behavior"), (6) *elements of the ultimate legal issue* (e.g., "although he was too anxious at the time of the offense to *reflect* on the consequences of his behavior, he *knew* the nature and consequences of his acts and *knew* that what he did was wrong"), and (7) *ultimate legal issue* (e.g., "he was sane at the time of the offense"). They recommend that mental health professionals ordinarily should refrain from giving opinions as to ultimate legal issues, but also present a framework that allows consideration of how close the forensic clinician wants to come in linking the findings of FMHA with the ultimate issue (Melton et al., 1997, p. 17).

There is an elaboration on the fifth or sixth of these levels that could be made, involving a description of the relationship between constructs that are relevant to the ultimate legal issue but do not define it. For example, one of the competence assessment tools developed by the MacArthur Research Network on Mental Health and Law measures capacities relevant to competence to consent to treatment (Appelbaum & Grisso, 1995; Grisso et al., 1995). Using this tool (the MacCAT-T) allows the evaluator to draw on empirical research in contextualizing an individual's capacities applicable to decision-making that is "knowing" (having, retaining, and communicating relevant information) and "intelligent" (reasoning about the costs and benefits of various alternatives). The evaluator can both compare such capacities with those demonstrated by others in similar diagnostic categories, and apply the level of demonstrated capacities to the demands of the present circumstances. Either of these conclusions would be at the fifth or sixth level, but would not address the ultimate issue ("is the person competent to consent to treatment?") or the penultimate issues ("are the capacities for knowing and intelligent reasoning sufficient to allow the individual to be considered competent to consent to treatment?"). Much of the most recent research and forensic instrument development is focused on the description and measurement of relevant capacities, but avoids classification in ultimate issue terms.

Again considering the survey conducted by Borum and Grisso (1996) of board-certified forensic psychologists and forensic psychiatrists on CST ($N = 102$) and CR ($N = 96$), it is helpful to focus on these results as an indicator of standard of practice as rated by highly specialized forensic clinicians. The majority of these respondents rated it either "essential" or "recommended" to include an ultimate issue opinion as part of an evaluation on CST or CR, although a higher percentage of respondents rated such a conclusion as "essential" or "recommended" for CST (78% of psychiatrists and 74% of psychologists) than for CR (71% of psychiatrists and 56% of psychologists).

The *Criminal Justice Mental Health Standards* (ABA, 1989) describes the contents of written reports of mental evaluations relevant to ultimate issue communication as follows: "The evaluator should express an opinion on a specific legal criterion or standard only if the opinion is within the scope of the evaluator's specialized knowledge" (p. 109). On the admissibility of expert testimony concerning a person's mental condition or behavior:

> Expert testimony, in the form of an opinion or otherwise, concerning a person's present mental competency or mental condition at some time in the past should be admissible whenever the testimony is based on and is within the specialized knowledge of the witness and will assist the trier of fact. However, the expert witness should not express, or be permitted to express, an opinion on any question requiring a conclusion of law or a moral or social value judgment properly reserved to the court or the jury. (p. 117)

This apparent inconsistency is interesting. If the *Standards* suggests, as it seems to, that ultimate issue communication is more objectionable in oral testimony than in a written testimonial form such as an FMHA report, it may be because the consumers of reports are judges and attorneys, while jurors, less legally knowledgeable than judges, are responsible for the decision in jury trials. Are judges better able than juries to disregard any

problems created by ultimate issue testimony? Is such bias better controlled in report form than in testimony? Certainly the report is the format
that better allows the forensic clinician to describe the findings and reasoning relevant to any opinions in all necessary detail, while testimony (even
direct testimony) may be a briefer and less effective means of conveying a
large amount of information. The questions of whether judges are less
influenced by ultimate issue testimony than juries, and whether reports
that address the ultimate issue are less compromising than testimony that
does so, are interesting questions for which we have no empirical answers.
Hopefully, evidence from empirical research will be forthcoming on these
questions in the coming years.

Rogers and Ewing (1989) present one of the strongest arguments
favoring answering the ultimate legal question directly. They examine the
criticisms of ultimate issue testimony and argue that attempts to eliminate
such testimony will not achieve their goals, but will instead obscure substantive issues inherent in insanity evaluations. They note that the proscription of ultimate issue opinions in the context of criminal mental state
evaluations is an attempt to remedy several interrelated problems: (1) professional taint in highly publicized cases, (2) expert opinions rendered
without sufficient clinical data, (3) undue influence of expert opinions on
the trier of fact, and (4) mental health experts' lack of expertise in moral
and legal issues. Calling the proscription of ultimate issue testimony a
"cosmetic fix," they suggest that it will have a limited effect on these four
areas. "Professional taint" will arguably occur when mental health professionals disagree in highly publicized cases, regardless of whether they
express an ultimate opinion. "Insufficient clinical data," a problem exacerbated when an ultimate opinion is expressed, may not be as common as
some criticisms would suggest (Petrella & Poythress, 1983; Poythress, 1982;
although cf. Heilbrun & Collins, 1995, and Heilbrun et al., 1994, for more
recent empirical data on this issue).[1] "Undue influence," it is argued, is not
actually undue; juries are "mildly interested" in mental health expert
testimony, but neither judges nor juries are invariably swayed by it. The
lack of "legal and moral" expertise is recast by asking whether the distinction between "right" and "wrong" refers to a moral dichotomy (regarding
which mental health professionals have no more expertise than lay witnesses) or to criminal behavior (implicitly "bad" and by definition "wrong"),

---

[1] If this criticism were phrased "insufficient clinical data that are relevant and reliable,"
combining several of Grisso's (1986a) frequently applied criticisms of forensic assessment,
then it probably continues to apply to FMHA as it is currently practiced. The limited
availability of normative data means this cannot be addressed empirically. My anecdotal
observations and informal communications with judges, attorneys, and forensic clinicians,
however, suggest that this area remains problematic.

which is simpler and falls more easily within the domain of the psychole-gal question.[2] They conclude by suggesting that the expression of ultimate insanity opinions are an "inevitable outcome" of FMHA, and no meaning-ful distinction can be made between ultimate opinions and ordinary expert opinions. Further, the more pressing problems for FMHA (professional bias, knowledge of legal standards, and the valid measurement of psycho-legal constructs) are those that should receive the empirical research atten-tion of the field.

The nature of the legal proceedings in which the results of the FMHA are presented is important, according to another analysis. Slobogin (1989) distinguishes between ultimate issue testimony (e.g., "she is committa-ble") and penultimate issue language (e.g., "she presents a danger to herself as a result of grave disability, although she does not present a danger to others, nor does she present a danger to herself through sui-cide"). He also considers legal context. Two of the important arguments against ultimate issue testimony—that forensic clinicians are not moral experts and that there may be "undue influence" over the decision-maker—are more likely to apply in proceedings that are less formal (such as civil commitment) than those such as insanity, considered as part of a trial and characterized by adversarial proceedings, evidentiary formality, and possibly opposing experts. Slobogin argues strongly against answer-ing the ultimate legal question directly in less formal legal proceedings. Although the "harm" may be minimized in more formal proceedings, Slobogin cautions (although less strongly) against ultimate issue testi-mony in these contexts as well.

The *Guidelines for Child Custody Evaluations in Divorce Proceedings* (APA, 1994) summarizes the issue as follows:

> Recommendations, if any, are based on what is in the best psychological interests of the child. Although the profession has not reached consensus about whether psychologists ought to make recommendations about the final cus-tody determination to the courts, psychologists are obligated to be aware of the arguments on both sides of this issue and to be able to explain the logic of their position concerning their own practice.
>
> If the psychologist does choose to make custody recommendations, these recommendations should be derived from sound psychological data and must be based on the best interests of the child in the particular case. Recommenda-tions are based on articulated assumptions, data, interpretations, and infer-ences based upon professional and scientific standards. Psychologists guard against relying on their own biases or unsupported beliefs in rendering opin-ions in particular cases. (p. 679)

---

[2]Rogers and Ewing argue that the legal question of insanity is conceptually closer to the included forensic issues than others have suggested.

Here, the *Guidelines* refers to one of the most troublesome aspects of ultimate issue communication: the potential that such communication will incorporate material other than "sound psychological data" and be based on considerations other than "the best interests of the child." When psychologists offer an opinion on child custody, or other ultimate legal questions in other kinds of FMHA, the challenge is to respect this dictum—to avoid incorporating nonclinical and nonscientific considerations—into the opinion.

Can this realistically be done? Some of the most compelling arguments against answering the ultimate legal question directly were originally provided by Morse (1978a,b), who clearly delineated the areas of expertise that mental health professionals could provide to the courts from those that were entirely beyond the scope of clinical and scientific expertise. There is some disagreement regarding where Morse draws this line. His conclusion that forensic clinicians should limit their evaluation and testimony to relevant areas of observed behavior, and avoid diagnoses, inferences, and "informed speculation" (1982a; cf. Bonnie & Slobogin, 1980) may be somewhat conservative, particularly when there are relevant, validated measures of forensic capacities that are available. However, there is much less disagreement that Morse identified a crucial distinction between the expertise needed to draw a conclusion about a legal question (with considerations reflecting political, moral, and community values) and that needed to describe relevant clinical symptoms and legal abilities. His caution that the former kind of expertise is neither possessed by the forensic clinician nor a part of the expert's role has had an important influence on the debate about the ultimate legal question.

One of the basic criticisms that has historically been applied to FMHA is "intrusion" (Grisso, 1986a). His discussion of this issue concerns both the quality of the expert's scientific evidence (something also discussed at length by Morse, 1978a,b) and the "fact-value" distinction between science and morality (see Stone, 1984). Science or clinical expertise may tell us "what is," but cannot tell us "what ought to be." Values are inevitably a part of the ultimate legal decision, and in some cases a very significant part. Grisso has subsequently summarized his position on this issue, based on considering the question over 25 years, and reduced it to five points:

1. The ultimate legal question (e.g., is the person competent or incompetent to stand trial) really means this: Does the person have enough ability (of the *Dusky* type) to put him or her to trial?
2. Answering that question requires deciding how much ability is enough to meet the legal standard.
3. How much ability is legally enough? However much it takes to be

able to say, "Putting this person to trial would be *fair*." There is no
other meaningful way to decide how much is legally enough.
4. Therefore, testifying to the ultimate legal question requires that one
   stand in judgment of what is fair and just.
5. Clinicians have no special expertise with which to interpret what is
   just or fair. (Grisso, personal communication, September 1998)

Melton et al. (1997) recommend that forensic clinicians resist answering the ultimate legal question. This recommendation is made with full
awareness that there can be many pressures toward answering the ultimate legal question: (1) legal professionals may view this as one of the most
important aspects of the expert's report or testimony, (2) legal or policy
requirements may dictate that the question be answered, with the possibility that the entire evaluation could be excluded if it is not, (3) economic
incentives may be present, such that forensic clinicians who avoid such
testimony may lose business to others who do not, (4) the dynamics of the
courtroom may make it difficult to avoid answering an important question, and (5) clinicians may believe there is no ethical or legal prohibition
against answering the ultimate legal question. These considerations not-
withstanding, Melton et al. argue that it is sufficiently important to avoid
this practice that they recommend strongly against it and offer strategies
for resisting answering various aspects of the ultimate legal question (1997,
pp. 543–545).

Discussion

The controversy about the role of the ultimate legal opinion on FMHA
has been active for over 20 years. This is reflected in a somewhat uneven
literature on the area. There is no direct reference to ultimate issue opinions among the sources of ethics authority reviewed, for example. In
contrast, there is relevant information in each of the areas of legal, empirical, and standard of practice areas on this topic. While the expression of an
ultimate legal issue was barred under common law, there is currently some
inconsistency among sources of legal authority on this issue. It remains
established legal principle that no witness should instruct the jury in
applicable principles of law; moreover, no opinion on any point should be
given unless within the expert's area of "specialization." However, the
Federal Rules of Evidence currently does not bar testimony containing an
ultimate issue opinion, except on the question of a defendant's mental
state at the time of the offense.
     There is limited empirical research available on ultimate issue opin-
ions in FMHA. However, the few studies that have been done support the
observation that legal and forensic practitioners are inclined to favor the

inclusion of ultimate issue opinions in reports and testimony; these studies included the preferences of judges, the values of experienced forensic psychiatrists and psychologists, and the reports of psychologists and psychiatrists. This evidence was confined to criminal issues, particularly CST and CR, so it is unclear whether the same preference would be shown as part of juvenile and civil litigation.

Several useful contributions to the standard of practice literature allow this discussion to be framed with greater attention to the intricacies of this debate. Ultimate opinions may be viewed as the highest level of directness (and perhaps intrusiveness) in relation to the legal question, but there are a number of other levels that range from only relevant observations of behavior up to the addressing of "penultimate" issues. The practice of addressing the latter, which may include relevant constructs that have more meaning for the behavioral and medical sciences, may be paralleling the research trend toward investigating such constructs in different populations and developing and validating tools to measure the constructs. The context in which an "ultimate opinion" is expressed may be useful to consider—when there are more procedural protections in place, such an opinion may be less objectionable—but it has also been argued that the improvement of FMHAs is more likely to result from the focus on other empirical and theoretical needs than from banning or voluntarily refraining from giving an ultimate opinion.

My own attempt to resolve this debate focuses first on the other principles that have been discussed in this book. To the extent that a forensic clinician performs an FMHA that is reasonably consistent with these other principles, the resulting report and testimony will provide a description of the data, reasoning, and conclusions about the individual's relevant capacities. Whether the conclusion is then expressed in penultimate or ultimate issue language, the entire effort will not simply provide the decision-maker with a conclusion that is unsupported by the available information. There are also ways in which to limit the intrusiveness of ultimate issue conclusions. If such an opinion is given in a report, it may be accompanied by cautionary language indicating that it is recognized that the responsibility for legal decision-making lies with the court, that the opinion should be regarded as "advisory only," that it is a clinical opinion relevant to a legal question, or other such indications that the forensic clinician recognizes and respects the decision-making role of the court and the jury. Similar caveats can be offered in testimony, and the connection can be immediately drawn between the opinion and its basis. When this is done, some of the potential harms of an ultimate issue opinion are reduced, while the report or testimony may be complying with an expectation, or even a requirement, of the court.

However, the preferable (although not easier) alternative is to avoid answering the ultimate legal question altogether. When the forensic clinician sets this as a goal, then some of the more practical justifications in favor of ultimate issue communication can be managed more easily. Focusing on facts, and limiting the role of values in FMHA, is the important larger goal that is served by this option.

This controversy does not appear to be settled. Consequently, this principle will be classified as *emerging*. In some respects, this seems odd. The question has been vigorously debated in the field for over two decades, and many of the basic arguments remain the same. There are two changes that may occur in FMHA, however, that could result in this principle being reconsidered as "established" some time in the future. First, empirical research addressing the extent to which decision-makers see this as an essential part of FMHA, as well as controlled research on the impact of decision-making when ultimate issue opinions are and are not provided, would be helpful. Second, if the current trend in the direction of empirically investigating relevant forensic issues, and using such research to provide the basis for the description of such capacities (but not the larger legal question) continues, then the FMHA field and its legal consumers may eventually come to expect that facts, but not values, will form the overwhelming basis for FMHA.

DESCRIBE FINDINGS AND LIMITS SO THAT THEY NEED CHANGE LITTLE UNDER CROSS-EXAMINATION

This is a principle taken from the maxims for expert testimony offered by Brodsky (1991). It is so important to the process of FMHA that it will be discussed in a full principle. Particularly when the forensic clinician is performing an evaluation that may result in a report and testimony (as contrasted with consultation), it is important to consider how the limits of the results will be described. There are a number of ways in which limitations on FMHA findings can be considered. Both data and reasoning can be discussed in a way that not only conveys their support for the FMHA conclusion(s), but also conveys their weaknesses. For example, there may be inconsistency in the evaluator's observations, or between observations, testing, and third-party information. Some testing tools, even when reliable and valid for the purpose toward which they are applied, yield results that must be considered cautiously because of varied other considerations, such as response style, reading problems, fluctuating attention and concentration, and the like. Reasoning through to conclusions may be fully and consistently supported by findings on all points, but this is unlikely; when reasoning is somewhat speculative or not parsimonious, this can be brought out. There are sometimes reasonable alternative explanations or conclusions that would be possible within the context of a single case; this information is important as well.

Another principle that appears as a maxim in Brodsky's (1991) book on expert testimony involves indicating some version of "I don't know" under some circumstances. This also will be discussed in the present section, with the justification that the forensic clinician "not knowing" something is a logical extension of the need to clarify the limits of knowledge in an evaluation or testimony. In the present context, its meaning is broader than for use in testimony (the context in which it is discussed by Brodsky). It does not refer to the use of "I don't know" in testimony to avoid larger issues in cross-examination that are of marginal relevance to the present case or even the underlying science (e.g., "what causes schizophrenia?"). Instead, the present discussion will focus on instances in which questions about relevant forensic issues do not, after the evaluation is completed, have clear or consistently supported answers. In addition to the reasons of inconsistent information and at least two plausible competing hypotheses, described earlier in this section, there is a third possible reason why a forensic clinician might conclude "I don't know" as part of FMHA: limited information.[3] Such circumstances will be distinguished from times in which relevant information is available, but is not included in the evaluation for other reasons.[4]

The question of *how* limitations on findings should be conveyed will

[3]A distinction should be drawn between cases in which relevant additional information is available but not collected, and cases in which such information is not available in response to reasonable or even intensive effort. Forensic clinicians can sometimes become involved in cases in which the needed effort to collect the appropriate information is much greater than it initially appeared; because of limited time, no expectation of additional compensation, pressure to complete the evaluation within a certain period, and the like, they may become tempted to speculate beyond what their available data can support rather than collect the additional information. An example of this may be seen in the following reasoning about mental state at the time of the offense: "The defendant is actively psychotic at present. Within the limits of medical probability, his condition was similar at the time of the alleged offense three months ago and, as a result, his delusions interfered with his ability to conform his conduct to the requirements of the law." With the information actually available to that forensic clinician, it would have been far more accurate to acknowledge that he did not know about the defendant's mental state at the time of the offense. Collection of relevant reconstructive information would have allowed an analysis of past mental state without the unsupported speculation, eliminating the need for "I don't know."
[4]Such reasons might include the status of third-party information as uncorroborated hearsay (despite reasonable attempts to corroborate it), or the attempt to ensure that the information provided in the evaluation would not create a "fruit of the poisonous tree" problem by inappropriately influencing the gathering of evidence at the guilt phase of the case, or in another criminal case.

also be discussed in this section. To the extent that limitations are applicable, their description will have implications for the consumers of FMHA.

ETHICS

The *Ethical Principles of Psychologists and Code of Conduct* (APA, 1992) provides the following commentary about assessment, particularly with special populations (often relevant to FMHA, as the individual being assessed frequently is a member of a "special population" as a result of being assessed for legal decision-making purposes rather than treatment purposes):

> Psychologists recognize limits to the certainty with which diagnoses, judgments, or predictions can be made about individuals. Psychologists attempt to identify situations in which particular interventions or assessment techniques or norms may not be applicable or may require adjustment in administration or interpretation because of factors such as individuals' gender, age, race, ethnicity, national origin, religion, sexual orientation, disability, language, or socioeconomic status. (p. 1603)

When the results of such assessments are being interpreted, and such interpretations are communicated to others, additional steps are to be considered regarding accuracy and its limitations:

> When interpreting assessment results, including automated interpretations, psychologists take into account the various test factors and characteristics of the person being assessed that might affect psychologists' judgments or reduce the accuracy of their interpretations. They indicate any significant reservations they have about the accuracy or limitations of their interpretations. (p. 1603)

Next, the *Ethics Code* addresses the circumstance, which can occur in the forensic context, when a personal examination cannot be conducted:

> When, despite reasonable efforts, such an examination is not feasible, psychologists clarify the impact of their limited information on the reliability and validity of their reports and testimony, and they appropriately limit the nature and extent of their conclusions or recommendations. (p. 1610)

Finally, the importance of truthfulness and candor, when necessary to avoid misleading, is explicitly noted:

> Whenever necessary to avoid misleading, psychologists acknowledge the limits of their data or conclusions. (p. 1610)

In the *Specialty Guidelines for Forensic Psychologists* (1991), there are a number of observations about the importance of clarifying limits. First is the need to test "plausible rival hypotheses":

> As an expert conducting an evaluation, treatment, consultation, or scholarly/empirical investigation, the forensic psychologist maintains professional integ-

rity by examining the issue at hand from all reasonable perspectives, actively seeking information that will differentially test plausible rival hypotheses. (p. 661)

Some particular kinds of information that may play an important part in FMHA—third-party information that would be hearsay—are particularly important to corroborate. When they cannot be corroborated, but are still used, it may be particularly important to indicate the "uncorroborated" status of such information:

> While many forms of data used by forensic psychologists are hearsay, forensic psychologists attempt to corroborate critical data that form the basis for their professional product. When using hearsay data that have not been corroborated, but are nevertheless utilized, forensic psychologists have an affirmative responsibility to acknowledge the uncorroborated status of those data and the reasons for relying upon such data. (p. 662)

Another form of third-party information often used in FMHA is mental health information, in the form of notes, reports, depositions, and interviews, that has been gathered by other mental health professionals. It is important to have general knowledge of the standard of practice of such professions, in order to determine whether the information was gathered in a standard manner. If it was not, then there must be appropriate observation about the possible limitation on accuracy that may result:

> When a forensic psychologist relies upon data or information gathered by others, the origins of those data are clarified in any professional product. In addition, the forensic psychologist bears a special responsibility to ensure that such data, if relied upon, were gathered in a manner standard for the profession. (p. 662)

Finally, there is discussion about clarifying limitations on findings when, despite reasonable efforts, it has not been possible to examine the individual personally, or for an adequate period of time:

> Forensic psychologists avoid giving written or oral evidence about the psychological characteristics of particular individuals when they have not had an opportunity to conduct an examination of the individual adequate to the scope of the statements, opinions, or conclusions to be issued. Forensic psychologists make every reasonable effort to conduct such examinations. When it is not possible or feasible to do so, they make clear the impact of such limitations on the reliability and validity of their professional products, evidence, or testimony. (p. 663)

The *Principles of Medical Ethics with Annotations Especially Applicable to Psychiatry* (APA, 1998) has nothing that is specifically applicable to this principle. However, the *Ethical Guidelines for the Practice of Forensic Psychiatry* (AAPL, 1995) provides several relevant points. First, there is the broad emphasis on the importance of honesty and striving for objectivity:

The adversarial nature of our Anglo-American legal process presents special hazards for the practicing forensic psychiatrist. Being retained by one side in a civil or criminal matter exposes the forensic psychiatrist to the potential for unintended bias and the danger of distortion of his opinion. It is the responsibility of the forensic psychiatrist to minimize such hazards by carrying out his responsibilities in an honest manner striving to reach an objective opinion. The practicing forensic psychiatrist enhances the honesty and striving for objectivity of his work by basing his forensic reports and his forensic testimony on all the data available to him. He communicates the honesty and striving for objectivity of his work and the soundness of his clinical opinion by distinguishing, to the extent possible, between verified and unverified information as well as between clinical "facts", "inferences" and "impressions." (p. 3)

Next, there are two specific examples provided about circumstances under which the accuracy of an opinion might be limited. First is the instance in which a personal examination of the individual being evaluated has not been possible, and the importance of the report and testimony reflecting such limitation:

While there are authorities who would bar an expert opinion in regard to an individual who has not been personally examined, it is the position of the Academy that if, after earnest effort, it is not possible to conduct a personal examination, an opinion may be rendered on the basis of other information. However, under such circumstances, it is the responsibility of forensic psychiatrists to assure that the statements of their opinion and any reports of testimony based on those opinions, clearly indicate that there was no personal examination and the opinions expressed are thereby limited. (p. 3)

Second is the particular example (a child custody FMHA) of an instance in which personal contact with all relevant parties is important but not obtained, and the comparable need to describe the resulting limitations (if the opinion can even be reached):

In custody cases, honesty and striving for objectivity require that all parties be interviewed, if possible, before an opinion is rendered. When this is not possible, or if for any reason not done, this fact should be clearly indicated in the forensic psychiatrist's report and testimony. Where one parent has not been seen, even after deliberate effort, it may be inappropriate to comment on that parent's fitness as a parent. Any comments on that parent's fitness should be qualified and the data for the opinion be clearly indicated. (p. 3)

LAW

There are two ways in which descriptions of limits on FMHA data and reasoning may occur. The first arises if the expert expresses findings with a "reasonable degree of medical certainty" or a "reasonable degree of professional certainty." The second encompasses the issue of whether, under the relevant evidentiary standard, the findings are admissible. Each will be discussed in this section.

Somewhere between absolute certainty and speculation is the "reasonable medical certainty" or "reasonable professional certainty" standard. The latter has been applied to nonmedical experts in a way that is comparable to the former, indicating that "[w]hile the law does not require [the expert] to state his expert opinion with unwavering certainty, it does require him to state his expert opinion with a reasonable degree of professional certainty" (*In re TMI Litigation Consolidated Proceedings*, 1996, pp. 867–868). Without a reasonable degree of certainty being expressed, expert evidence may be excluded (see, e.g., *Rosen v. Ciba-Geigy Corporation*, 1995, in which a medical expert acknowledged in his deposition that he could not state with a reasonable degree of medical certainty that use of a nicotine patch caused the plaintiff's heart attack, or *Rutigliano v. Valley Business Forms*, 1996, in which a physician's causation testimony was not admitted when she was unable to exclude other possible explanations with a reasonable degree of medical certainty).

The legal implications for the expression of limitations on FMHA data and reasoning may be first considered either under a *Daubert* or a *Frye* analysis, according to the applicable evidentiary standard. In a *Frye* jurisdiction, the relevant question for the court would concern whether the technique was generally accepted in the field to which it belongs. As may be seen from the material presented in the Ethics and Standard of Practice sections on this principle, it seems clear that psychiatrists and psychologists are expected to clarify the limitations in accuracy regarding their conclusions for a variety of reasons. The question of whether a technique is "generally accepted" in the field involves the need for information not only about the technique itself, but the purpose and the population for which it is used. Under such reasoning, the need to clarify FMHA limits would seem supported under *Frye*.

The importance of conveying limits on FMHA findings under *Daubert* seems even more straightforward. The *Daubert* framework, casting the judge in the role as "gatekeeper" for the admissibility of scientific evidence, provides the court with different questions with which to consider the larger issue of the scientific status of potential evidence.[5] When the

[5]The considerable disagreement as to whether FMHA is "scientific," "technical," or "other specialized knowledge" under the *Federal Rules of Evidence*, which *Daubert* affirmed, continues as of this writing. Some courts have seemingly held that FMHA is not scientific, within the meaning of *Daubert* as it was originally decided, referring to "Newtonian" or "hard" science; see, e.g., *Jenson v. Eveleth Taconite Co.* (1997), *Moore v. Ashland Chemical, Inc.* (1997), and *U.S. v. Bighead* (1997). Another court has argued that *Daubert* and the *Federal Rules of Evidence* require that the court scrutinize the methods, analysis, and principles of the expert evidence, whether it is "scientific," "technical," or "other specialized knowledge" (*McKendall v. Crown Control Corp.*, 1997), and yet another has observed that the list of factors relevant under *Daubert* to assess scientific methodology, testing, peer review, and general acceptance is also relevant to technical and other specialized knowledge (*Watkins v. Telsmith, Inc.*, 1997, but cf. *U.S. v. Jones*, 1997).

court must address the question of whether the method, analysis, and principles associated with a given FMHA are admissible under *Daubert*, it seems even clearer that the limitations of the included techniques should be brought to the court's attention. This pertains only to the importance of these limitations, and not the obligation of the forensic clinician to affirmatively bring out limitations by including them in a report or testimony; no explicit legal guidance could be located on the latter point. However, it is important to note that the majority of FMHA evaluations do not result in testimony, and that the court therefore cannot rely on testimony as a vehicle for eliciting the weaknesses and limitations of most evaluations. Accordingly, the more desirable course of action would involve addressing limitations affirmatively and explicitly as part of reports as well as in testimony.

EMPIRICAL

No empirical evidence on the normative frequency or the impact of communicating limits in FMHA was located. One study describing the perceived importance of communicating certain kinds of limits is available, however. In a survey of forensic psychiatrists ($N = 43$, 95% of whom were board certified in forensic psychiatry) and forensic psychologists ($N = 53$, 74% of whom were board certified in forensic psychology), Borum and Grisso (1996) had respondents rate a number of elements of FMHA as "essential," "recommended," "optional," or "contraindicated." Two such elements that are relevant to this principle are Alternative Explanations (defined as "discussion of any reason other than mental illness that could explain deficiencies in defendant's performance during assessment of CST abilities," pp. 315–316) and Malingering ("a statement addressing the question of malingering of mental illness at the time of the evaluation, or dissimulation by defendant when providing information about mental state at the time of the alleged offense," p. 316). The Alternative Explanation element of FMHA was perceived as "essential" by 38% of psychiatrists and 51% of psychologists, while another 38% of psychiatrists and 32% of psychologists called it "recommended." The Malingering statement was also seen as quite important. A total of 37% of responding psychiatrists rated the Malingering element as "essential," with another 32% describing it as "recommended." Responding psychologists emphasized its importance even more strongly, with 50% rating the inclusion of such a statement as "essential" and another 33% describing it as "recommended."

The issues of alternative explanation for relevant legal deficits and inaccurate self-report regarding mental health symptoms are clearly two examples of influences that could be important to the nature of conclusions and consistency of supporting findings in FMHA. However, it is also apparent that this is an area with virtually no empirical research available for guidance in drawing conclusions. Important empirical questions regarding the extent to which FMHA data and reasoning are accompanied by limiting language, when presented in either reports or testimony, remain to be investigated. In addition, the question of the *impact* of communicating in the context of limiting language has apparently not been studied. Both areas are ripe for investigation.

STANDARD OF PRACTICE

It is possible to identify two distinct positions regarding the way in which FMHA results are communicated. They might be described as (1) advocacy for one's own position versus (2) a "friend of the court." An expanded version of these positions, considering both the substance and style of communication, is described by Saks (1990): (1) educator (the priority involves communicating the contents of one's field), (2) the Philosopher-Ruler (focusing on the cause, but being largely indifferent to the contents of the field), and (3) the hired gun (indifferent to both the cause and the contents of the field). As is often the case, these can be identified most readily in discussion about expert testimony, but actually apply to the communication of FMHA results in both reports and testimony.

The *Guidelines for Child Custody Evaluations in Divorce Proceedings* (APA, 1994) contains two recommendations that are relevant to this principle. First, it is observed that

> The psychologist neither overinterprets nor inappropriately interprets clinical or assessment data. The psychologist refrains from drawing conclusions not adequately supported by the data. The psychologist interprets any data from interviews or tests, as well as any questions of data reliability and validity, cautiously and conservatively, seeking convergent validity. The psychologist strives to acknowledge to the court any limitations in methods or data used. (p. 679)

Using this particular guideline, a forensic clinician performing a child custody FMHA would communicate the results in a conservative fashion that is supported by data, in a way that makes clear the limits of the methods, data, and conclusions. Second, it is also noted that

> The psychologist does not give any opinion regarding the psychological functioning of any individual who has not been personally evaluated. This guideline, however, does not preclude the psychologist from reporting what an

evaluated individual (such as the parent or child) has stated or from addressing
theoretical issues or hypothetical questions, so long as the limited basis of the
information is noted. (p. 679)

Limits on the nature of the communication regarding an individual are
addressed by this guideline. If there is any communication at all regarding
an individual not evaluated, it is recommended that such communication
is made carefully and with the limitations of the communication clearly
described.

In a discussion of "aspirations for the forensic examiner" in the
context of civil FMHA, Greenberg and Brodsky (in press) offer a number of
suggestions that are relevant to this principle. First, they argue that the
primary role of the forensic evaluator is that of expert to the court, meaning that any communication as part of FMHA should be advocacy only for
the best available scientific and case-specific knowledge. Second, they
advocate a rigorous approach to communication accuracy, including the
accurate recording of all statements made by the litigant in the course of
the FMHA and the avoidance of any selectivity, unless the quotation
would be out of context and might actually distort the nature of the
presentation. Third, they suggest avoiding obvious limitations on the
accuracy of data-gathering by using tests and measures that are standardized, reliable, and valid. Fourth, they promote the consideration of both
the strengths *and* limitations of psychological tests and other measures
used in the FMHA, including statements as to the meaning, weight, applicability, and limitations of the tests. Fifth, ambiguous test results are to be
identified as such, with consideration given to additional testing if potentially helpful in resolving the ambiguity. Sixth, they recommend that no
partial opinions or recommendations be offered until the entire evaluation
has been completed. Seventh, they promote the use of "at least a substantial paragraph" making the best reasonable argument supporting the position of the party *against* whom the recommendation is made, and then
explaining why this position is outweighed by the conclusion(s) ultimately
reached by the evaluator. Finally, they suggest that examiners present
fairly and completely all information that might assist opposing counsel to
persuade the court to act contrary to the examiner's recommendations;
this is not to preclude arguing for one's own position, but to avoid the
omission or distortion of information that may be contrary to the examiner's opinion.

How should limitations on findings be conveyed in the report and
communicated in testimony, and how are these two related? Under the
Greenberg and Brodsky aspirations (which apply as well to criminal and
juvenile FMHA as to civil FMHA, the context in which they are offered,
when discussing this principle), the forensic clinician clearly has an ongo-

ing obligation to be comprehensive, evenhanded, and accurate about both strengths and limitations throughout all stages of FMHA. While they emphasize that the "friend of the court" model is useful, their application of this model through all stages of FMHA means that the evaluator must explicitly consider such limitations prior to reaching any conclusions and certainly prior to any communication in a report or testimony. When the "friend of the court" model is applied to the entire process of FMHA, therefore, it can effectively incorporate *both* the need to describe limits on findings *and* the importance of advocating for one's own conclusions, through an inclusive process that presents all relevant information but draws conclusions (both in report and in testimony) based on well-described data and articulated reasoning.

DISCUSSION

There are several reasons why the data and reasoning associated with FMHA may be limited in their accuracy. These include the unavailability or inconsistency of relevant information, the application of testing instruments with limited reliability or validity, the response style of the individual being evaluated, the frequent circumstance in which reasoning is not fully supported by data, and the existence of reasonable alternative explanations for conclusions. The sources of authority in ethics and standard of practice, in particular, strongly emphasize the importance of describing such limitations on accuracy in FMHA.

The *Ethical Principles of Psychologists and Code of Conduct* (APA, 1992) recognize the importance of addressing "limits to certainty" in professional activities such as diagnosis, judgments, and predictions. Particular limitations may be introduced when the individual being evaluated is different with respect to gender, age, race, ethnicity, national origin, religion, sexual orientation, disability, language, or socioeconomic status than the population(s) on which the applicable tests or techniques have been standardized. Given that limitations in the accuracy and applicability of data and procedures are present, it is important for the forensic clinician to be open about them. One option is to be reactive in expressing such limitations: providing appropriate cautions about the strength of conclusions, but leaving it to the court and attorneys to uncover the specific reasons for the cautions. A more desirable option, however, is to be proactive about acknowledging both limitations and the reasons for them. This is consistent with the ethical recommendations from other ethics authority, such as the *Specialty Guidelines*.

The *Specialty Guidelines* (1991) describes more specific instances in which limitations on the accuracy of data and reasoning may arise in the forensic context. When "uncorroborated hearsay" is used as one of the sources of information, there may be both accuracy and legal implications to be considered. Whether plausible "rival hypotheses" have been tested, third-party information collected by other professionals has been gathered in a "standard" fashion for that profession, and sufficient information available when there is limited or no personal contact with an evaluee are among the issues specifically addressed by the *Specialty Guidelines* that should be brought forward affirmatively and considered as part of FMHA. The *Ethical Guidelines* (AAPL, 1992) also speaks of the importance of honesty and striving for objectivity, accomplished by distinguishing between "facts" and "inferences" and providing specific examples of instances in which the adequacy of information collected would probably be impaired by the failure to personally evaluate all necessary parties.

Both a *Frye* and a *Daubert/Federal Rules of Evidence* analysis of what the court must consider when deciding to admit FMHA evidence would support the importance of limitations on FMHA accuracy being provided to the court. There is no explicit guidance on whether it is the responsibility of the forensic clinician to affirmatively provide information about such limitations, or merely to respond truthfully when questioned about such limitations in testimony. However, since the great majority of FMHA evaluations do not result in testimony, it would follow that the court would be unable to elicit such weaknesses through testimony in most cases, making it preferable to address limitations explicitly and affirmatively in reports.

Very limited empirical evidence is available on this point, and clearly much more work is needed. The one study cited, involving the great majority of responding psychologists and psychiatrists endorsing "alternative explanation" and "malingering" elements of FMHA as either "essential" or "recommended," might be replicated with experienced forensic clinicians in a variety of jurisdictions and forensic settings. Further, data on both the normative practice and the impact of addressing limitations need to be gathered in a systematic fashion.

The available standard of practice literature seems fairly consistent on the point that limitations should be addressed, but mixed on the question of how and when. The positions of "advocate for one's opinion" versus "friend of the court" were identified, and a blended modification emerged from the discussion of more recent standard of practice literature. When the forensic clinician is in the role of "impartial expert," then he or she can serve as a "friend of the court" by clearly and affirmatively identifying limitations and weaknesses throughout the FMHA process. At the point at which the relevant information is gathered, and conclusions drawn in consideration of both the data and their limitations, however, then it is reasonable to shift to a position in which the forensic clinician is an advocate for these conclusions. While this certainly does not preclude the continuing acknowledgment of limitations, it does provide attorneys and courts with a better reasoned and more helpful final product.

Given the consistency of the ethics authorities and the standard of practice literature on this principle, it seems to be *established*. Very limited empirical evidence is available, however, so this should clearly be a priority for FMHA researchers in years to come.

V

Communication

10

Communicating Clearly

The communication of FMHA results is a crucial step in the larger forensic assessment process. Whether these results are communicated in writing or orally,[1] the perceived value and the effectiveness of the entire FMHA is affected by the way in which it is communicated. In this chapter, three principles relevant to FMHA communication will be considered. The first two—attributing information to sources and using plain language—are applicable to both written and oral communication. The third principle, involving writing the report in sections, is less directly applicable to testimony. However, to the extent that it serves an organizing function, and provides a detailed reference for the forensic clinician during expert testimony, it also has some applicability to both written and oral communication.

ATTRIBUTE INFORMATION TO SOURCES

One of the most basic questions that is associated with FMHA is "How do you know that?" Conclusions or broader reasoning that are not based on accurate factual information are likely to be flawed, and one way to diminish the credibility of opinions is to attack the "facts" on which they are based. There is, accordingly, a high value in FMHA on gathering factual information that seems more accurate because it has been verified through comparison across sources. However, this painstaking process

---

[1] Forensic clinicians should be attentive to the variety of ways in which FMHA results are communicated. Even the less formal ways of communicating (e.g., telephone calls to attorneys, summary letters) are a formal part of the process, and the approaches to effective communication discussed in this chapter may apply to them as well. However, the more formal means of communication, such as reports, depositions, and testimony, are the primary focus of the principles discussed in this chapter.

241

will be largely in vain if the source of the information is not cited, and hence is not available to the court, or attorneys, who are interested in determining the sources of various kinds of information. This is an important difference between forensic and therapeutic assessment. In the latter, it is the conclusions (diagnoses, recommendations, and the like) that are of primary interest to clinicians and clients, the consumers of such evaluations. In FMHA, however, there is an emphasis on *both* the information itself and the associated reasoning and conclusions.

ETHICS

There is nothing specifically relevant to this principle in the *Ethical Principles of Psychologists and Code of Conduct* (APA, 1992). In contrast, the *Specialty Guidelines for Forensic Psychologists* (Committee on Ethical Guidelines for Forensic Psychologists, 1991) contains several applicable sections. First, there is the emphasis on particularly detailed documentation in FMHA:

> Forensic psychologists have an obligation to document and be prepared to make available, subject to court order or the rules of evidence, all data that form the basis for their evidence or services. The standard to be applied to such documentation or recording anticipates that the detail and quality of such documentation will be subject to reasonable judicial scrutiny; this standard is higher than the normative standard for general clinical practice. (p. 661)

One example of documentation that attributes to sources involves the use of data or information gathered by others:

> When a forensic psychologist relies upon data or information gathered by others, the origins of those data are clarified in any professional product. In addition, the forensic psychologist bears a special responsibility to ensure that such data, if relied upon, were gathered in a manner standard for the profession. (p. 662)

The importance of communicating so as to facilitate the understanding of the material is also cited. In the legal context, such "understanding" is reached through the adversarial process, so it should be expected that data presented in FMHA will be scrutinized:

> Forensic psychologists make reasonable efforts to ensure that the products of their services, as well as their own public statements and professional testimony, are communicated in ways that will promote understanding and avoid deception, given the particular characteristics, roles, and abilities of various recipients of the communications. (p. 663)

Finally, the issue of attribution is addressed in the *Guidelines*:

> Forensic psychologists, by virtue of their competence and rules of discovery, actively disclose all sources of information obtained in the course of their professional services; they actively disclose which information from which

source was used in formulating a particular written product or oral testimony. (p. 665)

The *Principles of Medical Ethics with Annotations Especially Applicable to Psychiatry* (APA, 1998) has nothing that is directly relevant. The *Ethical Guidelines for the Practice of Forensic Psychiatry* (AAPL, 1995) offers the following:

> The practicing forensic psychiatrist enhances the honesty and striving for objectivity of his work by basing his forensic reports and his forensic testimony on all the data available to him. He communicates the honesty and striving for objectivity of his work and the soundness of his clinical opinion by distinguishing, to the extent possible, between verified and unverified information as well as between clinical "facts," "inferences" and "impressions." (p. 3)

This is relevant to attribution by source because the distinction between "verified" and "unverified" information cannot be made without an indication of the source(s) of the information. Presumably, "unverified" information would consist of a litigant's self-report only, while "verified" information would incorporate documentation and third-party interviews regarding that individual's relevant history and current behavior to assess (and compensate for) the possibility of inaccurate self-report. Attribution of observations to source allows the evaluator (and the reader) to weigh the credibility of information used in this verification process, and draw conclusions about the extent to which the self-report actually does appear to be "verified."

LAW

No legal authority was located relevant to this principle.

EMPIRICAL

No empirical research is apparently available relevant to this principle.

STANDARD OF PRACTICE

Considering the importance of this principle, there is surprisingly little written about it in the standard of practice literature. The relationship between the FMHA report and expert testimony has been discussed elsewhere in this book. It has been noted by others (e.g., Melton et al., 1997) that a well-written report may facilitate effective testimony, while a poorly written report may be used to discredit or embarrass the forensic clinician.

One of the reasons for the potentially variable impact of the report involves the importance of documenting source(s) of the factual information presented in this report. Often there is conflicting information in basic areas (e.g., age, mental health history), and sometimes the contradictions cannot be resolved. Assuming that the forensic clinician has made a reasonable effort to obtain multiple sources of information,[2] however, it is important to document each source and the information that it yields.

Such documentation is important for several reasons. As noted in the Ethics section earlier on this principle, there is a responsibility to provide attorneys who might challenge the FMHA findings with a reasonable basis for understanding what the forensic clinician has considered and how it has shaped the conclusions. Second, a forensic clinician without a good command of the sources of various kinds of information is not an impressive witness. It is much easier and more efficient to facilitate the recall (during testimony) of sources of factual information by attributing them (in the report) to their respective source(s). Finally, such attribution may decrease the likelihood of testimony that is needed largely to clarify what has been communicated in the report. Testimony on substantive matters is an important part of FMHA. Testimony that serves mainly to clarify what has already been communicated is wasteful and inefficient, particularly if such testimony would have been unnecessary if the report had been written more clearly.

This is reflected most clearly in continuing education programs and workshops on FMHA. Part of the training in such workshops, such as those provided in Virginia and Florida and by the American Academy of Forensic Psychology, involves attributing information to sources when writing FMHA reports; this in turn promotes FMHA testimony that is more specific about sources.

DISCUSSION

There is relatively little in the literature that is relevant to this principle. One of the few indications of its importance in forensic evaluation (although not necessarily therapeutic evaluation) is seen in the way in which ethics authorities address it. Neither of the two major ethics codes

---

[2]A serious error occurs when the forensic clinician does not obtain multiple sources of information. In such cases, there may be factual inconsistencies that the clinician has not even considered. An effective cross-examination strategy when there is information that is inconsistent with the clinician's facts, reasoning, or conclusions is to ask a series of questions in the following form: "Doctor, are you aware that _____?" When the forensic clinician is aware of such information, and has explicitly considered it in the FMHA, then the damage inflicted by such cross-examination may be minimal. However, imagine the decision-maker's reaction to testimony in which the clinician responded "no" to a number of these questions—and could offer no plausible explanation for why the information had not been considered.

for psychology and psychiatry, respectively, allude to this principle—but both forensic specialty codes for psychology and psychiatry address it. There are several broad categories of information obtained in FMHA: self-report (e.g., mental status examination, unstructured clinical interview, self-reported history, description of critical incidents), formal testing (including psychological and neuropsychological testing, structured interviews, and medical testing, for example), and third-party information (e.g., interviews with relevant individuals and review of documents; see Table 7.1 for more detail). A list of sources at the beginning of an FMHA report should include sufficient information about each source so that it is clear to the reader what the source is, where and when it was obtained, and, in some instances, the duration of the procedure (e.g., "interview with defendant Samuel Jones for 3 hours on 2-9-97 and for 2 hours on 2-18-97," "interview with Mr. Jones's mother for 45 minutes on 2-20-97"). When attribution to source occurs in the report, the reader can then obtain the necessary information about the source from its description in the beginning of the report, facilitating access to that source if needed.

With no relevant legal authority or empirical data available, and relatively little in the standard of practice literature, it is tempting to describe this principle as emerging, and to diminish its current importance for FMHA. That would be a mistake. The attribution of information to sources is one of the most important principles underlying the communication of FMHA results. These can be seen most clearly by imagining FMHA communication *without* source attribution. Relevance and reliability, two of the cornerstones of evidence law, cannot be assessed as readily without source attribution. The accuracy of factual information from various sources cannot be assessed without knowing these sources; such knowledge is important for the preparation of cross-examination and the court's decision-making. Accurate factual information provides one basis for good reasoning in FMHA, so both factual information and reasoning (as well as the conclusions drawn) may be suspect without source attribution.

This is a principle for which the FMHA literature has lagged well behind good practice. FMHA training has emphasized this principle for some time, but the field is missing needed research and descriptive literature on its meaning and implementation. Such research might address the impact of attribution by source on how the information is understood, how it is weighed, its credibility, its facilitation of access to source and preparation of direct and cross-examination, and the perceived value of this practice to FMHA reports and testimony. Consumers of FMHA such as judges and attorneys would be ideal participants in such research. It seems best to conclude that this principle is *established*, but that it also must become much better elaborated through a significant expansion of the relevant literature.

USE PLAIN LANGUAGE; AVOID TECHNICAL JARGON

Many of the consumers of FMHA are not trained as mental health professionals. Judges and attorneys, who are trained in law, may have little or no formal training in psychopathology, personality, human development, diagnosis, treatment, or research methodology. Forensic and correctional administrators, parole officers, case managers, and others who play important roles in the larger systems that evaluate, treat, and make decisions about individuals with mental disorder in the criminal justice system may have differing levels of training in these areas. Even the mental health professions such as psychiatry, psychology, social work, and psychiatric nursing are trained somewhat differently in these areas, and there are a number of different theoretical orientations within these groups that may assign different meanings to the same terms. A common language is needed.

One approach to such a "common language" involves the attempt to remove any technical terms. When such terms cannot be avoided entirely, they can be defined as clearly as possible. The process of FMHA, in broad terms, involves the attempt to build a bridge between mental health findings and legal decision-making. There is often no simple or straightforward way to translate from one to the other, and legal decisions are driven only partly by relevant behavioral scientific and clinical evidence. Accordingly, when FMHA findings are communicated accurately but without the embellishment of technical terminology, the legal decision-maker should better understand such evidence and consider it with minimal distortion.

Ethics

The *Ethics Code* (APA, 1992) indicates that

> psychologists ensure that an explanation of the results is provided using language that is reasonably understandable to the person assessed or to another legally authorized person on behalf of the client. (p. 1604)

In the legal context, the "legally authorized person on behalf of the client" is typically the attorney, who is a primary client of FMHA.

The *Specialty Guidelines for Forensic Psychologists* (Committee on Ethical Guidelines for Forensic Psychologists, 1991) addresses the style of communication as well:

> Forensic psychologists make reasonable efforts to ensure that the products of their services, as well as their own public statements and professional testimony, are communicated in ways that will promote understanding and avoid deception, given the particular characteristics, roles, and abilities of various recipients of the communications. (p. 663)

The respective "characteristics" of many consumers of FMHA, such as judges and attorneys, include training in law but not necessarily in mental health. In this context, the use of plain language should promote a better understanding of findings by the consumers.

Neither the *Principles of Medical Ethics with Annotations Especially Applicable to Psychiatry* (APA, 1998) nor the *Ethical Guidelines for the Practice of Forensic Psychiatry* (AAPL, 1995) contains anything directly relevant to this principle.

LAW

No legal authority was located relevant to this principle.

EMPIRICAL

Little empirical study has investigated the use of technical language in FMHA. One exception involves a study by Petrella and Poythress (1983) who found that experienced forensic clinicians used a number of technical terms and phrases that judges and lawyers rated as unclear; such as "delusional ideation," "affect," "neologisms," "loosening of association," "flight of ideas," "blocking," "paranoid ideation is nonspecific, completely unsystematized," "oriented to time, place, and person," "lability," "loose associations and tangentiality," "flat affect," "grandiosity," "personality deficit," "hysterical amnesia," "lack of registration amnesia," and "psychotic mentation."[3] If this study were representative of FMHA practice more broadly, it would be easy to understand the frustration of legal professionals and other FMHA consumers in attempting to determine what these terms described in language that could be understood and, for purposes of legal decision-making, applied to the relevant questions of law. It is also worth noting that such communication was made by experienced forensic clinicians, who presumably would be familiar with the importance of clear communication with legal actors and attempt to minimize unnecessary jargon to facilitate such communication. The severity of the communication problems created by the use of technical language

---

[3]The results of this unpublished study are described briefly in Melton et al. (1997). The current summary is taken from that description.

might well be increased among clinicians who are less experienced in FMHA and, hence, less familiar with this problem.

STANDARD OF PRACTICE

Several commentators have directly addressed the importance of using plain language in FMHA communication. Melton et al. (1997) observe that the recipients of FMHA reports are not mental health professionals but legal personnel and laypersons; technical jargon should therefore be minimized and explained. This observation refers to all forms of FMHA, across a range of legal questions and forensic issues. It has been made by others as well, however, who refer more specifically to juvenile evaluations (Grisso, 1998a) and civil forensic evaluations (Greenberg & Brodsky, in press). Although it is best to avoid technical terminology whenever possible, there may be times when such usage cannot be avoided. At such times, terms should be defined and concepts explained in nontechnical language. Also, the use of a Glossary of Terms, such as those appearing in Melton et al. (1997) and Grisso (1998a), can help an attorney or a judge to better understand the meaning of the technical language of the mental health professions.

Kennedy (1986) has also addressed this principle in a chapter on expert testimony. His comments clearly apply to report-writing as well as testimony. He notes that

> Too sophisticated a style of speech in the courtroom also detracts from the witness's presentation. Experience and knowledge tend to make some psychologists speak in a manner too sophisticated, too technical, too complex for the jury to understand fully. Using plain, common language is highly important; taking minute care to make sure that issues are competently but simply stated makes an enormous difference in effective communication on the stand ....
>
> Too jargony speech, on the other hand, is worse in a psychological expert ... a jargony presentation simply leaves the jury confused and hostile, because jargon implies an "inside" language contemptuous of the intelligence of the jury.... Jargon must be avoided as much as possible in expert testimony. (p. 508)

DISCUSSION

The importance of this principle is underscored by the reality that many consumers of FMHA have little or no formal training in mental health. The attempt to create a "common language" has thus relied on either removing technical terms from written or oral communication, or defining such terms carefully when they are used. Both sources of ethics authority in psychology emphasize the need for language that is reasonably understandable to the consumer of the evaluation, with the *Specialty*

Guidelines particularly stressing communication that considers the characteristics and abilities of those who are recipients of the communication. However, despite the conceptual importance and commonsense value attached to this principle, there has apparently been no legal authority or empirical research that has addressed it directly. In contrast, the standard of practice literature is quite clear about the necessary emphasis on clarity of communication being facilitated by plain language; major works in FMHA, including both civil and juvenile assessment, support this principle directly. In addition to communicating with legal professionals and those who may have some training in mental health (e.g., parole officers, teachers), it is important to be able to communicate clearly with those (e.g., jurors) who may have no formal training in either law or mental health, and perhaps no experiences in cases in which technical terms in either discipline are relevant. This principle appears to be *established*, but needs to be addressed more directly in the legal and empirical research areas.

WRITE REPORT IN SECTIONS, ACCORDING TO MODEL AND PROCEDURES

In the discussion of previous principles, a number of points have been emphasized: the use of a model, the importance of cross-checking factual information, and the clarification of the relationship between data, reasoning, and conclusions. In the majority of cases, the FMHA product will be the report, and the forensic clinician will not have the opportunity to provide additional information through testimony. All of these considerations underscore the importance of the report's organization, making it as clear as possible what was done, for what purpose, with what results, and leading to what conclusions. This can be facilitated by a report that is presented in sections. Finally, the communication of FMHA results in testimony is, to a large extent, a matter of presenting what has already been documented in written form (a point that will be discussed in greater detail in Chapter 11). When the written report can also be used to promote organized, well-supported testimony, then it can be useful in this context as well.

Ethics

The *Ethical Principles of Psychologists and Code of Conduct* (APA, 1992) contains little that is relevant to this principle. The only language that is even indirectly relevant concerns the explanation of assessment results "using language that is reasonably understandable" (p. 1604). If this were broadened somewhat into "a form" or "a structure" that facilitates understanding, then it would be consistent with the attempt to communicate FMHA results by writing the report in sections.

The *Specialty Guidelines for Forensic Psychologists* (Committee on Ethical Guidelines for Forensic Psychologists, 1991) addresses the structure of the FMHA report only indirectly, and with the same language that applied to the previous principle:

> Forensic psychologists make reasonable efforts to ensure that the products of their services, as well as their own public statements and professional testimony, are communicated in ways that will promote understanding and avoid deception, given the particular characteristics, roles, and abilities of various recipients of the communications. (p. 663)

Since the expectation is that the results of FMHA will be provided to individuals in legal contexts, a report structure that efficiently summarizes and organizes the necessary information for direct examination, cross examination, and legal arguments and decisions in the absence of an expert witness, should be helpful.

Again, neither the *Principles of Medical Ethics with Annotations Especially Applicable to Psychiatry* (APA, 1998) nor the *Ethical Guidelines for the Practice of Forensic Psychiatry* (AAPL, 1995) contains language that is directly relevant to this principle.

LAW

No legal authority was located relevant to this principle.

EMPIRICAL

No empirical studies were located that are relevant to this principle.

STANDARD OF PRACTICE

The FMHA report, and the clinician writing it, will receive close scrutiny during adversary proceedings. A report that is well written and organized may facilitate effective testimony, while poor organization or imprecise language in a report may be used to discredit and embarrass the forensic clinician (Melton et al., 1997). Melton and colleagues also observe that

> the act of creating the report forces the clinician to impose some organization on his or her data. Data are often gathered from widely diverse sources and may often be inconsistent. Drafting a report requires the examiner to weigh this

information, find a theme that best integrates the various findings, consider
alternatives, and recognize vulnerabilities. (p. 523)

Further, on the relationship between report and testimony, they comment
that

Organizing data and thoughts for the report also helps the mental health
professional covertly prepare and rehearse the essence of any direct and cross-
examination testimony that may be given. (p. 523)

In the course of a deposition or testimony given in a hearing or trial,
the forensic clinician may be asked questions ranging from the highly
specific to the very broad. The written report should function as an organizing tool during such testimony. Having already allowed the expert to
condense a great deal of information into an efficient preparation period
by reviewing the report prior to testimony, a well-organized report then
allows the expert to quickly locate information that is needed to respond
with precision and detail to a question.

According to Melton et al. (1997), the following areas need to be
contained in the report at all times: (1) circumstances of the referral, (2) date
and nature of clinical contacts, (3) collateral data sources, (4) relevant personal background information, (5) clinical findings, and (6) psychological-
legal formulation. In a description of juvenile evaluations, Grisso (1998a)
recommends the use of a consistent outline for report writing. Some of the
sections in such an outline include purpose, sources of data, and opinions
on matters directly pertaining to the legal questions (what are called
forensic issues in this book).

Another description of recommended sections for a report on an
FMHA topic—in this case, insanity evaluations—has been provided by
Rogers and Shuman (2000). They recommend that all reports contain the
following sections: (1) referral (a clear description of the referral source and
the purpose of the evaluation, as well as the relevant legal standard for
insanity in the jurisdiction), (2) description of the evaluation (all tests and
procedures used, including a nontechnical explanation of any unfamiliar
measures), (3) defendant's behavior at the time of the offense (a thorough
description of behavior immediately before, during, and following the
offense, summarizing each source of information separately unless descriptions of this behavior are highly consistent across sources), (4) clinical
description (a thorough and accurate description of the defendant's clinical functioning at present and at the time of the offense), (5) consultations
(professional input obtained specifically for this evaluation, such as computerized test scoring and interpretation for instruments such as the
MMPI-2 or the MCMI-III), (6) clinical conclusions (the defendant's diagnosis at the time of the offense and the time of the evaluation, and the

relationship of the mental disorders/psychopathology at the time of the offense to the defendant's criminal behavior), and (7) opinions (applying the clinical data to the relevant CR standard). Rogers and Shuman differ with some others in their contention that the ultimate legal question can be answered at the clinician's discretion, as opposed to being avoided whenever possible (see the discussion in Chapter 9 for more detail). However, the other sections in their report structure are quite consistent with those recommended by others, for different kinds of FMHA.

Generally, then, the sections of a report recommended in the present book are consistent with the structure provided by the various sources of FMHA that have been described in this section. Convergent validity is suggested for a report structure that includes the following for FMHA: referral, procedures, relevant history, clinical condition, functional legal performance or capacities (depending on the particular legal question toward which the evaluation is oriented), and conclusion. Such a structure is also consistent with the use of either the Morse or Grisso models described in Chapter 4. In particular, these sections and both models require that the evaluator describe relevant symptoms or characteristics, functional legal capacities, and the relationship between these two areas.

Finally, the *Guidelines for Child Custody Evaluations in Divorce Proceedings* (APA, 1994) offers the following on the issue of maintaining written records:

> All records obtained in the process of conducting a child custody evaluation are properly maintained and filed in accord with the APA Record Keeping Guidelines (APA, 1993) and relevant statutory guidelines.
>
> All raw data and interview information are recorded with an eye toward their possible review by other psychologists or the court, where legally permitted. Upon request, appropriate reports are made available to the court. (p. 679)

DISCUSSION

Since the report may be the sole product of an FMHA, in cases in which neither depositions nor expert testimony are used to communicate results, it is particularly important that the report function as a form of communication that can stand alone. Despite the importance of the FMHA report, however, there is relatively little available on its structure from several sources of authority reviewed for this principle. Ethics authority in psychology cite the importance of "reasonably understandable" language, and the promotion of understanding and avoidance of deception considering the roles, characteristics, and abilities of the recipients of the communication, but nothing more specific. Relevant sources of ethics authority within psychiatry provide even less applicable comment. No relevant legal authority was located, nor was there applicable empirical research that could provide information about the impact of a particular structure in FMHA reports.

There is discussion of the FMHA report in different areas from those addressing the role of the report in forensic practice. Several commentators, discussing FMHA applicable to different legal questions, provide converging evidence that the structure of the forensic report should contain sections that include referral information, procedures, relevant history, clinical condition, functional legal performance or capacities, and conclusions. These sections can be elaborated for some kinds of evaluations, such as retrospective FMHAs, but should appear at a minimum in most FMHA reports. Such structure imposes organization on the evaluation and the communication of results, reveals inconsistencies in the findings, and facilitates preparation for testimony when it is needed. It also allows the application of a model, as discussed in Chapter 4, and facilitates the communication of such important model components as clinical characteristics, functional legal capacities, and causal relationship between them.

The importance of the FMHA report and its structure is sufficient, by itself, to consider this principle to be *established*. However, it is very clear that the field must expand its consideration of the FMHA report, particularly through empirical research, to increase our understanding of how FMHA data and reasoning can be communicated most effectively to legal and lay consumers.

11

Testifying Effectively

Expert testimony is the most visible part of FMHA. Indeed, judging from what appears in the media, it sometimes seems to be the *only* part. This is inaccurate, of course, but it is not uncommon to have even referring attorneys use language consistent with this stereotype (e.g., "Doctor, I'd like to hire you to appear as an expert witness for my client").

There are two particular reasons why this perception is inaccurate. First, just as the vast majority of criminal and civil litigants never come to trial, the majority of FMHA reports are not presented in testimony[1] by the evaluator.[2] Considering only those cases in which expert testimony has occurred is likely to yield an unrepresentative view of the larger FMHA process. Second, for a variety of reasons, it is preferable to view expert testimony as an integral part of FMHA, rather than a separate procedure. The ethical and scientific reasons for considering this linkage are compelling; unless testimony is based on a solid foundation built from both relevant research and applicable FMHA findings, the information provided to the decision-maker is likely to be incomplete, inaccurate, and misleading. This approach allows the "data to shape the conclusions," and limits the impact of preexisting biases that might result in "*a priori* conclu-

---

[1]While I am aware of no formal empirical study relevant to this point, I can cite anecdotal experience and observations from three states—Florida, Virginia, and Pennsylvania—in both hospital and community settings that suggest that across a range of criminal forensic issues and settings, testimony (whether in a deposition, hearing, or trial) occurs in about 10% of cases in which FMHA is performed. This certainly may vary across jurisdictions and forensic issues, and would be more frequent in attorney-referred, high-visibility cases in which the FMHA findings are helpful to the referring attorney.

[2]Reports and oral testimony are both evidence, and the legal distinction between the two may not be clear, although some legal scholars (e.g., Melton et al., 1997) refer to reports and testimony as different forms of evidence. In this book, I advocate a very close substantive relationship between the two, so that testimony is based clearly and directly on the results of the FMHA evaluation as documented in the report.

sions shaping data."[3] This chapter will consider the principle describing the relationship between forensic assessment and testimony.

Good expert testimony should be persuasive. Substantively, it should be grounded in science and based on the individual assessment. However, there are other aspects to "persuasiveness" that relate to the expert's perceived knowledge, impartiality, and trustworthiness, as well as the clarity and authority of the communication and the overall credibility of the expert. These factors have been considered under the broad rubric of "impression management" (Melton et al., 1997); in this chapter, I will call them *stylistic* variables. They will be discussed under the second principle in this chapter.

It is important to be clear about the respective roles of both substantive and stylistic variables. Substantive areas include the data, reasoning, and conclusions of FMHA, and the associated support from science, standard of practice, ethics, and law. Stylistic variables involve the manner in which this information is presented, and how the individual communicates in both direct testimony and cross-examination, as well as personal characteristics (manner of speech, style of dress, believability) that are relevant to the forensic clinician's impact. It is important that both areas be mastered for maximal effectiveness in communicating FMHA results in testimony.

This relationship is depicted in Table 11.1. Forensic clinicians who have been thorough and principled in their approach to FMHA *and* who are effective in their style of communicating data and reasoning are described in Cell 1. Such individuals are excellent in their roles as expert witnesses; they are thorough and accurate, but also effective in the way in which they communicate such information. It is possible to be substantively strong in

[3]In an invited presentation to the American Psychology–Law Society Biennial Conference in 1990, U.S. Supreme Court Justice Harry Blackmun commented that he had observed two styles of decision-making in his fellow Supreme Court Justices. First, there were those whose *a priori* position on an issue before the court caused them to consider how they could incorporate the facts and the legal issues of the case to support their conclusion, which would be consistent with their *a priori* position. Second, there were those who would reason from the facts and the legal issues to a conclusion; these justices would be less predictable or consistent from case to case given the variations in such cases. This is a reasonably good way to illustrate approaches to decision-making in FMHA as well. When a certain conclusion in an FMHA case is more likely because of some *a priori* position held by the evaluator, or the strength of such a position would overwhelm the data so that the decision-making process involves "position shaping data and conclusions" rather than "data shaping conclusions," then there is a major problem with the testimony that will be provided. Even more distressing are cases in which data and conclusions are not shaped by an *a priori* position, but driven primarily by financial considerations. The latter would describe the kind of testimony to which the "opinion for hire" criticism could be fairly applied.

TABLE 11.1. CHARACTERISTICS OF EXPERT WITNESSES ACCORDING
TO SUBSTANTIVE STRENGTH AND STYLISTIC EFFECTIVENESS

		Stylistic effectiveness[a]	
		High	Low
Substantive strength[b]	High	Excellent witness: informative, thorough, ethical, persuasive	Marginal witness: thorough, informative, but ineffective communicator and limited credibility
		1	2
	Low	Deceptive witness: prone to inaccuracy due to bias or lack of thoroughness, communicates effectively, may seem more credible than merited	Poor witness: inaccurate, inconsistent, not persuasive, minimal credibility
		3	4

[a]Stylistic effectiveness involves a combination of professional dress and demeanor, courtroom familiarity, speech that is clear and largely free of technical jargon as well as fluid and variable in pace and directed toward the judge or jury as well as the attorney, and the capacity to handle the challenge of cross-examination well.
[b]Substantive strength is the extent to which the FMHA is consistent wtih principles 1–27, as described in Chapters 2–10 of this book.

the areas described in Chapters 2–10 but largely ineffective in communicating this information, for different possible reasons. One may appear
overly intellectual, "ivory towerish," arrogant, obtuse, hostile, rigid, or
uncertain, for example, with the result being a lessening of credibility
afforded to that witness in testimony (see Cell 2). Conversely, a forensic
clinician who does not use FMHA principles effectively or consistently
may provide testimony that is substantively weak, but communicate such
information effectively. Such witnesses (in Cell 3) may be seen as more
credible and persuasive than they deserve. Finally, witnesses who are
neither substantively strong nor stylistically effective (Cell 4) will either be
forced to improve, or avoid future involvement in forensic assessment.

BASE TESTIMONY ON RESULTS
OF PROPERLY PERFORMED FMHA

This principle will describe the relationship between properly performed FMHA and expert testimony, and the need to clearly and explicitly
base testimony on the results of the FMHA. However, it is important to
emphasize that the FMHA must be performed well, or this principle

cannot be meaningful—basing testimony on the results of FMHA that is irrelevant, insufficient, or invalid would not yield good expert testimony. Properly performed FMHA will consider forensic issues relevant to the legal question, be sufficiently detailed and thorough, and will use good-quality tools and reasoning to yield more accurate results.

It is unclear how often "expert testimony" is based on an evaluation that is inadequate to support the substance of the testimony.[4] Testimony must be based on an evaluation that includes relevant information that is both valid in a nomothetic way and applied to the individual, with carefully described reasoning that links the data with the conclusions. When it is not, such testimony will be of limited value. This will be discussed under the first principle in this chapter.

ETHICS

This principle is quite broad. It will be defined as the sum of the principles discussed in Chapters 2–10, and will tend to be addressed broadly by various sources of ethics authority. The *Ethical Principles of Psychologists and Code of Conduct* (APA, 1992) has several relevant components in the Preamble and General Principles (which are aspirational) as well as one in the Ethical Standards (the section of the *Ethics Code* that is enforceable). It is first observed in the Preamble that psychologists "work to develop a valid and reliable body of scientific knowledge based on research" with their "goal … to broaden knowledge of behavior and, where appropriate, to apply it pragmatically to improve the condition of both the individual and society" (p. 1599). They "also strive to help the public in developing informed judgments and choices concerning human behavior" (p. 1599). Each of these broad goals is consistent with the use of a set of principles developed from the FMHA literature, informed by scientific data and reasoning, professional standards, and legal and ethical authority ["Psychologists make appropriate use of scientific, professional, technical, and administrative resources" (p. 1599)]. To the extent that a coherent body of such principles exists, it is important that they be applied to FMHA as described in Chapters 2–10 of this book:

> Psychologists rely on scientifically and professionally derived knowledge when making scientific or professional judgments or when engaging in scholarly or professional endeavors. (p. 1600)

---

[4]One of the ways in which the quality of an FMHA could be measured would involve considering it in light of the principles discussed in this book. This will be discussed further in Chapter 12, under "Implications for Research."

It is also ethically incumbent on psychologists to describe the basis for their opinions in both reports and testimony:

> In forensic testimony and reports, psychologists testify truthfully, honestly, and candidly and, consistent with applicable legal procedures, describe fairly the bases for their testimony and conclusions. (p. 1610)

One straightforward approach to satisfying this demand comes from the present principle. When reports and testimony are each considered as a form of FMHA communication, then testimony would involve describing the methods, findings, reasoning, and conclusions *that have already been described* if a report has been written.

Similarly, in a broad vein, the *Specialty Guidelines for Forensic Psychologists* (1991) indicates that

> Forensic psychologists make reasonable efforts to ensure that the products of their services, as well as their own public statements and professional testimony, are communicated in ways that will promote understanding and avoid deception, given the particular characteristics, roles, and abilities of various recipients of the communications. (p. 663)

One straightforward approach to "promoting understanding" is to conduct FMHA according to the principles described in Chapters 2–10. In this sense, the *Specialty Guidelines* is also consistent with the present principle.

The *Principles of Medical Ethics with Annotations Especially Applicable to Psychiatry* (APA, 1998) contains nothing relevant to this principle. The *Ethical Guidelines for the Practice of Forensic Psychiatry* (AAPL, 1995) addresses the importance of basing testimony on a solid foundation, and apply the same standard ("honesty and striving for objectivity") to both report writing and testimony:

> Forensic psychiatrists ... adhere to the principles of honesty and they strive for objectivity. Their clinical evaluation and the application of the data obtained to the legal criteria are performed in the spirit of such honesty and efforts to attain objectivity. Their opinion reflects this honesty and efforts to attain objectivity.... Practicing forensic psychiatrists enhance the honesty and objectivity of their work by basing their forensic opinions, forensic reports and their forensic testimony on all the data available to them. They communicate the honesty of their work, efforts to attain objectivity, and the soundness of their clinical opinion by distinguishing, to the extent possible, between verified and unverified information as well as between clinical "facts," "inferences," and "impressions." (p. 3)

LAW

The sources of legal authority most relevant to this principle appear to be the evidentiary standards for the admissibility of scientific expert testimony.[5] In jurisdictions in which the *Frye* (1923) standard applies, the admissibility of evidence will depend on whether the proposed evidence is of a kind sufficiently established to have gained general acceptance in the field to which it belongs. In such a jurisdiction, the question would be whether the testimony was based on data and techniques that were "generally accepted" in the field as applicable for assessment (particularly *forensic* assessment) purposes.

In the *Daubert* (1993) decision, the U.S. Supreme Court affirmed the applicability of the *Federal Rules of Evidence* to the admissibility of scientific evidence in the federal jurisdiction. There are two particular parts of the *Daubert* decision that are particularly relevant to this principle. First, Rule 703 of the *Federal Rules* indicates that the facts or data in the particular case, on which an expert bases an opinion or inference, may be either perceived by or made known to the expert *at or before the hearing* (italics added). If such facts or data are of a type reasonably relied on by experts in the particular field in forming opinions or inferences, then they do not need to be independently admissible.[6] Under Rule 703, there may be some legal basis for offering an expert opinion based in part on facts or data provided at the time of the hearing. While this could be interpreted as inconsistent with the contention within this principle that the larger evaluation and the expert testimony should be closely linked, it could also suggest that additional facts or data beyond those considered in the evaluation could contribute to what is considered during testimony.

The second part of the *Daubert* decision relevant to this principle is seen in the Court's dicta, which offered several factors that might be considered in weighing the admissibility of scientific evidence. These included whether the scientific method was applied to yield the inference forming the basis for the opinion, whether the reasoning or methodology underlying the testimony is scientifically valid, and whether it can be

[5]There is some question about whether FMHA should be considered "scientific" or "technical or other specialized knowledge" under the *Federal Rules of Evidence*. Reasoned arguments can be made for either position. What is clear, however, is that some appellate courts have cited the applicable standard for the admissibility of scientific evidence—*Daubert*, in the federal jurisdiction—in case law concerning FMHA. Since it is possible to consider FMHA as "scientific," and since some courts have done so, I will treat FMHA as though, for the purposes of admissibility, it were "scientific." This question is less important than it was prior to *Kumho v. Carmichael* (1999), however, since the Court in *Kumho* made it clear that the *Daubert* standard could be applied to expert evidence provided on the basis of "technical or other specialized knowledge" as well as on the basis of science.
[6]Some jurisdictions have held that evidence must be independently admissible in order to form part of the basis for expert testimony. See, e.g., *Mayer v. Baiser* (1986). This could result in the exclusion of an opinion based on clinical techniques, such as hypnosis or polygraph, that have not been established as admissible.

applied to the facts of the given case. Additional factors included the testability of the method forming the basis for the opinion, whether it has been tested, the associated error rate, and *Frye* considerations such as general acceptance and peer review approval. The Court emphasized that the inquiry was to be a "flexible" one. The important considerations of available nomothetic data and their individualized application to the case at hand can be readily observed in the Court's commentary.

Some jurisdictions have adopted *Daubert*, others have rejected it and retained the *Frye* standard, and yet others have yet to rule on the issue (Melton et al., 1997). Forensic clinicians should be attentive to the applicable standard in their own jurisdiction.

EMPIRICAL

No empirical studies were located that specifically addressed the relationship between the forensic assessment and the communication of results in expert testimony.

STANDARD OF PRACTICE

For several decades, Stanley Brodsky has presented workshops on expert testimony for various groups of mental health professionals. More recently, he has condensed many of his major points about expert testimony into a book that provides 62 "maxims" for the expert witness (Brodsky, 1991). Considering these maxims is particularly useful in the present context, because many of them are either "substantive" or "stylistic" as these were defined earlier in this chapter.[7] Substantive maxims, which will be discussed under this principle, describe ways to strengthen the relationship between the substantive FMHA findings and testimony. Stylistic maxims involve approaches to enhancing the credibility, persuasiveness, and perceived professionalism of the expert, including responses to cross-examination efforts to diminish these attributes.

What follows is my categorization of the "substantive" maxims described by Brodsky. I comment on each maxim as it relates to standard of practice in the area of expert testimony.

Respond to implications of being a bought expert by showing awareness of the issue and assertively presenting the foundations of your objectivity (p. 7). Two of the principles already discussed in this book involve the identification of the legal question(s) at the initial stage of the evaluation, and maintaining reasonable impartiality in the role of evaluator. Brodsky em-

---

[7]This distinction is made for the discussion in this chapter, not in Brodsky's book.

phasizes that both are important—and that the forensic clinician should be prepared to describe relevant information on each. Doing so can counter any mistaken impression that a forensic clinician's opinion is "for hire," or that the interpretation of data has been affected by *a priori* biases.

Check and recheck that routine pulls toward affiliation are not diminishing the impartiality of the expert role (p. 10). Achieving and maintaining a reasonably impartial stance is not only a matter of declining participation in cases when it is clear that the evaluator could not be impartial. Remaining impartial takes work. Part of this work is self-monitoring, in which the forensic clinician regularly "checks" to make sure that public scrutiny, competitiveness, fear of being attacked or embarrassed, the desire to please others, or the desire to avoid hurting others (among many possibilities) have not interfered with the needed impartiality. Describing this process is another way of ensuring that information is conveyed as accurately as possible.

Review current literature on the topic about which you will testify (p. 13). A good working knowledge of the relevant literature is important at all stages of FMHA. Reviewing this literature before testimony can help the expert to integrate relevant aspects of the literature with current findings, and testify about both.

Burdens of proof and degrees of defined certainty are legal concepts. Do not accept, define, or incorporate them into clinical, psychological, or scientific testimony (p. 17). Just as one of the arguments against directly answering the ultimate legal question involves the poor fit between clinical/scientific terminology and legal concepts, there are similar reasons to avoid using the concepts of burden of proof and standard of certainty in a report or testimony. The attempt to deconstruct the concept of "reasonable professional certainty" in testimony, for example, has been met with confusion and suspiciousness on the part of some decision-makers (see, e.g., Poythress, 1982). A smoother course may result from the effort to describe the findings and their basis, and (if asked) indicating that the expert does hold the opinion with "reasonable professional certainty" while again indicating the basis for this opinion.

Be prepared to present the bases for generalizability of findings and demographic communalities in your testimony (p. 23). This is an important consideration, because it encompasses not only the applicability of various tools, but their limitations as well. One of the questions that arises when applying nomothetic data to an individual case is whether that case is one to which the empirical findings could be reasonably generalized. This is another important part of "individualizing" the evaluation and testimony in a given case.

Challenges to professional experience should be met with a knowledge of the literature and affirmations of the worth of your own experience (p. 26). Awareness of the relevant empirical studies, combined with a knowledge of accepted practice standards and a reasonable amount of experience (including forensic experience) with individuals similar to the one being evaluated, should enhance both the quality of the evaluation and the credibility of the evaluator.

Do not change a professional opinion on the basis of a cross-examination. Your opinions should always arise from your data (p. 29). One of the most important justifications for the strong link between FMHA and subsequent expert testimony is that alternative interpretations are weighed, and decisions made about which conclusions are best supported, before testimony is ever given. When this occurs, then problems with a particular interpretation will have been considered and incorporated into reasoning toward a conclusion, with the findings and reasoning detailed in the report. A conclusion offered in testimony can be retained, therefore, because it appears strongest in light of all considerations, including those that may be inconsistent with that particular conclusion.

Questions about children's lying and fantasies should be answered with open acknowledgment of their existence and the ways in which the clinical examination ruled them out as causes of the allegations of abuse (p. 32). This is a specific example of the broader "hypothesis testing" process discussed in the previous maxim. Testimony should always acknowledge the potential inaccuracy of self-report. If the forensic clinician concludes that self-report appears accurate in a given case, then that clinician should be prepared to justify this conclusion by explaining how alternative explanations were not supported.

Challenges about clients faking bad or faking good should be met with affirmative statements of clinical validity, sensitivity, and vigilance for client dissimulation (p. 39). The importance of response style has been emphasized strongly in this book, as it is throughout the FMHA literature. The response style of an individual should have been carefully considered as part of the evaluation, and the findings conveyed as part of expert testimony. If the response style does not appear to be reliable, then the clinician should go on to describe the procedures used to minimize overall distortion. While this information can be provided again in response to challenge on cross-examination, such a challenge is more easily addressed when it is clear that the issue has been considered in the FMHA, and how it has been handled.

Research on client dissimulation should be known and used in clinical work and testimony. Enough of the research findings are equivocal that caution in evaluations and witness statements are always in order (p. 42). Advances in such research have continued since 1991, when Brodsky published this book, and are summarized in Chapter 7 of his book. Despite such advances, however, this maxim continues to apply. Indeed, it seems unlikely

that empirical research will, in the foreseeable future, provide dissimulation tools of such sensitivity and specificity that such cautions, along with
collateral information, would not be needed.

Good definitions are necessary but not sufficient bases for answering fundamental questions. Broader conceptual understanding is needed (p. 49). Definitions can be particularly important in FMHA, because the decision-maker
must be provided with the best available information in a given case when
making a decision that may not be subject to revision. However, many of
the concepts of science and clinical practice do not translate readily into
law. For example, there are a number of forensically relevant tools that
employ continuous scales rather than yielding simple dichotomous outcomes. When the court must reach a decision that is dichotomous, however, there can be pressure on an expert to present FMHA findings in a
dichotomous way. A broader understanding of FMHA, its tools, and the
legal context can facilitate testimony that will allow continuous variables
to inform dichotomous decision-making.

Prepare a list of professionally relevant and complete qualifying questions for
the attorney to use in the opening of the direct examination (p. 55). Concisely
conveying the nature and extent of one's relevant training and experience
can help to establish the expert's substantive competence to perform a
particular FMHA and testify as an expert about its results. Although many
of the questions on this list will be generic, establishing the expert's
credentials and training in a fairly nonspecific way, there should be other
questions that directly address the issues of forensic experience and
population-specific experience.

Culture does affect the assessment of psychopathology. Witnesses should be
culture educated while still clearly identifying and affirming the conventional
foundations of their testimony (p. 62). Part of being culturally sensitive in
FMHA involves having experience with those in a specific cultural group.
Another part is a genuine awareness of how the values, standards, norms,
and expectations within specific cultural groups differ, and the willingness
to consider broader questions of psychopathology and capacities within
cultural context. A broad set of principles does exist for FMHA, but
cultural considerations affect how some of these principles are applied.

Do not be befuddled if you do not know specific DSM cautions. Do affirm the
underlying principles of such cautions in which you believe (p. 71). The DSM-IV
is a widely accepted diagnostic manual, but it contains the following
caution about its applicability in legal contexts:

> The clinical and scientific considerations involved in categorization of these
> conditions as mental disorders may not be wholly relevant to legal judgments,
> for example, that take into account such issues as individual responsibility,
> disability determination, and competency. (American Psychiatric Association,
> 1994, p. xxvii)

Moreover, symptoms and diagnostic categories represent only part of the information relevant to legal questions involving forensic issues. In Morse's (1978a) model, they would be the mental disorder. However, the functional legal abilities and the causal connection must also be described. Nonetheless, forensic clinicians are well advised to be familiar with both the broad categories and their specific DSM-IV criteria when reaching a conclusion about diagnosis as part of FMHA.

Cross-examinations about examiner effects call for the witness to explain how training and standardized procedures diminish such effects (p. 83). In addition, examiner effects can be reduced through the incorporation of third-party information (both document review and collateral interviews). The attempt to verify the accuracy of information through multiple sources, discussed in an earlier principle, can both enhance the accuracy of the conclusions and serve as an effective response to the implication that impressions or conclusions may be overly influenced by the characteristics of the forensic clinician.

From the earliest stage of legal activity, be certain to have mastered the foundations of your knowledge and role (p. 99). When the role is clear from the beginning of the FMHA, and the forensic clinician is confident that she or he is sufficiently knowledgeable in relevant areas, then it is more likely that the substantive aspects of the evaluation will be addressed properly.

Agree to be an expert only when genuine expertise is present (p. 124). When there is any question about the appropriateness of the forensic clinician's relevant training, competence, familiarity with the population, or forensic experience, the clinician should decline the referral. If this simple dictum were followed consistently, it is likely that many of the unsatisfactory experiences reported by mental health professionals in forensic contexts, and the dissatisfactions of judges and attorneys with mental health professionals, would be dramatically decreased.

It is normal for psychotherapists to be reluctant or ambivalent when testifying about their clients. Testimony should include the strengths of the participant– observer role and the extended opportunities to observe their clients (p. 163). When psychotherapists are testifying as fact witnesses about their clients, then their reluctance can be reduced by ensuring that their clients have agreed to the testimony, and avoiding the expert role because the information they have gathered in this case does not justify assuming this role. If psychotherapists are considering testifying as experts about their clients, then reluctance is quite appropriate.

When you truly do not know, say so (p. 175). The limits of scientific evidence, and the tools used in FMHA, as well as the mixed findings that are observed in some cases, mean that some questions cannot be answered well. On certain points in the report, and at certain times in testimony, it is appropriate to indicate that the evaluator cannot answer the question.

The Ziskin and Faust reviews have an adversarial component and conse-
quently may not meet the respected minority test. Nevertheless, they have made us
more accountable and that can be acknowledged constructively (p. 203). Throughout the process of FMHA, the evaluator should consider challenges to
accuracy and reasoning. It is useful to consider the Ziskin and Faust works
(Ziskin, 1981; Ziskin & Faust, 1988) as a good source of such challenges. It is
less useful, however, to consider them as a balanced guide to data collection or reasoning, as they focus almost exclusively on data that are nonsupportive of various potential FMHA procedures.[8]

Discussion

The sources of authority are fairly consistent in support of this principle, although no empirical information was located. Sources of ethics
authority emphasize the importance of accurate evaluation, consistent
with professional standards, forming the basis for expert testimony. Conversely, when there are limitations on the availability of relevant data,
when the proper role has not been assumed, or when professional standards cannot otherwise be met, it is recommended that the expert *avoid*
providing expert testimony, or at least limit the testimony by clearly
describing what is absent, and adjusting the conclusions accordingly.

Under either the *Frye* "general acceptance in the field" or the *Daubert/*
Federal Rules of Evidence broader emphasis on relevance and reliability for

---

[8]In the third edition of *Coping with Psychiatric and Psychological Testimony*, Ziskin (1981) wrote:
"It is the plan of this book to supply the attorney with a systematic and methodical basis for
objecting to the admission of psychiatric and psychological evidence by utilizing the scientific literature in the experts' fields. In the event the objection fails and the testimony is
admitted, the same information can be utilized to educate judge and jury and to systematically and methodically reduce the credibility of psychiatrists and clinical psychologists to
the point where it is difficult to believe that a judge or jury would attach much, if any weight
to their testimony. For this reason, the book consists almost entirely of the literature which
negates the expertise of these professionals. The lawyer should be aware that there is some
literature supportive of psychiatric and psychological evaluation. I have not included such
literature because I view it as irrelevant in the legal context. Thus, if there is, for example, a
body of literature indicating that psychiatric diagnoses are made with a fairly high degree of
reliability and there is another body of literature of approximately equal quality indicating
that psychiatric diagnoses are not made with a high degree of reliability, the least that can be
said is that the issue is in doubt and is therefore unresolved within the profession itself.
Therefore, if the scientific and professional literature casts doubt on the reliability of psychiatric diagnoses, the fact that a portion of that literature supports it does not remove the
doubt. In the face of such doubts, the evidence should not be admitted, and if it is admitted,
no weight should be given to it. Therefore, from a legal perspective, I would view the
recitation of some supportive literature as an exercise in futility" (p. x). Similar language
appears in the fourth volume (Ziskin & Faust, 1988).

admissibility of expert scientific testimony, there is support for a close link between previous stages of the evaluation and testimony. The ethics and standard of practice literature described under this principle support the link between evaluation and testimony, and the "generally accepted" procedures within FMHA are described in the earlier principles of this book. The application of the *Daubert/Federal Rules of Evidence* standards of relevance and reliability highlights the connection between evaluative techniques and expert testimony even more sharply, as each individual technique as well as the nature of the reasoning may be scrutinized by the court for its scientific support.

The absence of empirical evidence on this principle is noteworthy. Studies of two kinds would be helpful: *prescriptive* (in which the particular FMHA techniques are studied for predictive, construct, and discriminant validity, and for face validity, to determine their persuasiveness to legal decision-makers) and *descriptive* (in which the connection between the assessment, report-writing, and testimony are examined in large, highly generalizable samples of forensic clinicians).

Finally, the standard of practice literature integrated into Brodsky's (1991) substantive maxims on expert testimony presents a strong basis for considering testimony as one stage of the larger FMHA process. This principle appears to be *established.*

TESTIFY IN AN EFFECTIVE MANNER

This principle will describe the importance of using stylistic effectiveness in testimony to enhance the value of the communication and make it more persuasive. There are several factors that are common to both report-writing and expert testimony in this respect (e.g., avoiding technical jargon, the organization of information, the use of examples and quotations to illustrate particular points), which will be considered in this discussion. However, there is also a certain uniqueness to the process of expert testimony that will shape the discussion as well.

Much of the criticism that has been directed at expert testimony provided by mental health professionals can be conceptualized through the organization in Table 11.1, which suggests that good expert testimony is stylistically effective as well as substantively strong. Testimony that is substantively weak yet stylistically strong may result when mental health professionals (1) are poorly informed about forensic assessment principles, although they are strong in the areas of assessment and treatment with a particular population and also communicate in a forceful, articulate way, (2) provide testimony that is little more than an "opinion for hire," or

(3) are primarily advocating a social position (e.g., "juveniles should never be treated as adults," "plaintiffs should receive compensation from wealthy defendants following an accident, regardless of the nature of the injuries incurred"). In such cases, an evaluator may be strongly disposed toward a certain conclusion before collecting any data, and have drawn conclusions and presented testimony in which the data are shaped by the conclusion. When testimony is substantively strong but presented ineffectively, then it may be accurate but unpersuasive for reasons that will be discussed under this principle. Finally, testimony that has neither a good substantive basis nor a stylistically effective presentation is likely to be neither helpful nor persuasive.[9]

This point is made somewhat differently by Saks (1990), who describes the extent to which the contents of an expert's substantive field are related to expert testimony. When substantive testimony is strongly linked to the field, Saks describes the expert as playing an "educator" role, while the "Philosopher-Ruler" role is more strongly associated with advocacy for a cause. He does not describe the style of testimony, however; expert testimony in either of these roles could be presented effectively or poorly.

ETHICS

The *Ethical Principles of Psychologists and Code of Conduct* (APA, 1992) emphasizes that all relevant provisions within the *Ethics Code* would apply to how expert evidence is communicated:

> Psychologists who perform forensic functions, such as assessments, interviews, consultations, reports, or expert testimony, must comply with all other provisions of this Ethics Code to the extent that they apply to such activities. (p. 1610)

When the results of assessment are communicated, this should be done using language that is clear:

---

[9]Testimony from a mental health professional that was neither substantively strong nor stylistically impressive might not be requested again. For a number of reasons, however, it might. Some courts may have a limited pool of experts from which to select, because (1) there are few individuals in the area with appropriate training and experience, (2) there is little professional interest because of limited available funding, and/or the circumstances of the work (including possible perceived undesirability of the conditions or the clientele), or (3) individuals doing the evaluations are permanent or contract employees of the court or of an agency. In such circumstances, there may be ongoing requests for evaluations even when the substantive *and* stylistic aspects of the expert testimony are deficient. Under such circumstances, those conducting FMHA nonetheless have an obligation to make their FMHAs relevant and useful to the decision-maker, and to resist the temptation to produce reports or provide testimony that may reflect the use of outmoded tools or long-discredited theories.

> psychologists ensure that an explanation of the results is provided using language that is reasonably understandable. (p. 1604)

Whatever approaches are taken to communicating more effectively and persuasively cannot cross the line by violating the letter (or, hopefully, the spirit) of other provisions of the *Ethics Code*. More specifically:

> Psychologists do not make public statements that are false, deceptive, misleading, or fraudulent, either because of what they state, convey, or suggest or because of what they omit, concerning their research, practice, or other work activities or those of persons or organizations with which they are affiliated. (p. 1604)

Here the importance of both accuracy and completeness in "public statements" is emphasized. It seems appropriate to consider expert testimony to be a kind of public statement, increasing the applicability of this section of the *Ethics Code*. This is even clearer when the topic of testimony and reports is addressed specifically:

> In forensic testimony and reports, psychologists testify truthfully, honestly, and candidly and, consistent with applicable legal procedures, describe fairly the bases for their testimony and conclusions. (p. 1610)

The *Specialty Guidelines for Forensic Psychologists* (1991) makes it clear that the effective presentation of information in testimony is not precluded by other parts of the *Guidelines*:

> When testifying, forensic psychologists have an obligation to all parties to a legal proceeding to present their findings, conclusions, evidence, or other professional products in a fair manner. *This principle does not preclude forceful representation of the data and reasoning upon which a conclusion or professional product is based* [italics added]. It does, however, preclude an attempt, whether active or passive, to engage in partisan distortion or misrepresentation. Forensic psychologists do not, by either commission or omission, participate in a misrepresentation of their evidence, nor do they participate in partisan attempts to avoid, deny, or subvert the presentation of evidence contrary to their own position. (p. 664)

The *Principles of Medical Ethics with Annotations Especially Applicable to Psychiatry* (APA, 1998) indirectly addresses this principle by describing the importance of honesty, and emphasizing the need to avoid misrepresenting information in testimony. It is observed that "a physician shall deal honestly with patients and colleagues, and strive to expose those physicians deficient in character or competence, or who engage in fraud or deception" (p. 2).

The *Ethical Guidelines for the Practice of Forensic Psychiatry* (AAPL, 1995) also addresses the need to accurately present information; it does so by stressing the importance of honesty and striving for objectivity. Beyond this, however, neither the *Principles of Medical Ethics* nor the *Ethical Guidelines* directly addresses the issue of communicating in an effective or persuasive way.

LAW

Nothing relevant to this principle was located among sources of legal authority.

EMPIRICAL

Broadly speaking, research on the social psychology of persuasive communication has identified three elements of credibility. These include expertise (training and experience, such as degrees, positions, and the like), trustworthiness (perceptions by the judge and jurors of trustworthiness), and dynamism (style, charisma, and nonverbal aspects of credibility) (Brehm, Kassin, & Fein, 1999; Melton et al., 1997). Moreover, there is evidence that expert testimony may be understood and processed differently depending on its complexity. The distinction between systematic versus heuristic processing of information (Chaiken, 1980) or central versus peripheral routes to persuasion (Petty & Cacioppo, 1986) suggests that decision-makers, such as judges or jurors, may resort to heuristic "shortcuts" in processing information that is presented in a style too complex to be reasonably understood, when under time pressure, or when unmotivated to deal with very complex material. Some ramifications of this distinction for communication style and other expert witness variables have been investigated and are described in a study (Cooper & Neuhaus, 2000) cited later in this section.

The importance of an expert's capacity to convey technical information in an understandable way was emphasized in two studies. In the first, a survey of jurors, judges, lawyers, and experts from 40 civil cases in Dallas County, Texas, over a period of three months, it was noted that communicating clearly and drawing firm conclusions was more important than educational credentials; attractiveness and a "pleasant personality" were of least importance (Champagne, Shuman, & Whitaker, 1991). In a second three-city study (Baltimore, Tucson, and Seattle), these investigators again found that clarity of presentation was the most important factor in expert believability. Importance was also attached to expert articulateness and firmness, as well as to the experts' reputations and educational credentials (Shuman, Champagne, & Whitaker, 1994).

Some support for a professional appearance (e.g., short hair, a suit) was seen in a small study involving interviews of 8 members of a 12-person

California jury (Rosenthal, 1983). Impartiality has also been viewed as important. Most believable experts had "independent involvement" (that is, professional experience with other cases) with the issue on which they were testifying, and had done independent research on the subject (ABA Special Committee, 1989), while "hired guns" were disregarded. Payment of the expert by the attorney also suggested biased testimony, according to 35% of jurors in one study cited earlier (Champagne et al., 1991).

In a series of three studies, published in a single article, Cooper and Neuhaus (2000) investigated the impact of expert witness variables such as compensation, frequency of testifying, and credentials on their credibility with, and influence on, mock jurors. A previous study (Cooper, Bennett, & Sukel, 1996) had demonstrated that mock jurors hearing complex scientific testimony in a civil case were influenced most in their verdicts and beliefs about experts by the experts' credentials—identical testimony was perceived as more persuasive when the expert was from a prestigious university. In Study 1 of the Cooper and Neuhaus (2000) article, the authors reported that jury-eligible residents of central New Jersey between the ages of 18 and 65 ($N = 80$) participated as mock jurors in small groups of two to seven and listened to a 30-minute audiotape of an expert biochemist testifying about the relationship between the chemical polychlorinated biphenyl (PCB) and the risk for colon cancer in a toxic tort case. They varied whether the expert was highly paid ($4800) or minimally compensated ($75), and highly credentialed (Ph.D. in biochemistry from a prestigious institution, author of several dozen articles, and teaching at another prestigious institution) versus modestly credentialed (less well known institutions at which the biochemist had been trained and currently taught, and published far fewer articles). They reported that the combination of pay and credentials affected jurors most; the highly credentialed, highly paid expert was much less effective in persuading mock jurors than the modestly credentialed, highly paid expert. The authors noted that the specific combination of high pay and high credentials rendered the expert less likeable [$F(1, 76) = 5.33, p < .05$], less believable [$F(1, 76) = 4.89, p < .05$], less trustworthy [$F(1, 76) = 8.84, p < .01$], less honest [$F(1, 76) = 5.26, p < .05$], and more annoying [$F(1, 76) = 10.18, p < .01$] than the expert in the other three conditions.

In Study 2, the impact of "frequency of the expert's appearance" was assessed using a similar design (Cooper & Neuhaus, 2000). A total of 40 jury-eligible residents of New Jersey communities between the ages of 19 and 72 were recruited to function as mock jurors, listening to the same audiotape of expert testimony based on the facts of a toxic tort case. All expert testimony was delivered by witnesses who were "highly credentialed," as described in Study 1, but half were described as inexperienced in providing expert testimony ("second time testifying") and the other half as experienced ("14th appearance"). The second variable was compensation (high versus low). The authors reported an interaction between frequency of testimony and compensation: The expert who produced the most confidence was the highly paid individual who testified rarely, while the expert who produced the least confidence was the highly paid and testified frequently. The authors suggested that mock jurors who were engaged in "peripheral processing" of this complex material were using cues such as pay, credentials, and frequency of testifying as heuristic guides to their decision-making concerning the substance of an expert's testimony.

They tested this in Study 3 (Cooper & Neuhaus, 2000), with 60 jury-eligible New Jersey residents between the ages of 19 and 53. Pay was again varied for the expert, although in this study it was described at three levels ("highly paid" was $750/hour, "moderately paid" was $350/hour, and "low-paid" was $100/hour) that were seen as more consistent with compensation for actual experts. The second expert variable involved the use of technical jargon. In one condition ("high complexity") the expert frequently used specialized technical jargon, while in the other ("low complexity") the use of jargon was minimized. The substance of the testimony was comparable, but the use of jargon presumably made the material more "complex" and hence more difficult to understand. The authors again reported an interaction, this time between complexity and pay: When complexity was low, the level of payment had no impact on juror findings; when it was high, level of payment was inversely related to juror findings consistent with the expert testimony (see Figure 11.1).

It is not clear how generalizable the Cooper and Neuhaus (2000) findings are to FMHA. Several important distinctions between their procedures and actual FMHA practice may limit such generalizability: (1) The expert was a scientist in a toxic tort case, (2) the mock jurors reviewed an audiotape of testimony and rendered their judgments individually, rather than deliberating as a group, and (3) the "experience" variable would not apply well (testifying on only 14 prior occasions would not define a "highly experienced" forensic clinician). However, to the extent that these results can be generalized to FMHA, they have some intriguing implications. First, they may suggest that strong credentials, greater experience, or high fees on the part of experts are not necessarily perceived as positive by jurors. Second, they may imply that such variables may be used as heuristic "shortcuts" by some decision-makers when testimony is overly complex or otherwise poorly understood. Finally, these results suggest that clear, jargon-free communication may not only facilitate better under-

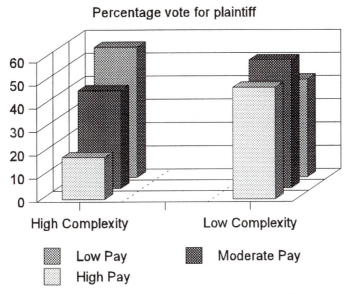

FIGURE 1.1. Effect of witness' pay and complexity of testimony on verdict for plaintiff (from Cooper & Neuhaus, 2000).

standing of the substance of testimony, but may also make jurors less inclined to use heuristic shortcuts to assess the credibility of the testimony.

STANDARD OF PRACTICE

Before discussing the literature in this area and its contributions to stylistically effective testimony, it is important to acknowledge the controversy in this area. One important basis for such controversy is the contention that "impression management" contains a significant element of deception. In a recent discussion of the "deceptions of psychiatrists," for example, Haroun and Morris (1999) described a number of areas in which there is the potential for psychiatrists (and other mental health professionals) to deceive attorneys and decision-makers in the context of expert testimony. These areas included the limitations on confidentiality, informed consent, impartiality, expertise, the sources from which information is drawn, the attributes of psychological tests, and the limits of accuracy in areas such as diagnosis and prediction. Such areas have been addressed elsewhere in this book, and their potential for yielding misleading FMHA results discussed. However, one broader point of the article is that deception, treated as evil by society and illegal within our judicial system, is adaptive in contexts such as evolution and war. What role is there for deception in FMHA?

There is no place for deception in FMHA. The principles described earlier in this book are oriented toward increasing the relevance, accuracy, comprehensiveness, and impartiality of FMHA. It would be inconsistent to suggest that such substantive results should be communicated in testimony in any way that involves deception, either in what is said or in what is omitted, *even if deception made such results more persuasive*. However, there are other stylistic approaches to enhancing the effectiveness of testimony that do not involve deception, and are more acceptable means of improving expert testimony.

These approaches are discussed in the remainder of this section. They are drawn from the larger literature and relevant experience of the authors (Brodsky, 1991; Melton et al., 1997), and are reasonably representative of current standard of practice.

Four particular recommendations in this area are made by Melton et al. (1997). The first is *style of dress*, which they suggest should be conservative, professional, neat, and not bright or flashy. It is also important that such attire should be comfortable, particularly over an extended period of time involving a lengthy hearing, and appropriate for comfort in summer air conditioning or winter heating. The second is *familiarity with courtroom protocol*, involving behaving in a manner that conveys familiarity and comfort with courtroom, pausing before answering questions, using a clear and even tone, not volunteering information, and knowing how to react when an objection is made. The third involves style of communication, in which the expert *speaks to the jury*, particularly during cross-examination, using understandable language, first making eye contact with the cross-examining attorney and then gradually shifting toward looking at the jury. The use of examples and hand gestures can help to keep the attention of the jury. The fourth also involves communication, with a particular *style of speech* that is fluid, conversational in tone, clear, and confident. Dramatic or hyperbolic tones should be avoided, as should intensifiers and qualifiers. Although the report and notes may be present, most of the testimony can be delivered without reading from (or even referring to) them. A brief reference to or quotation from the report can be made sufficiently often so that it is clear that the issue was considered, carefully evaluated, and addressed in the report, which can enhance the connection between the report and the testimony.

Some of the maxims for expert testimony provided by Brodsky (1991) appear more relevant to stylistic than substantive aspects of testimony.

Brodsky's principles that are particularly relevant in this area, along with brief comments of mine, appear as follows.

Handle loaded and half-truth questions by first admitting the true part in a dependent clause and then strongly denying the untrue part in an independent clause (p. 4). Using this "admit–deny" approach is one way of responding when the answer to the question, narrowly made, would provide only part of the information necessary for an accurate answer. When it is important to provide additional information, this approach to answering a question (beginning the response with a dependent clause, such as "While it is true that …," and finishing it with an independent clause, such as "it is also the case that …") can allow the expert to complete the entire response without being interrupted.

When challenged about insufficient experience, keep track of the true sources of your expertise (p. 20). Lack of experience in forensic assessment or with a given population is a reasonable basis for declining participation in a particular FMHA. Even when the forensic clinician's experience in both of these areas is reasonable to justify participation in a given case, however, there always remains some basis for challenging the clinician for lacking a very specific kind of experience (e.g., with a combination of population-specific characteristics like the number of "15-year-old African-American girls charged with murder" who have been evaluated). The appropriate response to such a challenge is to emphasize the sources of expertise that are generally relevant to expertise with an individual with these specific characteristics.

Criticize your field as requested, but be poised and matter of fact and look for opportunities to regain control (p. 45). Many of the criticisms of the mental health professions as they apply to legal proceedings should be antici-pated by the forensic clinician, and managed as part of the evaluation. In this respect, a weakness in the available tools, for example, can be de-scribed in a straightforward way. It can also be observed, however, that this weakness was considered in selecting the procedures for this particu-lar FMHA, and the weakness was managed by supplementing and inte-grating the findings with information from other sources, with resulting limitations described in the report. A response like this can enhance the perception that the expert is credible and knowledgeable.

Comfortably agree with accurate challenges to your credentials. Offer narra-tive explanations only when they are nondefensive and unforced (p. 59). Every expert has areas in which his or her credentials could be stronger. Ac-knowledging weakness is important.

Meet with the attorney prior to the direct examination and be involved in preparing the questions (p. 65). Like most other professional activities, expert testimony is improved by practice and through an explicit awareness of what will be asked (and how it will be asked) on direct examination. It may also be helpful to anticipate what might be asked on cross-examination. Both can be accomplished through a meeting with the attorney before the hearing or trial.

After a disaster during testimony, correct the error as soon as you can. If you cannot, let it go (p. 68). If it is possible to return to a reply that was misstated, then it is helpful to do so—simply indicate that the previous answer was in error, and that the expert would like to correct it. It may not be possible to do this, however. If not, it is preferable to simply move on, and resume concentrating on the current line of questioning.

Neither fraternize nor discuss any element of the case with opposing counsel, other witnesses, clients, or jurors (p. 89). The legal reasons for avoiding any discussion of the case with those involved in the litigation stem from the formal nature of the legal proceeding, which is conducted according to rules of evidence and provides for communication only within such rules. However, there are also the perceptions of others to be considered. More specifically, a mental health professional in the role of impartial expert, even when testifying on behalf of an individual, should *behave* in a way consistent with impartiality, and avoid being too closely allied with the litigant, or with the litigant's family or attorney. For this reason, individuals who testify as impartial experts should decline an attorney's invitation to sit at the counsel table,[10] and should also avoid sitting with litigants, victims, witnesses, or litigants' or victims' friends or family in the courtroom. While this need not be taken to an extreme—professional courtesy and politeness should be observed—the forensic clinician should carefully consider the perception that can result from observing even casual conversation or "body language" during interactions before or after testimony.

When testifying about something in which you believe, testify in a manner that shows that you believe in it (p. 93). The training of mental health professionals and behavioral scientists can often foster an interpersonal style that appears detached and dispassionate. While this orientation can be helpful during earlier steps in FMHA, it can be misleading and counterproductive if the forensic clinician does not appear firm and confident in the testimony that is provided. This must be conveyed in the manner as well as the substance of the testimony.

---

[10]A mental health professional who is serving in the role of consultant, with the goal of assisting the attorney only, is a member of the team and need not be concerned about appearance in the same way. However, it is worth noting that this role distinction may be lost on members of the media, observers, and jurors, who might conclude that this is how all behavioral scientists or mental health professionals behave in court.

The historic hysteric gambit is an indication that nothing else has worked for the attorney. Respond with poise, either declining to discuss the historical events or dismissing them as obsolete and not applicable (p. 97). The "historic hysteric gambit" involves the attempt to diminish the credibility of testimony by invoking a historical figure, typically in a scientific or professional area, who advocated a theory that was accepted at the time but subsequently shown to be inaccurate. The implication is that the forensic clinician, like this historic figure, might also be mistaken. This challenge can be handled in a variety of ways. Among the more effective are noting the differences between present scientific evidence and that available at the time of the example, or emphasizing the different possibilities that were considered in the present case, and the data and reasoning that yielded the conclusion(s) eventually reached.

Explicitly relax or engage in productive work just before your court appearance (p. 112). The time just before court testimony should be spent preparing as effectively as possible for such testimony. Different approaches to preparation have been observed. Some may find that relaxation works best. For others, concentration on a directly relevant task (either a review of the report or the planned questions and answers of testimony) may be preferable. As an additional part of such preparation, it can also be helpful to begin "warming up" the speaking voice by rehearsing responses to expected questions in a normal tone. (This works best when the forensic clinician is alone.) Still others, when confident that they are fully prepared, may work on other projects. The latter can be particularly useful when there is an extended period waiting to testify, and the concentration required for such tasks can distract the expert and make the wait seem shorter.

Effective language usage comes about when the witness personalizes answers, varies the format, uses narrative well, and produces convincing spoken and transcribed testimony (p. 115). One way to enhance the effectiveness of oral communication of complex material is to present this material in an interesting and understandable way. The reaction of the "audience" (in the case of testimony, the judge and jury) should be gauged in an ongoing way. If listeners appear distracted, bored, or confused, the expert should adjust the presentation accordingly. The use of examples, occasional explanations, and variability in voice tone and sentence structure can help to keep listeners' attention. For these reasons, it is unwise to read more than brief passages from a report, or the text of prepared answers. Preparation of "bullet items" or "talking points" is preferable, as this allows enough flexibility for the expert to pay appropriate attention to the audience.

Gain control of fluency on the witness stand by speaking slowly, stressing syllables, easing into your breath pattern, and varying the loudness of your speech (p. 118). Following this maxim keeps the expert from speaking too quickly, which can result from nervousness, or from thinking so rapidly that it seems necessary to talk quickly in order to "keep up" with the pace of thoughts. It can also prevent speaking in a monotone, or improve a speech pattern characterized by frequently interrupting the expression of a direct point with a qualifier or a contradictory thought.[11] Listening to the speech of radio journalists is illustrative of this maxim. Speaking in this way during testimony can also keep the court reporter from having to interrupt to ask a witness to repeat something, which can be disruptive to the continuity of the testimony.

Never accept the learned treatise as expertise unless you are master of it (p. 122). There are some "learned treatises" that are so basic to FMHA that the expert *should* have mastered them. For example, any expert using a diagnosis in the course of a report or testimony should be sufficiently familiar with DSM-IV so that the major categories and the internal diagnostic logic can be described.[12] However, there may be works with which the expert is only somewhat familiar, or entirely unfamiliar. To avoid being challenged by findings when the forensic clinician has not been able to review methodology *and* results, the preferable response is to indicate insufficient familiarity with the work to judge whether it is authoritative. To strengthen this response, it is also helpful to point out the relevant influential works with which the expert *is* familiar (Melton et al., 1997).

Listen with care to the wording of the attorneys' questions and use this knowledge in the interests of precision and control (p. 128). Just as experts should strive for precision in their use of language, so should they listen carefully to the precise questions they are asked. A vaguely or imprecisely

---

[11]Some clinicians who are bright and somewhat obsessive tend to speak using frequent qualifiers and self-interruptions. An example would be the following response to a question about whether a defendant was experiencing symptoms of a thought disorder around the time of an alleged offense: "Let me just respond to that. I think it's pretty likely—not certain, but likely—that Mr. Jones was having some problems with his thinking around the time you mention. He could have been having some problems with his perceptions, too, although there's not as much evidence for that as for problems with thinking; that evidence is strong, even though, as I said previously, I can't be certain about something like that." This style is annoying and confusing to the listener. Contrast this with a firm "Yes, he was. Both his own account and the descriptions of collateral observers indicated that he felt confused and frightened, and he also experienced the delusion that the Devil in human form was nearby."

[12]Other examples of strong candidates for learned treatise status include Melton et al. (1997) on forensic assessment, Grisso (1986a) on competencies, Rogers (1988, 1997b) on response style, and Monahan's work (1981; Monahan & Steadman, 1994) on violence risk assessment.

worded question can give the expert a chance to respond, truthfully, in a way quite different than the attorney might expect. For example, an attorney might have prepared her cross-examination by reading an article by Smith and Jones, who concluded that the diagnostic reliability of Disorder X is poor. If the attorney asked, "Doctor, isn't it true that, according to Smith and Jones, the diagnostic reliability of Disorder X is poor?", then the expert could indicate that the Smith and Jones article, in his view, was not authoritative, or could acknowledge the Smith and Jones conclusion but deny the larger implication of the diagnostic unreliability of Disorder X. However, if the question were phrased, "Doctor, isn't it true that the diagnostic reliability of Disorder X is poor?", then the expert has an additional option: simply responding "no," and elaborating if asked a follow-up question.[13]

When the time is right to disagree with cross-examination questions, do so with strength, clarity, and conviction (p. 131). Listening carefully can allow the expert to identify questions that are only partly accurate, but also those that convey an impression that is largely inaccurate. The responses to the latter kind of question can begin with a strongly worded phrase (e.g., "on the contrary" or "certainly not") that sets the tone for the remainder of the response. This should be used cautiously, however, and only when the response will contain information that is quite inconsistent with the question's implication. Experts who overuse this response can seem stubborn or argumentative, and hence less credible.

Effective witnesses are familiar with expected trial procedures, interpersonal transactions, and the dynamics of testifying (p. 136). As an expert becomes more familiar with legal procedures, she or he will be better able to decide when it is appropriate to respond, to pause, or to remain silent. Such procedures can vary considerably between courts (criminal versus juvenile, for example) and proceedings (e.g., deposition versus hearing versus bench trial versus jury trial). Observing such proceedings as a part of training, as well as being supervised in testimony, can help experts learn nuances and expectations, and respond accordingly.

Cross-examining attorneys will use substantive and psychological means to gain control over witnesses. Witnesses, in turn, need to be free of such control to perform well and feel good about their testimony (p. 139). Effective cross-examination by the opposing attorney should weaken the points made by

---

[13]Sometimes an attorney, surprised by a "no" when expecting an affirmative answer, will be thrown off-stride and follow up with a disbelieving "No?" This gives the expert the opportunity to disrupt the continuity of the questioning and to elaborate on why "no" is the better answer.

the expert during direct examination, and possibly strengthen alternative arguments favorable to the cross-examiner's case. One way to do this involves asking a series of questions, each calling for a short, affirmative answer. Experts can be drawn into the rhythm of responding "yes," resulting in the attorney doing most of the talking, and the expert affirming the points being made. To avoid this particular pattern, it is advisable to interrupt the rhythm. This can be done by pausing before replying, asking for a clarification, interspersing brief answers with narrative replies, and (if warranted) responding in an unexpected way.

Take a breath and explicitly think about questions that require thought (p. 142). Such a pause allows time to think. It also interrupts any pattern of responding too quickly.

Look at the jury during narrative answers and avoid being captured in eye contact by the cross-examining attorney (p. 146). The cross-examining attorney may attempt to maintain exclusive eye contact with the expert as a means to control the witness. If this is successful, then the expert pays attention to the attorney, not the jury, and therefore is less able to observe cues about the jurors' reactions, or to speak directly to the jurors. To avoid feeling controlled and responding only to the attorney, and to observe the reactions of members of the jury, the expert should shift her gaze between the attorney and the jury, spending most of her time during testimony looking at the jury.

When the cross-examination question is true but is asked in a pushy and negative manner, consider agreeing strongly (p. 166). Just as an unexpected "no" can be disorienting to an attorney, a strongly expressed agreement can unexpectedly change the tone of the cross-examination from adversarial to agreeable. The expert is less able to respond thoughtfully when kept off balance through verbal intimidation. An unexpected, strongly worded agreement can surprise the attorney, and allow the expert to regain control.

Dress for court in clothes that are familiar, comfortable, and professional (p. 191). Both Brodsky and Melton et al. (1997) make this point clearly. More detailed comments were offered earlier in this section.

Make the last impression a good one (p. 194). The completion of testimony, particularly when it has been long or grueling, can create such a feeling of relief that the expert may be tempted to leave the courtroom quickly. In addition, the forensic clinician may feel frustrated, confused, embarrassed, or angry if testimony has not gone well. Such feelings should be set aside temporarily. The expert should first thank the judge when she is dismissed. A pleasant nod to the jurors, and polite acknowledgment of both attorneys, will leave observers with the final impression of a professional who has been gracious, however the testimony has gone.

DISCUSSION

The available support for this principle is somewhat indirect for sources of ethical and legal authority. There is more direct support in the empirical and standard of practice areas, however.

The *Ethics Code* in psychology makes it clear that deception in expert testimony must be avoided, but it is not specific about the style of such testimony. However, in the *Specialty Guidelines*, it is noted that the "forceful representation" of data and reasoning in testimony is not precluded by the needs for accuracy and fairness. As long as the latter requirements are satisfied, however, there is nothing in the other psychology or psychiatry ethical standards to suggest that testifying in an effective manner, without deception, is problematic.

No statutes or case law relevant to this principle were located. Viewed broadly, however, our legal system is an adversarial one presuming that accurate decision-making is most likely when opposing positions are challenged. An attorney's or witness's persuasive style is an important element in litigation. As long as the expert is an advocate for her conclusions, and uses an effective style to present the substantive data and reasoning, there is practical support for such a style.

Empirical research has identified several ways in which experts may testify more effectively. Trustworthiness, expertise, and dynamism, as well as the abilities to communicate clearly and plainly, are all elements of an effective style. The ability to communicate complex material in an understandable way may promote "central" rather than "peripheral" decision-making among jurors, and minimize any tendency to rely on heuristic shortcuts. This is potentially an important link between substance and style in expert testimony. As well, these areas are related to a number of previous principles discussed in this book. Substantive expertise, impartiality, and clear communication of data and reasoning have each been incorporated into relevant principles, as have suggestions for how they might be operationalized. When such have already been considered at an earlier stage of FMHA, then conveying them in testimony is more straightforward.

Nonetheless, effective testimony involves more than communicating the results of the FMHA. The suggestions for stylistic effectiveness discussed in the present principle can contribute to the expert's ability to maintain credibility and control in testimony. A number of Brodsky's maxims are relevant to style, supporting the conclusion that a reasonable standard of practice for FMHA testimony involves stylistic as well as substantive components.

The classification of this principle will be conditional. To the extent that stylistic effectiveness in testimony is combined with substantive strength in FMHA, and deception is avoided, then this final principle appears *established*. However, when deception is involved in the style of testimony, or when the substance of testimony is not strong, then this principle is *neither established nor emerging*. It is actually inimical to the goal of better-informed legal decision-making to have expert testimony that is stylistically effective but substantively weak. Hence, the first 28 principles discussed in this book must be observed to make this final principle viable.

VI

Applying the Principles of Forensic Mental Health Assessment

12

Implications for Research, Training, Practice, and Policy

The principles described in this book have been derived from FMHA literature and standards that have evolved in significant ways during the last decade. However, there are important areas in which further work is needed. FMHA should become an applied activity that is strongly supported by a relevant empirical base, recognized realistically by the law for its potential strengths and limits, guided by applicable sources of ethics authority, and accompanied by a standard of practice literature that integrates these other areas with a realistic view of how FMHA is actually performed. This book provides some indication of the level of development in the FMHA field. It would have been different if it had been written 10 years ago, and it hopefully will be quite different 10 years hence.

The principles discussed in the last 10 chapters, and the support for each, have implications for research, training, practice, and policy that will be discussed in this chapter, moving from general to specific implications. Some research needs for FMHA are clear, particularly those seen in principles that are recognized by law and supported by ethics and practice literatures, but have little or no empirical support. Other research needs are apparent for principles with mixed support, but little empirical evidence regarding how the principle should be structured.

Training in FMHA has typically been structured by first exposing mental health professionals to relevant information about law, then describing the legal and forensic contours of various kinds of FMHA. There should be another step, however, focusing on the common aspects of various kinds of FMHA, and how forensic assessment is distinct from mental health evaluation that is done for diagnostic or treatment-planning purposes. The principles in this book provide the basis for this step. They allow trainees at levels ranging from the early exposure to FMHA in graduate school or residency, to continuing education for seasoned mental health professionals seeking to gain competence in FMHA. Even for clinicians who want to become competent in only one kind of FMHA, however, a mastery of the broad principles outlined in this book would be an important component of such competence.

The practice of FMHA includes both providing assessments and using them in litigation. Judges and attorneys play important roles in the effective use of FMHA, so the discussion of practice implications will include both legal and mental health professionals. Attorneys must decide whether to seek an FMHA for a client, how to frame the request, whether to use the results, and how to present or challenge the results in litigation. Judges must agree to authorize an FMHA, if the evaluation is requested under court order, and must also make important decisions regarding the use of FMHA. Under *Daubert*, judges are asked to play an even larger role, evaluating the scientific merit of various FMHA procedures used in the evaluation to determine their admissibility. The potential for mental health professionals to provide high-quality forensic assessment to attorneys and courts can be enhanced by a literature that provides guidance in relevant areas.

Finally, these principles have implications for policymakers. Such policy can range from administrative, involving agencies or courts which set standards concerning FMHA, to legislation that may have significant implications for FMHA, such as NGRI conditional release laws or sentencing laws concerning the assignment of "violent predator" status to convicted sexual offenders. Across this range of decisions, it is helpful for those who make or administer policy to receive guidance from the literature regarding the strengths, limitations, and applicability of FMHA.

IMPLICATIONS FOR RESEARCH

The contributions of science to FMHA include case-specific data and reasoning as well as empirical research, but there is no question that the field needs empirical scientific study in areas included in a number of FMHA principles. The "vision" for FMHA underlying this statement is the use of relevant, well-validated tools to assess forensic issues, persuading the law of the value of such tools. This does not imply that FMHA will be reduced to mechanistic proceedings with no role for reasoning or case-specific evidence. Rather, it suggests that important tools need to be added to the list from which forensic clinicians can select for a given case.

There are a number of research implications to be drawn from the review of the principles of FMHA. These will be discussed in terms of those ranging from the broadest implications to the most specific.

IDENTIFICATION OF RESEARCH QUESTIONS

The first observation about research needs is a general one. In reviewing the empirical research that was available for various principles, there were a number of instances in which there was no research available because it appeared that *the relevant research question(s) had not yet been identified.* A careful reading of this book, and others in the area of FMHA, will clearly yield a wealth of important questions, some of which can be operationalized and investigated scientifically. The areas under this discussion of research implications involve my perceptions of the important priorities for FMHA research, but other works on FMHA focusing in more detail on specific legal questions and forensic issues can provide a more fine-grained source of research questions.

IDIOGRAPHIC DATA, SCIENTIFIC REASONING, AND FMHA

Although it is primarily empirical research needs that are being described in this section, the potential respective roles of idiographic evidence and scientific reasoning that are discussed in Chapter 8 raise interesting questions about how such evidence and reasoning actually are applied. It is conceptually important to recognize these two separately, but it is equally important to assess how they are used, and their contributions to data gathering, reasoning, and drawing conclusions. Operationalizing the recognition and rating of these as research variables would be challenging. It might be approached through reviewing and rating a large number of FMHA reports and by interviewing experienced forensic clinicians in a semistructured way and content analyzing their responses on relevant questions.

EMPIRICAL DESCRIPTIONS OF NORMATIVE FMHA PRACTICE

Much of the debate concerning questions related to FMHA has occurred in the absence of virtually any good normative data on how FMHA is actually performed and perceived. Instead, such debate has given extraordinary weight to a relatively small number of cases (in the criminal context, typically those in which there has been a very serious alleged offense that is covered widely by the media) that are probably unrepresentative of the vast majority of cases in which FMHA is used.

The value of information about normative practice should be clear. The frequency and degree of poorly performed or misapplied FMHA could be gauged. As well, the frequency with which FMHA was performed well (using measures of quality discussed in the chapter) could be judged. This would allow criticisms to be made with more accuracy, and remedies planned more effectively, in the event of unacceptable findings. Investigations using multiple jurisdictions would also help to address questions concerning the specificity of some standards and procedures to a given jurisdiction versus the broader applicability of standards across jurisdictions. Normative data revealing differences between jurisdictions would not necessarily reflect problems in a given jurisdiction, but when "cross-jurisdictional" standards were not met, as revealed by normative research, then the conclusion regarding the existence of deficits would be clearer.

EMPIRICAL DESCRIPTIONS OF DESIRABLE FMHA PRACTICE

An important complement to research on normative FMHA practice is the investigation of desirable aspects of such practice. Such research involves obtaining perceptions of aspects of FMHA practice that are rated according to their value or appropriateness. In order to be particularly helpful, research like this should be done with individuals who are expert in FMHA, or with individuals who are frequent consumers of FMHA, such as judges or attorneys. It can also be helpful to do such research with participants who are responsible for a number of FMHAs performed under their auspices, a group such as forensic administrators.

Such research can serve two major purposes. First, it can help to identify potentially new measures of FMHA quality. A very comprehensive review of a large number of included factors in FMHA, such as that performed by Borum and Grisso (1996), can identify certain factors that may not have been considered or emphasized before in the literature. The forensic assessment field is still at a developmental stage in which the identification of such new components is feasible and helpful. Research such as the Borum and Grisso study should be performed with additional samples of forensic experts, legal consumers, and forensic administrators, and include FMHA in areas beyond their focus (CST and CR).

The second purpose of such research is to consider how the value assigned to certain FMHA procedures may vary across jurisdictions and across different kinds of evaluations. When such jurisdictional differences are observed, it might reflect the need for additional exposure to national standards to enhance consumers' understanding of the potential strengths and limits of FMHA. Alternatively, however, such findings could also reflect the need for a certain flexibility and capacity for accommodation in how FMHA (even as it becomes increasingly well defined with respect to core principles) is implemented in a given jurisdiction. The translation of FMHA research findings into jurisdiction-specific policy may not be straightforward, but having such research findings available would allow such policy to be empirically informed.

ASSESSING THE IMPACT OF TRAINING

One of the most important questions regarding FMHA is how it can be taught at various levels with the goal of improving the overall quality with which it is conducted. Such training is now available at graduate training, internship, and postdoctoral fellowship levels in psychology, and residency and fellowship levels in psychiatry. It is also available for both professions at the level of continuing professional education, which varies in intensity from single-day workshops on a few specific aspects of FMHA up to the multiday training and subsequent mentoring leading to a "certified forensic" designation that is available in a few U.S. states. Also, a workshop series in relevant FMHA topics is sponsored by the American Academy of Forensic Psychology for those preparing for diplomate examination in forensic psychology. Likewise, a review course of several days' duration, and relevant forensic workshops, are also available for psychiatrists pursuing board certification in forensic psychiatry from the American Board of Psychiatry and Neurology.

To what extent is such training effective in improving the quality of FMHA practice? The limited available evidence suggests that training can help to make forensic assessments more legally relevant, but many questions remain to be investigated. As the mental health professions become increasingly specialized, there will be attempts to define expertise at various levels (this will be discussed under "Implications for Training" later in this chapter). What would be the empirically developed criteria for demonstrating expertise at various levels? How can training be configured most efficiently to allow mental health professions to achieve a desired level of specialization? Questions such as these can be investigated empirically using good quality measures to operationalize FMHA outcome.

ASSESSING THE IMPACT OF FORENSIC SYSTEMS

Relatively little research has been conducted on the nature and configuration of the forensic system on the quality of FMHA products. Questions such as the source and level of funding for different services, the distribution of resources within a system, whether funding is public, private, or some combination, the number of evaluations funded for a single case, the disciplines of the evaluators, and a number of other possible influences can have an impact on FMHA reports and testimony. Some groundbreaking research has been performed in this area (see Grisso et al., 1994), but the potential strength of system-level variables should justify much more research. The ultimate question for policymakers who would be informed by such research is how forensic services can be delivered most efficiently within a system, considering that there are rarely sufficient resources to hire many highly specialized clinicians to deliver all forensic assessment services.

Measuring FMHA Quality

One of the most important needs for research involves measuring the quality of FMHA. Certainly this need applies to training, practice, and policy areas as well. But it is an important research question in the sense that a reliable and valid approach to measuring FMHA quality could be applied to addressing these questions in other areas. Moreover, such a measure would allow researchers to obtain information on the quality of service in this area being provided to courts and attorneys across a number of jurisdictions. The impact of such influences as how forensic services were organized within a jurisdiction, whether forensic training was available and at what levels, the characteristics of evaluators, the characteristics of those being evaluated, the nature of the litigation, the form in which evidence is presented (report only versus report and testimony), and a number of other factors could be influenced. One of the most important outcomes, however, is FMHA quality; when this is measured effectively, it will facilitate some of these other investigations.

Good measures of FMHA quality should incorporate the principles discussed in this book, the perceptions of legal professionals, and the perceptions of FMHA experts. They should be applied primarily to FMHA work products (reports and testimony). Research on the perceptions of quality add to this area in important ways, and may inform the development of measures of the quality of the product. However, there are often differences between what mental health professionals perceive they do, or report that they value, and what they actually do. Research on the quality of actual FMHA products can function as a crucial outcome variable for a variety of other factors that may be related to this outcome.

Expertise and Its Relation to FMHA Practice

The working assumption about expertise, in the absence of much data on the topic, is that the greater the expertise in the forensic area, the better the products. This broad assumption (which remains to be tested empirically) actually covers a series of questions, many of which seem amenable to empirical investigation. Expertise can be acquired in different ways, and it has only been relatively recently that specialized training at the graduate, internship, residency, and fellowship levels has become more widely available to those seeking it. Expertise in FMHA may also be acquired less formally, through a combination of experience, informal mentoring, surveying the literature in law and mental health, and continuing education. Many current forensic specialists, particularly those completing their formal training prior to 1980, have acquired their expertise in the latter fashion.

However, even a good awareness of law and forensic issues does not convey expertise across the range of evaluations, civil and criminal, that constitute the current domains of FMHA. In this book, I have argued that a two-part definition of expertise is appropriate: competence and experience in working with a particular population, and experience and awareness of legal and forensic matters. If such a definition were adopted, then the question would arise as to what proportion of FMHAs are currently performed by those meeting these criteria. Further, the field is moving toward implementing "levels" of expertise (see discussion under "Implications for Training" in this chapter). Can these be operationalized, and an intermediate level of quality or high level of quality in a more limited area be demonstrated?

These are important questions for legal decision-makers and policymakers as well. Knowing that FMHA services can meet a designated standard is valuable in deciding whether such services should be publicly funded, and at what level. Quality indicators, derived from the FMHA literature and tested for reliability, provide a reasonable basis for making such decisions. Before relevant law and policy are implemented that require FMHA to assist courts in decision-making, however, it would also be useful to provide information to legislators about the relationship between expertise (perhaps operationalized by such criteria as written tests of knowledge, observation of practice, board certification, and the like) and quality in FMHA, and the limits as well as the reasonable expectations that might apply.

COMMUNICATING FMHA FINDINGS AND LIMITS

How are FMHA data, reasoning, and conclusions communicated? The assertion of findings accompanied by limitations, the use of nontechnical language, and the relationship between the content of the report and that of expert testimony are each important areas for investigation. Moreover, how well are such findings understood by judges and attorneys? It may be that a certain style (e.g., one using frequent examples to illustrate data and reasoning) might be particularly effective. In this respect, research in this area could provide important clues about how an already-effective style of communication in FMHA could be altered to make it even better.

Research in this area should again investigate both normative practice and perceived effectiveness, as rated by the primary consumers of FMHA (legal professionals). The former investigation might involve a survey of forensic clinicians (involving descriptions of practice, ratings of desirability, or both) or review of work products (reports or testimony). The second area of study might by pursued through surveys of the primary consumers of FMHA—attorneys and judges. It would also be amenable to the use of experimental designs with future legal professionals (law students), who might be more readily available and willing to participate in such research.

THIRD-PARTY INFORMATION

Third-party information is one of the most important domains from which FMHA data are drawn, yet the empirical investigation of this area has been virtually nonexistent. To some extent this may reflect the perception that interviewing collateral observers and reviewing records and other documents is more of an art (akin to investigative journalism) than an area that can be investigated scientifically. Yet some have argued that such investigative reporting can itself be considered a kind of research method (Levine, 1980), and this book discusses the role of both idiographic evidence and reasoning as scientific contributions to FMHA.

It may be, therefore, that research on the use of third-party information will be facilitated by employing approaches that are sensitive to the ways in which third-party information is actually used. For example, rather than seeking a high degree of internal validity through controlling the information that is presented, a researcher might choose to maximize the external validity of a study on third-party information by providing sanitized material from actual cases. However, other approaches to the empirical study of third-party information could use more controlled designs that maximize internal validity. For example, one could measure the level of interrater agreement on certain structured questions following the review of documents, in the same way that one examines interrater reliability on items included on instruments such as the Psychopathy Checklist-Revised (which requires the evaluator to review relevant background records before making item ratings, and suggests that the PCL-R should not be used if such records are unavailable). Approaches to increasing the validity of the ratings of certain forensic issues from third-party information could be studied by considering the contribution of each collateral source separately; alternatively, reliability and validity could be assessed using a structured approach to rating whatever information (within certain defined limits) is available. Empirical study is badly needed in this area, and it is possible that some research strategies that have been used in the development of other forensically relevant tools might be applicable.

Measuring the Capacities Relevant to Notification of Purpose and Informed Consent

There has been little empirical work on the measurement of capacities relevant to the notification of purpose or informed consent step in FMHA. Researchers in this area must be particularly careful in designing studies and generalizing results, however, as the nature of the notification or consent is different depending on several considerations. For example, when the evaluation is court-ordered, the individual being evaluated has no legal right to refuse participation; when it is an attorney-requested consultation, there is an absence of any kind of legal coercion to participate.

Drawing on recent research in the area of treatment consent would be particularly helpful. Several areas need investigation. First, there is the question of whether an appropriate measure can be developed for the capacity to understand FMHA notification of purpose. This notification varies somewhat across different kinds of evaluations, so the measure would need to be sufficiently flexible to accommodate such variability. However, the understanding of such information would be an integral part of a second measure, which would address the capacity to consent to FMHA when informed consent is needed. A measure of informed consent in this area would also need to address the ability to rationally manipulate information to make a decision about participation. Thus, it might be possible to develop two flexible measures, the first for notification of purpose (measuring the capacity to understand relevant information) and the second for informed consent (measuring both capacity to understand and capacity for rational decision-making).

It would require considerable research effort to develop such tools well. Prior to undertaking it, therefore, it would be useful to obtain data about the need for such tools. We currently have no empirical guidance on the questions of (1) how frequently individuals undergoing court-ordered FMHA seem to have difficulty understanding the notification of purpose, (2) what currently happens when an individual does not appear to understand this notification under this circumstance, (3) whether it would therefore be helpful to evaluate the issue more formally, (4) how frequently individuals being evaluated for attorney-requested consultation apparently have difficulty with either the understanding or reasoning relevant to the decision to participate, (5) what occurs when they do not appear to have these capacities, and (6) whether it would be helpful to measure such capacities more formally.

ROLE CLARIFICATION AND DUAL ROLES

Ethics authorities are quite clear in recognizing the importance of considering one's role in FMHA, and actively discourage playing multiple roles. However, we have little available data regarding the entire process of role selection, reasoning about single versus multiple roles, or the frequency with which an initial role (e.g., that of impartial evaluator), when rendered moot by FMHA results that are not helpful to the referring attorney, might be abandoned, but another role assumed (e.g., that of consultant) in the course of a single case.

As health-care system changes make fee-for-service clinical practice increasingly difficult, there will be additional attention paid to "new markets." FMHA may represent an area to which some practitioners may turn, however poorly prepared or lacking in relevant knowledge and experience they may be. One particularly abused "back door" into FMHA and expert testimony is reportedly the child custody area, in which treating therapists agree to testify in custody proceedings, although we have no systematic data regarding this or other kinds of potential dual-role conflicts. There is a pressing need for empirical data and other attention to this particular issue, if the attempt to improve the overall quality of FMHA practice is not to be badly impeded by changing market forces. However, the literature on the relevant principles reviewed in this area did not yield a consensus about the established status of this principle, and the role of empirical data in addressing some of the current questions is crucial.

IMPARTIALITY

The assumption that a mental health professional will approach and carry out FMHA in an impartial way seems quite important, but has not been investigated. Indeed, there has been much discussion (on ethical grounds) about such importance, but very little attempt to even describe how it *might* be investigated. This would clearly be a difficult and sensitive topic to investigate with rigor. One of the major impediments to using a measure of impartiality and outcome measures of quality in actual work products is the problem with self-report; most forensic clinicians are well aware of the importance of impartiality in FMHA, and would probably be reluctant to fully describe instances in which impartiality may not have been achieved.

Nonetheless, there are approaches that might provide some useful answers to some of the questions in this area. For example, most forensic clinicians, in response to survey questions, would probably have no difficulty in identifying and prioritizing factors that potentially could interfere with impartiality. In a related vein, such participants might be able to describe factors that emerged in the course of the FMHA process (as opposed to those that were apparent at the time the referral was considered). Third, there is an important question about "bias management" that should be addressed. Impartiality is, of course, a goal that can never be fully realized in any evaluation, and one important question involves how potential challenges to impartiality are recognized and managed.

Other research strategies might capitalize on approaches that are less likely to induce defensiveness, such as hypothetical questions, vignette rating, and condensed case results involving other professionals. A possible two-part broad test of impartiality is suggested in this book: (1) a reasonable balance between favorable and unfavorable results rendered to referring sources and (2) reasonable consistency with available base rates. Also, researchers might employ different populations of participants, employing advanced graduate students in psychology (as did Otto, 1989), interns, fellows, or residents to investigate whether potential biasing influences remain constant from trainee to practicing clinician.

USING A MODEL

The use of a model in FMHA is neither discussed nor investigated empirically with any frequency. Yet the use of a good model in FMHA can probably have a favorable impact on the structure and organization of the report, and perhaps on the associated reasoning and subsequent testimony. Does using a model in FMHA increase the relevance of the way in which forensic issues are selected? Does it clarify reasoning, and promote improved structure in the written report? If it accomplishes these goals, then using a model might also have a favorable impact on the way in which FMHA reports are understood by judges and attorneys.

While this question has apparently not been investigated empirically, it would not be difficult to do so. Providing participants with mock (or sanitized) FMHA data and asking some to communicate the results using a model, while others would be designated to communicate in whatever fashion they chose, could begin to address the question of whether the use of a model has a favorable organizing impact at the time the report is being written. Its use could also be investigated at other stages of the process. Alternatively, reports at various levels of rated quality could also be rated as to whether a model was apparently employed. Such investigation could focus more attention on the use of a model, perhaps resulting in its more active consideration at various levels of training.

SPECIFYING THE FORENSIC ISSUES

As part of a larger deficit in normative data regarding FMHA, we know little about how well the relevant forensic issues are specified in reports and testimony by mental health professionals doing this work. In a related vein, we do not know how well the legal questions are identified. Several possible outcomes from research on these issues might be observed. The best kind of outcome would involve finding that evaluators were doing a reasonably good job of specifying both the legal question and the included forensic issues. It is also quite possible that research would reveal that the legal question is usually specified, but the relevant forensic issues are not identified well. Finally, it is conceivable that research across a range of jurisdictions and types of FMHA would suggest that neither the legal question(s) nor the included forensic issues are identified as frequently as they should be.

The findings in this area would have significant implications. Is the trend in FMHA practice paralleling that seen in research in the last 5–10 years? This research trend has involved measuring functional capacities primarily, with the implication that such information can be provided to the decision-maker, who considers it (along with other evidence and influences) in rendering a decision on the legal question. Without normative data on whether such functional capacities are being specified and addressed in FMHA, however, we cannot conclude that this approach has become part of forensic practice. If "capacity focus" has not become a part of FMHA, it could be because specifying and focusing on relevant forensic issues either requires a tool to guide such consideration, or a careful awareness of the legal context and demands and an attempt to translate those demands into measurable criteria. Since there are still relatively few specialized tools in FMHA, there is currently a considerable demand on the practitioner to identify forensic issues and structure the FMHA accordingly.

The more straightforward approach to specifying relevant forensic issues and structuring the FMHA around them involves the development of additional forensic tools. The movement in this area has been positive and encouraging during the last 5–10 years, with empirically based tools developed in the areas of competence for trial, competence to consent to treatment, risk assessment, malingering of mental health symptoms, and malingering of cognitive deficits, among others. If this trend continues, and such tools are well developed, validated, and commercially available with appropriate levels of documentation, then the focus on appropriate forensic issues in FMHA should be facilitated.

FEES

No research is available at present on the issues of fee clarification, fee setting, or the impact of professional fees on FMHA. How do fees compare with those from other kinds of mental health practice? How do forensic clinicians determine fees? Some clinicians may charge at a higher rate for testimony than for evaluation time. How frequent is this, and what is the difference? How do forensic clinicians control the potential bias introduced by having one party in litigation responsible for the entire fee? Other influence may be introduced by charging very high fees. How is potential bias controlled under this circumstance?

The issue of whether expert mental health testimony as part of FMHA can be "bought" or "influenced" is actually two different questions. The prospect that a forensic clinician would fabricate or distort the results of FMHA obviously exists, but hopefully this phenomenon is relatively rare. (Some critics of FMHA claim otherwise, but it's difficult to envision the kind of research design that would yield valid empirical data on this issue.) What is undoubtedly more frequent is the influence of financial considerations on the way in which FMHA is conducted and communicated. More open discussion of this issue, as well as empirical investigation, would be helpful.

VISIBILITY OF CASES

One of the ways in which FMHA differs from other kinds of mental health assessment is in its public visibility, as reflected in media coverage, public awareness, and potential consequences for elected officials involved in the legal process. Even within FMHA, however, there is a range in case visibility from routine cases of low visibility to cases of very high visibility, typically involving individuals who are already well known to the public and/or offenses of extreme seriousness, accompanied by intense media coverage. The latter kind of cases, although only a small percentage of the overall number of cases to which FMHA is applied, tend to receive a grossly disproportionate share of public attention, and are probably highly influential in shaping the public's views regarding FMHA.

Yet there are doubtless a number of important differences between high- and low-visibility cases for FMHA. Considerations such as the time invested in the evaluations, the fees provided to experts, the selection process for such forensic clinicians, the probability of testimony following the evaluation, and the intensity of preparation by attorneys for both sides as well as the forensic clinicians involved are some such differences. These may be the inevitable correlates of events that are perceived as very important by all involved. Would the principles outlined in this book apply in the same way in high-visibility cases? Are there potential sources of bias for participating forensic clinicians that are stronger in high-visibility cases than in low? Empirical investigation in this area would promote a better understanding of the decision-making process in such cases relevant to FMHA, and the indicated adjustments necessary for the forensic clinician to preserve impartiality and respect the integrity of the FMHA process.

THE ULTIMATE LEGAL ISSUE

In its most basic form, the ultimate issue debate concerns whether data and reasoning forming the basis for conclusions will be provided to the decision-maker, and whether the focus of FMHA will be on areas within the forensic clinician's expertise. Simply keeping experts from addressing the ultimate issue may not improve the overall quality of FMHA, however, and may also frustrate practicing judges, who (according to the limited available research) report a preference for ultimate issue testimony (and as much other relevant FMHA information as they can possibly receive).

If this debate is to continue, it must be better informed by empirical data. One alternative to ultimate issue testimony involves the focus on the relevant forensic issues, which should be well described and helpful to the court, and the attempt to avoid an ultimate opinion on the grounds that good evaluation and testimony regarding included forensic issues is as far as FMHA can go in approaching the ultimate issue. Will this compromise, which would involve an evaluation approach consistent with the recent development of tools to empirically measure forensic capacities, satisfy courts that might prefer ultimate issue testimony? Can the rationale for such an approach and limit in evaluation and testimony persuade legal decision-makers? Is ultimate issue testimony, although theoretically undesirable, a necessary step in having other aspects of FMHA admitted by courts? If research were framed to address not simply the question of whether ultimate issue testimony is valued by courts, but also to determine whether the "focus on forensic issues" approach just discussed might be an acceptable compromise, then perhaps some real progress could be made in this debate.

IMPLICATIONS FOR TRAINING

LEVELS OF SPECIALIZATION

There has been recent effort within the forensic psychology field to describe expertise at the levels of the *informed*, the *proficient*, and the *specialized* clinician. If the basis for the first largely involves an awareness of relevant laws guiding practice, in the same way that a clinician should be aware of appropriate ethical standards, research, and practice literature, then training such individuals in the principles described in this book—applicable to various forms of FMHA—would not be indicated.

However, proficient and specialized clinicians should be aware of general principles applicable to FMHA, and their implications for practice across a variety of kinds of forensic evaluations. In turn, this has implications for how and when such training should be provided. It would seem preferable to begin training forensic clinicians broadly, and then move subsequently toward more specific areas. Combining training in broad principles with didactic exposure to a text (such as Melton et al., 1997) that provides a comprehensive overview of relevant law, research, and practice considerations for a number of kinds of FMHA, would provide a needed overview for those beginning the process of specialization. Following this level of training, the curriculum or mentor could provide more specific training in areas that are now beginning to be covered in books as well (e.g., juvenile forensic evaluations, risk assessment, civil forensic evaluations, assessing response style). When accompanied by supervised experience, such didactic training, provided over several years, could establish a solid base for the developing forensic specialist.

ROLE OF PRINCIPLES

When the principles discussed in this book are used in training, they can serve several purposes. First, they will introduce the trainee to relevant sources of authority in ethics, law, empirical research, and standards of practice. As part of this exposure, it will become clear that there are gaps in the support provided for some principles in some of these areas, which should help to engender a realistic perception of how the field has developed and important ways in which such development must continue. Second, considering these principles will help trainees learn about the clear differences between FMHA and therapeutic assessment; however, if they have some training or experience in the latter area already, it may also allow them to assess common ground and build on their existing strengths. Moreover, these principles are not described at a level that would allow anyone, without further training, to begin to conduct FMHA. However, *with further training,* they should provide a context for more specific forms of FMHA that are ultimately mastered by demonstrating the relationship between different forms of FMHA. Finally, they should provide (in a fairly concentrated way) a guide for how a trainee can begin to think like a forensic clinician. Ultimately, if that trainee should pursue board certification in forensic psychology or psychiatry, or should conduct research in FMHA, an awareness of the common elements of FMHA should allow more sophisticated thinking about any of its particular variations, leading to research and practice that is more relevant and legally sensitive.

EXPANDING TRAINING OPPORTUNITIES

Training in FMHA principles could be integrated into a formal curriculum as part of graduate, residency, or fellowship training. However, the demand for relevant forensic training for individuals who are already practicing clinicians will undoubtedly produce more training offerings in this area. Designing training that provides the opportunity for a clinician to expand his or her competence into the forensic area will need to be done carefully, to avoid the problem of "clinically competent but forensically naive" individuals beginning to provide services to the courts on a large-scale basis. However, for some such individuals, reality constraints will not allow taking a year away from practice to complete a full-time fellowship in forensic psychiatry or forensic psychology. An acceptable compromise might involve a half-time fellowship (if it were available), or a contractual, part-time mentoring relationship with a forensic specialist who agreed to provide supervision with some didactic training, sufficient to allow a competent clinician to provide appropriate FMHA in targeted areas at the completion of a mentoring period.

TRAINING IN FMHA-RELEVANT PROCEDURES

An additional component of forensic training at several levels would involve the exposure to certain specialized inventories and tools that have been developed to measure forensic issues. It is important to gain competence with such tools at the same level one might become competent to administer and interpret a traditional psychological test (for psychologists) or a mental status interview (for psychiatrists). Additionally, psychiatrists who wished to use such tools would need some formal training in the area of test development, validation, administration, and interpretation.

However, beyond an awareness of the nature of the tool, its purpose, and how to administer, score, and interpret it, there is more required for the trainee to integrate such tools into the larger FMHA context. Specialized tools are one part of FMHA. They may be a very important part, particularly if they are appropriately developed and validated, and have respectable psychometric properties. However, an understanding of how the results of the specialized tool can be integrated with other sources of information, how these results should be communicated, and a number of other considerations about FMHA must be integrated with training in specialized tools for the most meaningful development of sophistication in FMHA.

INTEGRATING SCIENCE AND PRACTICE

Many clinicians are trained to consider research findings and integrate them into practice. However, the respective roles of idiographic and nomothetic evidence and scientific reasoning, as they are applied to FMHA, are applied in somewhat different ways than in therapeutic assessment. They represent a "way of thinking" as much as an exposure to relevant empirical research. As such, the development of these capacities for the trainee learning about FMHA depends both on supervised experience and on didactic learning. It can be particularly valuable to work with a mentor who can model the use of each.

IMPLICATIONS FOR PRACTICE

MEASURING FMHA QUALITY IN PRACTICE

The possible application of these principles to the development of "FMHA quality indicators" for use in empirical study was discussed earlier in this chapter. However, these principles represent a distillation of what currently exists in the literature; as such, they could be applied to the development of "quality indicators" for monitoring FMHA practice in the same way that any literature review could yield such criteria. FMHA products, such as reports, testimony, and related products (e.g., consultation that does not yield a written report), may be evaluated according to their degree of "fit" with these principles. Clearly some flexibility and accommodation to jurisdiction-specific law and policy would be needed if this were done. However, supervisors and agency administrators should not necessarily assume that "local practice convention" should trump a principle if the two are inconsistent. Instead, it would be advisable to carefully consider the reason for the inconsistency; there is always the possibility that local practice might be inconsistent with the standards of the field, and could benefit by moving in the direction of such standards.

Answering Specific Questions

One of the reasons that this book is structured as it is involves access to specific information concerning a principle. Anyone wanting to know whether the AAPL *Ethical Guidelines*, for example, addresses the issue of informed consent in FMHA can locate this information readily. Once the reader is familiar with the book's structure, then comparably specific questions can be researched quickly. The book also reflects the absence of relevant information from a given source of authority on a specific point, which can sometimes be as useful as knowing what *is* available.

Threats to FMHA Integrity

A number of influences can diminish the quality of a given FMHA. Experienced forensic clinicians who are highly competent have almost always developed ways of recognizing and managing these influences to protect the "integrity" of the FMHA process (as well as others' perceptions of the clinician's integrity). However, such knowledge has often been gained through the unfortunate experience of having one or more of these problems arise in the course of an evaluation, and in a way that was more difficult to handle than would have been the case if primary prevention or early detection had been operative.

Readers who are not highly experienced forensic clinicians, however, can find a description of many of these problems discussed, as well as their possible impact on FMHA. Potential difficulties such as lack of impartiality, limited time, poor evaluation circumstances, irrelevant and unreliable procedures, nonparsimonious or otherwise inappropriate interpretation, and poor communication are among the most important. Perhaps this accounting will allow some evaluators to avoid the problems that can come from learning about these "integrity threats" firsthand.

Dual Roles

The literature is not entirely clear about the avoidance of dual roles in FMHA. However, this question might be considered as follows. The risk to a forensic clinician's reputation for impartiality that is created by dual-role problems is never a problem if dual roles are strictly avoided. Conversely, while some apparent advantages may accrue to the attorney or client who asks a treating therapist to testify as an expert about a legal issue (a forensic role), there is relatively little to be gained for the therapist. The exception to this, of course, is that a therapist would be paid for such testimony (and perhaps at a higher rate than the hourly therapy fee, as well as being paid out-of-pocket rather than through a third-party provider). However, therapists who provide treatment to families and children can certainly pursue additional forensic training (if needed) that would make them sufficiently competent to perform child custody evaluations, and perform such evaluations with children and families who are not therapy patients. There is risk associated with performing such dual-role evaluations: It is almost always unethical, and they could be sued as a result.

My recommendation, therefore, is to avoid dual roles strictly and entirely. In order to carry this out, a clinician will need to anticipate that, at times, a therapy patient might request a therapist's involvement in a forensic role. There are certainly cases in which this seems more likely (e.g., cases in which a single parent requests treatment for a child, is in the process of a divorce, and has already retained an attorney). Clinicians can then notify patients at the beginning of a therapeutic relationship about how they will serve as therapists but not for other purposes, perhaps even specifying what other purposes are sometimes requested, and indicate their willingness to refer the individual or family to another individual for forensic evaluation if that should become important.

FROM TREATING CLINICIAN TO INVESTIGATIVE JOURNALIST

Some significant reconsideration of the contours of role is important as a psychologist or psychiatrist conducts FMHA. As the respective fields of forensic psychology and forensic psychiatry mature, the injunction to "think like a forensic mental health professional" may develop a clear, specific meaning. However, these fields have probably not yet reached the stage at which this kind of phrase has a generally accepted meaning even within the broader fields of psychology and psychiatry, let alone with the general public.

What can be helpful is the consideration of an analogous profession in which many of the tasks are comparable to those undertaken in FMHA. The field of investigative journalism has served this function well, both because it has a more consensually accepted meaning and because it is so visible in the public eye. Examining the principles derived and discussed in this book underscores this point—in many important respects, psychologists and psychiatrists in a forensic role do not behave like treating therapists, nor should they be expected to. In particular, the skills involved in "truth seeking," checking facts through the use of multiple sources of information, assessing the contribution of any given source and eliminating those with little or no credibility, accessing documents, and reviewing third parties are as essential to FMHA as they are to good investigative journalism.

NOTIFICATION OF PURPOSE AND INFORMED CONSENT

The issues of notification of purpose and informed consent in FMHA are complex. They also vary across kinds of FMHA and associated legal circumstances, as well as the age and other capacities of the individual(s) being evaluated. Forensic clinicians should therefore take steps to help ensure that the notification delivered prior to beginning the evaluation is appropriate to the circumstances, and that the client's understanding of the information can be assessed and described. When it is appropriate to go beyond notification of purpose and obtained informed consent, the forensic clinician should also be prepared to assess the reasoning capacity underlying the decision about participation.

This means that the practicing forensic clinician should consider these questions and develop an appropriate form or checklist containing the relevant points of information to be delivered for each kind of FMHA that is to be performed. It is probably not necessary to deliver this in written form and ask for a client's signature by way of acknowledgment. Although this is preferable in some respects, it also may increase problems in comprehension (verbal notifications are easier to use interactively, and the forensic clinician can use cues about the client's responding to help gauge whether the wording and concepts have been understood). It may also make some individuals even more suspicious than they might have been initially. However notifications and requests for informed consent are administered, there should certainly be a set of written prompts for the evaluator's use, and at least some brief discussion of the information to assess how well it was understood.

ADMINISTRATION CONDITIONS

Many times FMHAs are conducted in settings or under circumstances in which an individual is in custody, or there are related issues involving security. Certainly these priorities must be respected. However, the need for security must be balanced with the need for a setting in which there is privacy and relative freedom from distraction. The failure to obtain an evaluation setting in which these features are present can invalidate or severely bias the results of the FMHA. Diplomacy and flexibility in working with facility staff can often yield improved conditions without having to resort to the more draconian solution of contacting the referring attorney or the court in the attempt to resolve difficulties in this area.

FORENSIC ISSUES AND ULTIMATE LEGAL QUESTIONS

At present, forensic clinicians may not be forced to choose between refusing to give an ultimate legal opinion (on ethical or theoretical grounds) versus reporting and testifying in a way that exceeds the bounds of the forensic clinician's expertise. Forensic clinicians observing the research trend involving the measurement of forensic issues rather than ultimate legal questions can justifiably focus their evaluation efforts on assessing the functional legal capacities that are the focus of "forensic issues." In some cases, they may be assisted by the use of specialized forensic tools, which will be applied in the same way they were developed (e.g., the measurement of capacities relevant to competence rather than competence as a larger construct). In order to perform evaluations and communicate results in this way, however, forensic clinicians will need to develop a convincing justification for why they are avoiding the ultimate legal question. As an increased number of specialized forensic tools are developed, it may be that the justification for avoiding the ultimate issue is given less in theoretical and ethical terms than with the explanation that the primary focus of the FMHA, and the supporting relevant research, is on measuring relevant capacities rather than reaching conclusions about ultimate legal questions.

Expert Testimony

Skilled expert testimony depends to some extent on communicating effectively and persuasively in general, and other "impression management" skills. These skills should be developed by all forensic clinicians, and honed until they are at least reasonably good. However, another large part of testifying effectively as a mental health expert involves performing FMHA well, and conveying the evaluation's procedures and results in testimony. In this respect, forensic clinicians' efforts to incorporate these principles in FMHA will pay consistent dividends, whether testimony is required or not. In those cases in which no testimony is needed, the report serves as a means of conveying the procedures and results; an impressive report may sometime be sufficiently persuasive or otherwise sufficient so that testimony is not required when it otherwise would have been. However, no effort is wasted by applying these principles to the FMHA report when testimony is needed, as the forensic clinician will be attempting to convey in testimony much of what has already been communicated in the report.

IMPLICATIONS FOR POLICY

Identifying Areas Relevant to FMHA

Legislators or legal decision-makers may pass or implement law that involves the contribution of FMHA without recognizing this. This may occur, for example, when states pass sentencing laws concerning "sexual predators," allowing the sentencing court the prospect of a significant upward departure on the finding that a convicted offender is a "sexually violent predator." Mental health professionals may become involved in such determinations through nomination to a "board" or assigned list of evaluators. When such mental health professionals are selected for their treatment expertise with sexual offenders, but have little or no expertise in FMHA, then the result can be having reports sent to sentencing courts that would violate many of the principles described in this book.

Two oversights are illustrated by this kind of experience. The first is that of the policymakers who passed the law but failed to identify the decision-making assistance from mental health professionals as FMHA rather than therapeutic evaluation, and of the administrative support provided to the implementation of this law, where the same failure occurred. The second oversight is on the part of those mental health professionals who became associated with the board's evaluation process while not realizing that the demand for evaluating convicted sexual offenders at the sentencing stage was a somewhat different form of an FMHA sentencing evaluation. Policymakers and administrative support staff might use the principles described in this book to make such a distinction, or to remedy existing problems as they begin to occur.

Setting Standards for FMHA

Just as these principles might be used by agencies or clinics to evaluate the quality of FMHA services that they provide, they could also use them in prescriptive fashion. By specifying in their own policy how these principles should be operationalized in reports, that agency could come closer to ensuring that their FMHA services are consistent with the broader standards and sources of authority described in the existing literature. Agency policy could also be written to accommodate differences between their goals or resources and those that would be implied by the implementation of these principles. Like individual practitioners seeking to monitor their own FMHA performance, however, changes should be carefully considered. Further, the evaluation of adherence to and monitoring of compliance with prescribed areas will help such agencies to ensure that policy is being carried out consistently.

Potential Contributions of FMHA

Assessing the potential contributions of FMHA in a reasonable fashion requires a working knowledge of the current state of the field. There are some respects in which the FMHA has made significant, even dramatic, progress in the kind of information that can be provided to assist legal decision-makers and attorneys. Areas such as risk assessment, response style, and the capacities underlying various legal competencies now feature research support, specialized tools, and considerably more sophisticated theoretical underpinnings than existed a decade ago. FMHA has now reached a level of development where it is reasonable to talk about prescriptive standards for its practice, to develop guidelines to assist practitioners in various FMHA areas, and to identify a broad set of principles characterizing the entire process.

Certainly the strengths and potential contributions of this field are more apparent as it has matured. To the extent that related policy has not kept pace with the developments in the field, it should be updated to reflect such advances.

LIMITS OF FMHA

The principles in this book and their discussion also provide important indications of areas in which FMHA has not yet developed an adequate empirical base, resulting in the inability to provide empirical data as part of evaluation of certain forensic issues. There remain disagreements concerning ultimate issue testimony and multiple roles as part of FMHA. It would be helpful to have specialized tools developed in more areas for which capacities must be measured. It is important to have these limits reflected as well in policy relevant to FMHA. The history of the discipline of forensic psychology and psychiatry reflects the premature and somewhat naive enthusiasm for the application of mental health concepts and research to the practice of law, resulting in the disillusionment of some who had to consider inconsistent, intrusive, and irrelevant testimony stemming from inapplicable theory and the absence of good data. As the forensic specialty fields mature in the early twenty-first century, commentators and policymakers should combine critical thinking with cautious optimism to establish limits as well as opportunities that are both dictated by genuine advances and demonstrable areas of limitation.

REASONABLE BALANCES FOR POLICY

The need for such limits is driven not only by scientific and ethical constraints, but also by practical considerations that must influence policy relevant to FMHA. Questions such as reasonable expectations for quality, balanced against existing constraints in staffing, funding, and other resources and competing against other time demands must be considered.

However, efficiency is one of the considerations of investigators developing forensic specialty tools as well. Policymakers should pay particular attention to developments in this area, for empirically developed screening tools and specialty applications are likely to be both cost effective and frequently better in many other respects than some procedures that require the labor intensive participation of a forensic specialist.

However, there is no immediate prospect for the obsolescence of forensic specialty practitioners. Quite the contrary; despite significant advances in FMHA, its quality remains dependent to a large extent on the skills of the individual practitioner. When such skills are elaborated in systematic form, using quality measures, decision trees, and more structured measures, and are reflected in the policy of an agency or administration that has been reviewed by those with specialized knowledge, then such policy is most likely to appropriately balance the dual goals of quality and efficiency in FMHA.

References

Achenbach, T. (1991). *Manual for the Child Behavior Checklist/4-18 and 1991 Profile*. Burlington: University of Vermont Department of Psychiatry.

Achenbach, T.M., & Edelbrok, C. (1983). *Manual for the Child Behavior Checklist and Revised Child Behavior Profile*. Burlington: Department of Psychiatry, University of Vermont.

Ackerman, M. (1999). *Essentials of forensic psychological assessment*. New York: John Wiley & Sons.

Ackerman, M., & Kane, A. (1998). *Psychological experts in divorce actions* (3rd ed.). New York: Aspen Law & Business.

Ackerman, M., & Schoendorf, K. (1992). *The Ackerman–Schoendorf Parent Evaluation of Custody Tests (ASPECT)*. Los Angeles: Scales for Western Psychological Services.

American Academy of Child and Adolescent Psychiatry. (1997). Practice parameters for child custody evaluation. *Journal of the American Academy of Child and Adolescent Psychiatry, 36* (10 Supplement), 57S–68S.

American Academy of Psychiatry and the Law. (1995). *Ethical guidelines for the practice of forensic psychiatry*. Bloomfield, CT: Author.

American Academy of Psychiatry and the Law, Association of Directors of Forensic Psychiatry Fellowships. (2000). *Directory of forensic psychiatry fellowships*. Bloomfield, CT: Author.

American Bar Association. (1980). *Standards for criminal justice* (2nd ed.). Washington, DC: Author.

American Bar Association. (as amended 1980). *Model code of professional responsibility*. Washington, DC: Author.

American Bar Association. (1984). *Criminal justice mental health standards*. Washington, DC: Author.

American Bar Association. (1989). *Criminal justice mental health standards*. Washington, DC: Author.

American Bar Association Special Committee on Jury Comprehension. (1989). *Jury comprehension in complex cases*. Washington, DC: Author.

American Psychiatric Association. (1994). *Diagnostic and statistical manual of mental disorders* (4th ed.). Washington, DC: Author.

American Psychiatric Association. (1998). *The principles of medical ethics with annotation especially applicable to psychiatry*. Washington, DC: Author.

American Psychological Association. (1978). Report of the task force on the role of psychology in the criminal justice system. *American Psychologist, 33*, 1099–1113.

American Psychological Association. (1985). *Standards for educational and psychological testing*. Washington, DC: Author.

American Psychological Association. (1986a). *Brief amicus curiae*, in *Colorado v. Connelly* (1986). Washington, DC: Author.

American Psychological Association. (1986b). *Guidelines for computer-based tests and interpretations*. Washington, DC: Author.

American Psychological Association. (1992). Ethical principles of psychologists and code of conduct. *American Psychologist, 47*, 1597–1611.

American Psychological Association. (1994). Guidelines for child custody evaluations in divorce proceedings. *American Psychologist, 49*, 677–680.

American Psychological Association. (1995, April). APA recognizes areas of expertise in practice. *APA Monitor*, p. 45.

Anastasi, A. (1988). *Psychological testing* (6th ed.). New York: Macmillan.

Andersen, S.M., & Harthorn, B.H. (1989). The Diagnostic Knowledge Inventory: A measure of knowledge about psychiatric diagnosis. *Journal of Clinical Psychology, 45*, 999–1013.

Anderten, P., Staulcup, V., & Grisso, T. (1980). On being ethical in legal places. *Professional Psychology, 11*, 764–773.

Appelbaum, K. (1990). Criminal defendants who desire punishment. *Bulletin of the American Academy of Psychiatry and the Law, 18*, 385–391.

Appelbaum, K., & Zaitchik, M. (1995). Mental health professionals play critical role in presentencing evaluations. *Mental and Physical Disability Law Reporter, 19*, 677–683.

Appelbaum, P.S. (1983). Death, the expert witness, and the dangers of going Barefoot. *Hospital and Community Psychiatry, 34*, 1003–1004.

Appelbaum, P.S. (1984a). Hypotheticals, psychiatric testimony, and the death sentence. *Bulletin of the American Academy of Psychiatry and Law, 12*, 169–177.

Appelbaum, P.S. (1984b). Psychiatric ethics in the courtroom. *Bulletin of the American Academy of Psychiatry and Law, 12*, 225–231.

Appelbaum, P.S. (1985). The role of the mental health professional in court. *Hospital and Community Psychiatry, 36*, 1043–1044, 1046.

Appelbaum, P.S. (1987). In the wake of *Ake*: The ethics of expert testimony in an advocate's world. *Bulletin of the American Academy of Psychiatry and Law, 15*, 15–25.

Appelbaum, P.S. (1990). The parable of the forensic psychiatrist. *International Journal of Law and Psychiatry, 13*, 249–259.

Appelbaum, P.S. (1993). *Godinez v. Moran*: The U.S. Supreme Court considers competence to stand trial. *Hospital and Community Psychiatry, 44*, 929–930.

Appelbaum, P.S. (1998). Missing the boat: Competence and consent in psychiatric research. *American Journal of Psychiatry, 155*, 1486–1488.

Appelbaum, P.S., & Grisso, T. (1995). The MacArthur Treatment Competence Study. I: Mental illness and competence to consent to treatment. *Law and Human Behavior, 19*, 105–126.

Appelbaum, P.S., & Gutheil, T.G. (1991). *Clinical handbook of psychiatry and the law* (2nd ed.). Baltimore: Williams & Wilkins.

Arkes, H.R. (1981). Impediments to accurate clinical judgment and possible ways to minimize their impact. *Journal of Consulting and Clinical Psychology, 49*, 323–330.

Ash, P., & Guyer, M. (1986). The functions of psychiatric evaluation in contested child custody and visitation cases. *Journal of the American Academy of Child Psychiatry, 25*, 554–561.

Audubon, J.J., & Kirwin, B.R. (1982). Defensiveness in the criminally insane. *Journal of Personality Assessment, 46*, 304–311.

Bagby, R., Gillis, J., Toner, B., & Goldberg, J. (1991). Detecting fake-good and fake-bad responding on the Millon Clinical Multiaxial Inventory-II. *Psychological Assessment, 3*, 496–498.

Bagby, R.M., Nicholson, R.A., Rogers, R., & Nussbaum, D. (1992). Domains of competency to stand trial: A factor analytic study. *Law and Human Behavior, 16*, 491–507.

Bagby, R.M., Rogers, R., Nicholson, R., Buis, T., Seeman, M., & Rector, N. (1997). Effectiveness of the MMPI-2 validity indicators in the detection of defensive responding in clinical and nonclinical samples. *Psychological Assessment, 9*, 406–413.

Bank, S., & Poythress, N. (1983). The elements of persuasion in expert testimony. *Journal of Psychiatry and Law, 10*, 173–204.

Barnard, G.W., Nicholson, R.A., Hankins, G.C., Raisani, K.K., Patel, N.R., Gies, D., & Robbins, L. (1992). Itemmetric and scale analysis of a new computer-assisted competency assessment instrument (CADCOMP). *Behavioral Sciences and the Law, 10*, 419–435.

Bartol, C., & Bartol, A. (1987). History of forensic psychology. In I.B. Weiner & A. Hess (Eds.), *Handbook of forensic psychology* (pp. 3–21). New York: Wiley.

Bazelon, D.L. (1978). The role of the psychiatrist in the criminal justice system. *Bulletin of the American Academy of Psychiatry and Law, 6*, 139–146.

Beaber, R.J., Marston, A., Michelli, J., & Mills, M.J. (1985). A brief test for measuring malingering in schizophrenic individuals. *American Journal of Psychiatry, 142*, 1478–1481.

Beckham, J., Annis, L., & Bein, M. (1986). Don't pass go: Predicting who returns from court as remaining incompetent for trial. *Criminal Justice and Behavior, 13*, 99–109.

Bell, F., Hoff, A., & Hoyt, K. (1964). Answer sheets do make a difference. *Personnel Psychology, 17*, 65–71.

Bem, D., & Allen, A. (1974). On predicting some of the people some of the time: The search for cross-situational consistencies in behavior. *Psychological Review, 81*, 506–520.

Bem, D., & Funder, D. (1978). Predicting more of the people more of the time: Assessing the personality of situations. *Psychological Review, 85*, 485–501.

Bemporad, J.R., & Schwab, M.E. (1986). The DSM-III and child clinical psychiatry. In T. Millon & G.L. Klerman (Eds.), *Contemporary directions in psychopathology* (pp. 135–150). New York: Guilford Press.

Bennett, G., & Kish, G. (1990). Incompetency to stand trial: Treatment unaffected by demographic variables. *Journal of Forensic Sciences, 35*, 403–412.

Bennett, G.T., & Sullwold, A.F. (1985). Qualifying the psychiatrist as a lay witness: A reaction to the American Psychiatric Association petition in *Barefoot v. Estelle. Journal of Forensic Sciences, 30*, 462–466.

Berry, D.T., Baer, R., & Harris, M.J. (1991). Detection of malingering on the MMPI: A meta-analysis. *Clinical Psychology Review, 11*, 585–598.

Bersoff, D. (1995). *Ethical conflicts in psychology.* Washington, DC: American Psychological Association.

Bersoff, D., Glass, D., Dodds, L., Eckl, L., & Peters, L. (1999). *The admissibility of forensic psychological and social science evidence.* Currently unpublished paper, Villanova Law School, Villanova, PA.

Bersoff, D., Goodman-Delahunty, J., Grisso, T., Hans, V., Poythress, N.G., & Roesch, R. (1997). Training in law and psychology: Models from the Villanova Conference. *American Psychologist, 52*, 1301–1310.

Binder, L. (1990). Malingering following minor head trauma. *Clinical Neuropsychologist, 4*, 25–36.

Binder, L., & Kelly, M. (1996). Portland Digit Recognition Test performed by brain dysfunction patients without financial incentives. *Assessment, 3*, 403–409.

Binder, L., & Willis, S. (1991). Assessment of motivation after financially compensable minor head trauma. *Psychological Assessment: A Journal of Consulting and Clinical Psychology, 3*, 175–181.

Black, H.C. (1983). *Black's law dictionary.* St. Paul, MN: West.

Blau, T. (1984a). Psychological tests in the courtroom. *Professional Psychology: Research and Practice, 15*, 176–186.

Blau, T. (1984b). *The psychologist as expert witness*. New York: Wiley.

Blumberg, S. (1967). The MMPI F Scale as an indicator of severity of psychopathology. *Journal of Clinical Psychology, 23,* 96–99.

Bonnie, R. (1989). *Competency in the criminal process*. Unpublished paper presented at the meeting of the MacArthur Network for Research on Mental Health and the Law, New York, NY.

Bonnie, R. (1990). The competence of criminal defendants with mental retardation to participate in their own defense. *Journal of Criminal Law and Criminology, 81,* 419–446.

Bonnie, R. (1992). The competence of criminal defendants: A theoretical reformulation. *Behavioral Sciences and the Law, 10,* 291–316.

Bonnie, R., Hoge, S.K., Monahan, J., Poythress, N.G., Eisenberg, M., & Feucht-Haviar, T. (1997). The MacArthur Adjudicative Competence Study: A comparison of criteria for assessing the competence of criminal defendants. *Journal of the American Academy of Psychiatry and the Law, 25,* 249–258.

Bonnie, R., & Slobogin, C. (1980). The role of mental health professionals in the criminal process: The case for informed speculation. *Virginia Law Review, 66,* 427–522.

Borum, R., & Grisso, T. (1995). Psychological test use in criminal forensic evaluations. *Professional Psychology: Research and Practice, 26,* 465–473.

Borum, R., & Grisso, T. (1996). Establishing standards for criminal forensic reports: An empirical analysis. *Bulletin of the American Academy of Psychiatry and the Law, 24,* 297–317.

Borum, R., Swartz, M., & Swanson, J. (1996). Assessing and managing violence risk in clinical practice. *Journal of Practical Psychiatry and Behavioral Health, 4,* 205–215.

Brehm, S., Kassin, S., & Fein, S. (1999). *Social psychology* (4th ed.). Boston: Houghton Mifflin.

Bricklin, B. (1992). Data-based tests in custody evaluations. *American Journal of Family Therapy, 20,* 254–265.

Brigham, J. (1999). What is forensic psychology, anyway? *Law and Human Behavior, 23,* 273–298.

Brodsky, S.L. (1991). *Testifying in court: Guidelines and maxims for the expert witness*. Washington, DC: American Psychological Association.

Brodsky, S.L., & Robey, A. (1972). On becoming an expert witness: Issues of orientation and effectiveness. *Professional Psychology, 3,* 173–176.

Brodzinsky, D.M. (1993). On the use and misuse of psychological testing in child custody evaluations. *Professional Psychology: Research and Practice, 24,* 213–219.

Brown, J.W. (1987). The microstructure of action. In E. Perecman (Ed.), *The frontal lobes revisited* (pp. 251–272). New York: IRBN Press.

Bursten, B. (1982). The psychiatrist-witness and legal guilt. *American Journal of Psychiatry, 139,* 784–788.

Bursten, B. (1985). Detecting child abuse by studying the parents. *Bulletin of the American Academy of Psychiatry and the Law, 13,* 273–281.

Butcher, J., Dahlstrom, W., Graham, J., Tellegen, A., & Kaemmer, B. (1989). *MMPI-2: Manual for administration and scoring*. Minneapolis: University of Minnesota Press.

Campbell, D., & Fiske, D. (1959). Convergent and discriminant validation by the multitrait–multimethod matrix. *Psychological Bulletin, 56,* 81–105.

Carbonell, J.L., Heilbrun, K., & Friedman, F.L. (1992). Predicting who will regain trial competency: Initial promise unfulfilled. *Forensic Reports, 5,* 67–76.

Carlin, A., & Hewitt, P. (1990). The discrimination of patient-generated and randomly generated MMPIs. *Journal of Personality Assessment, 54,* 24–29.

Cecil, J., Hans, V., & Wiggins, E. (1991). Citizen comprehension of difficult issues: Lessons learned from civil jury trials. *American University Law Review, 40,* 727–774.

Cecil, J., & Willging, T. (1994). Court–appointed experts. In Federal Judicial Center, *Reference Manual on Scientific Evidence*. Washington, D.C.

Chaiken, S. (1980). Heuristic versus systematic information processing and the use of source versus message cues in persuasion. *Journal of Personality and Social Psychology, 39*, 752–766.

Champagne, A., Shuman, D., & Whitaker, E. (1991). An empirical examination of the use of expert witnesses in American courts. *Jurimetrics Journal of Law, Science, and Technology, 31*, 375–392.

Ciccone, J.R., & Clements, C.D. (1984). The ethical practice of forensic psychiatry: A view from the trenches. *Bulletin of the American Academy of Psychiatry and Law, 12*, 263–277.

Clark, C.R. (1982). Clinical limits of expert testimony on diminished capacity. *International Journal of Law and Psychiatry, 5*, 155–170.

Cofer, C.N., Chance, J., & Judson, A.J. (1949). A study of malingering on the MMPI. *Journal of Psychology, 27*, 491–499.

Coggins, M., Pynchon, M.R., & Dvoskin, J. (1998). Integrating research and practice in federal law enforcement: Secret Service applications of behavioral science expertise to protect the President. *Behavioral Sciences and the Law, 16*, 51–70.

Colbach, E.M. (1981). Integrity checks on the witness stand. *Bulletin of the American Academy of Psychiatry and the Law, 9*, 285–288.

Committee on Ethical Guidelines for Forensic Psychologists. (1991). Specialty guidelines for forensic psychologists. *Law and Human Behavior, 15*, 655–665.

Committee on Government Policy, Group for the Advancement of Psychiatry. (1994). *Forced into treatment: The role of coercion in clinical practice*. Washington, DC: American Psychiatric Association.

Conte, J., Sorenson, E., Fogarty, L., & Rosa J. (1991). Evaluating children's reports of sexual abuse: Results from a survey of professionals. *American Journal of Orthopsychiatry, 61*, 428–437.

Coons, P. (1989). Iatrogenic factors in the misdiagnosis of multiple personality disorder. *Dissociation: Progress in the Dissociative Disorders, 2*, 70–76.

Cooper, D., & Grisso, T. (1997). Five year research update (1991–1995): Evaluations for competence to stand trial. *Behavioral Sciences and the Law, 15*, 347–364.

Cooper, J., Bennett, E., & Sukel, H. (1996). Complex scientific testimony: How do jurors make decisions? *Law and Human Behavior, 20*, 379–394.

Cooper, J., & Neuhaus, I. (2000). The "hired gun" effect: Assessing the effect of pay, frequency of testifying, and credentials on the perception of expert testimony. *Law and Human Behavior, 24*, 149–171.

Cronbach, L.J. (1971). Test validation. In R.L. Thorndike (Ed.), *Educational measurement* (2nd ed., pp. 443–509). Washington, DC: American Council on Education.

Cruise, K., & Rogers, R. (1998). An analysis of competency to stand trial: An integration of case law and clinical knowledge. *Behavioral Sciences and the Law, 16*, 35–50.

Curran, W., McGarry, A., & Shah, S. (Eds.). (1986). *Forensic psychiatry and psychology: Perspectives and standards for interdisciplinary practice*. Philadelphia: Davis.

Curran, W., McGarry, A., & Shah, S. (Eds.). (1987). *Modern legal psychiatry and psychology*. Philadelphia: Davis.

Dahlstrom, W.G., Welsh, G.S., & Dahlstrom, L.E. (1972). *An MMPI handbook: Vol. I. Clinical interpretation* (rev. ed.). Minneapolis: University of Minnesota Press.

Dammeyer, M. (1988). The assessment of child sexual abuse allegations: Using research to guide clinical decision making. *Behavioral Sciences and the Law, 16*, 21–34.

Daniel, A., & Resnick, P. (1987). Mutism, malingering, and competency to stand trial: A conceptual model for its proper assessment. *Bulletin of the American Academy of Psychiatry and the Law, 15*, 85–94.

Dawes, R., Faust, D., & Meehl, P. (1989). Clinical versus actuarial judgment. *Science, 243*, 1668–1674.

Dennis, D., & Monahan, J. (Eds.). (1996). *Coercion and aggressive community treatment: A new frontier in mental health law.* New York: Plenum Press.

Diamant, J.J., & Hijmen, R. (1981). Comparison of test results obtained with two neuropsychological test batteries. *Journal of Clinical Psychology, 37,* 355–358.

Diamond, B.L. (1983). The psychiatrist as expert witness. *Psychiatric Clinics of North America, 6,* 597–609.

Dietz, P. (1978). Forensic and non-forensic psychiatrists: An empirical comparison. *Bulletin of the American Academy of Psychiatry and the Law, 6,* 13–22.

Dietz, P., Matthews, D., Martell, D., & Stewart, T. (1991). Threatening and otherwise inappropriate letters to members of the United States Congress. *Journal of Forensic Sciences, 36,* 1445–1468.

Dietz, P., Matthews, D., Van Dayne, C., Martell, D., Parry, C., Stewart, T., Warren, J., & Crowder, J. (1991). Threatening and otherwise inappropriate letters to Hollywood celebrities. *Journal of Forensic Sciences, 36,* 185–209.

Drob, S., Berger, R., & Weinstein, H. (1987). Competency to stand trial: A conceptual model for its proper assessment. *Bulletin of the American Academy of Psychiatry and the Law, 15,* 85–94.

Duncan, J. (1995). *Medication compliance in schizophrenic patients.* Unpublished dissertation, University of North Texas, Denton.

Ekman, P., & O'Sullivan, M. (1991). Who can catch a liar? *American Psychologist, 46,* 913–920.

Elwork, A. (1984). Psychological assessments, diagnosis and testimony: A new beginning. *Law and Human Behavior, 8,* 197–203.

Emery, R.E., & Rogers, K.C. (1990). The role of behavior therapists in child custody cases. *Progress in Behavior Modification, 26,* 60–88.

Endicott, J., & Spitzer, R.L. (1978). A diagnostic interview: The Schedule for Affective Disorders and Schizophrenia. *Archives of General Psychiatry, 35,* 837–844.

Everington, C.T. (1990). The Competence Assessment for Standing Trial for Defendants with Mental Retardation: A validation study. *Criminal Justice and Behavior, 17,* 147–168.

Ewing, C.P. (Ed.). (1985). *Psychology, psychiatry, and the law: A clinical and forensic handbook.* Sarasota, FL: Professional Resource Exchange, Inc.

Ewing, C.P. (1987). *Battered women who kill: Psychological self defense as legal justification.* Lexington, MA: Heath.

Ewing, C.P. (1990). Psychological self-defense: A proposed justification for battered women who kill. *Law and Human Behavior, 14,* 579–594.

Faigman, D. (1995). The evidentiary status of social science under Daubert: Is it "scientific," "technical," or "other" knowledge? *Psychology, Public Policy, and Law, 1,* 960–979.

Fairbank, J.A., McCaffrey, R.J., & Keane, T.M. (1985). Psychometric detection of fabricated symptoms of Posttraumatic Stress Disorder. *American Journal of Psychiatry, 142,* 501–503.

Faust, D. (1989). Data integration in legal evaluations: Can clinicians deliver on their premises? *Behavioral Sciences and the Law, 7,* 469–483.

Faust, D. (1995). The detection of deception. *Neurological Clinics, 13,* 255–265.

Faust, D., Hart, K., & Guilmette, T. (1988). Pediatric malingering: The capacity of children to fake believable deficits of neuropsychological testing. *Journal of Consulting and Clinical Psychology, 56,* 578–582.

Faust, D., & Ziskin, J. (1988). The expert witness in psychology and psychiatry. *Science, 241,* 31–35.

Faust, D., & Ziskin, J. (1991). *Forensic neuropsychology: Challenging the assessment of brain damage.* Marina Del Rey, CA: Law and Psychology Press.

Federal Judicial Center. (1994). *Reference manual on scientific evidence.* Washington, DC: U.S. Government Printing Office.

Federal Rules of Evidence for United States Courts and Magistrates. (1987). St. Paul, MN: West.

Fein, R.A., Appelbaum, K.L., Barnum, R., Baxter, P., Grisso, T., & Leavitt, N. (1991). The designated forensic progressional program: A state government–university partnership to improve forensic mental health services. *Journal of Mental Health Administration, 18,* 223–230.

Fein, R., & Vossekuil, B. (1998). Preventing attacks on public officials and public figures: A Secret Service perspective. In R. Meloy (Ed.), *The psychology of stalking: Clinical and forensic perspectives* (pp. 175–191). San Diego: Academic Press.

Felner, R., Rowlison, R., Farber, S., Primavera, J., & Bishop, T. (1987). Child custody resolution: A study of social science involvement and impact. *Professional Psychology: Research and Practice, 18,* 468–474.

Felthous, A.R. (1986). Schizotypal personality disorder and the insanity defense. *Journal of Forensic Sciences, 31,* 1016–1022.

Fisher, D. (1994). *Daubert v. Merrell Dow Pharmaceuticals*: The Supreme Court gives federal judges the keys to the gate of admissibility of expert scientific testimony. *South Dakota Law Review, 39,* 141–158.

Fitch, W.L., Petrella, R.C., & Wallace, J. (1987). Legal ethics and the use of mental health experts in criminal cases. *Behavioral Sciences and the Law, 5,* 105–117.

Florida Mental Health Institute. (1989). *Florida forensic evaluator training manual.* Tampa, FL: Author.

Flynn, J. (1987). Massive IQ gains in 14 nations: What IQ tests really measure. *Psychological Bulletin, 101,* 171–191.

Frazen, M., Iverson, G., & McCracken, L. (1990). The detection of malingering in neuropsychological assessment. *Neuropsychology Review, 1,* 247–279.

Frazier, P.A., & Borgida, E. (1992). Rape trauma syndrome: A review of case law and psychological research. *Law and Human Behavior, 16,* 293–311.

Frederick, R. (1997). *Validity Indicator Profile manual.* Minneapolis, MN: National Computer Systems.

Freedman, A., Kaplan, H., & Sadock, B. (1980). *Comprehensive textbook of psychiatry* (Vol. 3, 3rd ed.). Baltimore: Williams & Wilkins.

Gannon, J. (1990). Validation of the Competency Assessment Instrument and elements of competency to stand trial. *Dissertation Abstracts International, 50-B,* 3875.

Garb, H.N. (1984). The incremental validity of information used in personality assessment. *Clinical Psychology Review, 4,* 641–655.

Garb, H.N. (1989). Clinical judgment, clinical training, and professional experience. *Psychological Bulletin, 105,* 387–396.

Garb, H.N. (1992). The *trained* psychologist as expert witness. *Clinical Psychology Review, 12,* 451–467.

Geller, J., & Lister, E. (1978). The process of criminal commitment for pre-trial psychiatric examination: An evaluation. *American Journal of Psychiatry, 135,* 53–63.

Giannelli, P. (1983). *Frye vs. United States. Federal Rules Decisions, 99,* 189–202.

Giannelli, P., & Imwinkelried, E. (1993). *Scientific evidence* (2nd ed.). Charlottesville, VA: The Michie Company.

Glassman, J. (1998). Preventing and managing board complaints: The downside risk of custody evaluation. *Professional Psychology: Research and Practice, 29,* 121–124.

Golding, S. (1990). Mental health professionals and the courts: The ethics of expertise. *International Journal of Law and Psychiatry, 13,* 281–307.

Golding, S. (1993). *The Interdisciplinary Fitness Interview-Revised.* Salt Lake City: University of Utah.

Golding, S., Eaves, D., & Kowaz, A. (1989). The assessment, treatment, and community outcome of insanity acquittees: Forensic history and response to treatment. *International Journal of Law and Psychiatry, 12,* 149–179.

Golding, S., & Roesch, R. (1987). The assessment of criminal responsibility: An historical approach to a current controversy. In I. Weiner & A. Hess (Eds.), *Handbook of forensic psychology* (pp. 396–436). New York: Wiley.

Golding, S., Roesch, R., & Schreiber, J. (1984). Assessment and conceptualization of competency to stand trial: Preliminary data on the Interdisciplinary Fitness Interview. *Law and Human Behavior, 3,* 321–334.

Goldstein, A., & Burd, M. (1990). Role of delusions in trial competency evaluations: Case law and implications for forensic practice. *Forensic Reports, 3,* 361–386.

Goldstein, R. (1988). Psychiatrists in the hot seat: Discrediting doctors by impeachment of their credibility. *Bulletin of the American Academy of Psychiatry and the Law, 16,* 225–234.

Goldstein, R. (1989a). Spying on psychiatrists: Surreptitious surveillance of the forensic psychiatric examination by the patient himself. *Bulletin of the American Academy of Psychiatry and the Law, 17,* 367–372.

Goldstein, R. (1989b). The psychiatrist's guide to right and wrong: Part IV: The insanity defense and the Ultimate Issue Rule. *Bulletin of the American Academy of Psychiatry and the Law, 17,* 269–281.

Goldstein, R., & Stone, M. (1977). When doctors disagree: Differing views on competency. *Bulletin of the American Academy of Psychiatry and Law, 5,* 90–97.

Goodman–Delahunty, J., & Foote, W. (1995). Compensation for pain, suffering, and other psychological injuries: The impact of Daubert on employment discrimination claims. *Behavioral Sciences and the Law, 13,* 183–206.

Goodwin, D.W., Alderson, P., & Rosenthal, R. (1971). Clinical significance of hallucinations in psychiatric disorders. *Archives of General Psychiatry, 24,* 76–80.

Gothard, S., Rogers, R., & Sewell, K. (1995). Feigning incompetency to stand trial: An investigation of the Georgia Court Competency Test. *Law and Human Behavior, 19,* 363–373.

Gough, H.G. (1950). The F minus K dissimulation index for the MMPI. *Journal of Consulting Psychology, 14,* 408–413.

Gough, H.G. (1987). *Manual for the California Psychological Inventory* (2nd ed.). Palo Alto, CA: Consulting Psychologists Press.

Greenberg, J., & Wursten, A. (1988). The psychologist and the psychiatrist as expert witnesses: Perceived credibility and influence. *Professional Psychology: Research and Practice, 19,* 373–378.

Greenberg, S., & Brodsky, S. (in press). *The civil practice of forensic psychology: Torts of emotional distress.* Washington, DC: American Psychological Association.

Greenberg, S., & Shuman, D. (1997). Irreconcilable conflict between therapeutic and forensic roles. *Professional Psychology: Research and Practice, 1,* 50–57.

Greene, R.L. (1978). An empirically derived MMPI carelessness scale. *Journal of Clinical Psychology, 34,* 407–410.

Greene, R.L. (1979). Response consistency on the MMPI: The TR index. *Journal of Personality Assessment, 43,* 69–71.

Greene, R.L. (1980). *The MMPI: An interpretive manual.* New York: Grune & Stratton.

Greene, R.L. (1988). Assessment of malingering and defensiveness by objective personality inventories. In R. Rogers (Ed.), *Clinical assessment of malingering and deception* (pp. 123–158). New York: Guilford Press.

Greene, R. (1991). *The MMPI-2/MMPI: An interpretive manual.* Boston: Allyn & Bacon.

Greene, R.L. (1997). Assessment of malingering and defensiveness by multiscale inventories. In R. Rogers (Ed.), *Clinical assessment of malingering and deception* (2nd ed., pp. 169–207). New York: Guilford Press.

Grisso, T. (1981). *Juveniles waiver of rights: Legal and psychological competence.* New York: Plenum Press.

Grisso, T. (1986a). *Evaluating competencies: Forensic assessments and instruments.* New York: Plenum Press.

Grisso, T. (1986b). Psychological assessment in legal contexts. In W. Curran, A.L. McGarry, & S. Shah (Eds.), *Forensic psychiatry and psychology: Perspectives and standards for interdisciplinary practice* (pp. 103–128). Philadelphia: Davis.

Grisso, T. (1988). *Competency to stand trial evaluations: A manual for practice.* Sarasota, FL: Professional Resource Exchange.

Grisso, T. (1992). Five-year research update (1986–1990): Evaluations for competence to stand trial. *Behavioral Sciences and the Law, 10,* 353–369.

Grisso, T. (1993). The differences between forensic psychiatry and forensic psychology. *Bulletin of the American Academy of Psychiatry and the Law, 21,* 133–145.

Grisso, T. (1996). Pretrial clinical evaluations in criminal cases: Past trends and future directions. *Criminal Justice and Behavior, 23,* 90–106.

Grisso, T. (1998a). *Forensic evaluation of juveniles.* Sarasota, FL: Professional Resource Press.

Grisso, T. (1998b). *Instruments for assessing and understanding appreciation of Miranda rights.* Sarasota, FL: Professional Resource Press.

Grisso, T., & Appelbaum, P.S. (1995). The MacArthur Treatment Competency Study: III. Abilities of patients to consent to psychiatric and medical treatments. *Law and Human Behavior, 19,* 149–174.

Grisso, T., & Appelbaum, P.S. (1996). Values and limits of the MacArthur Treatment Competency Study. *Psychology, Public Policy, and Law, 2,* 167–181.

Grisso, T., & Applebaum, P.S. (1998a). *Assessing competence to consent to treatment: A guide for physicians and other health professionals.* London: Oxford University Press.

Grisso, T., & Appelbaum, P.S. (1998b). *MacArthur Competence Assessment Tool for Treatment (MacCAT-T).* Sarasota, FL: Professional Resource Press.

Grisso, T., Appelbaum, P.S., & Hill-Fotouhi, C. (1997). The MacCAT-T: A clinical tool to assess patients' capacities to make treatment decisions. *Psychiatric Services, 48,* 1415–1419.

Grisso, T., Appelbaum, P.S., Mulvey, E., & Fletcher, K. (1995). The MacArthur Treatment Competence Study: II. Measures of abilities related to competence to consent to treatment. *Law and Human Behavior, 19,* 127–148.

Grisso, T., Cocozza, J., Steadman, H., Fisher, W., & Greer, A. (1994). The organization of pretrial forensic evaluation services: A national profile. *Law and Human Behavior, 18,* 377–393.

Grisso, T., Miller, M., & Sales, B. (1987). Competency to stand trial in juvenile court. *International Journal of Law and Psychiatry, 10,* 1–20.

Grove, W.M. (1987). The reliability of psychiatric diagnosis. In C.G. Last & M. Hersen (Eds.), *Issues in diagnostic research* (pp. 99–119). New York: Plenum Press.

Grove, W.M., Andreasen, N.C., McDonald-Scott, P., Keller, M.B., & Shapiro, R.W. (1981). Reliability studies of psychiatric diagnosis. *Archives of General Psychiatry, 38,* 408–413.

Grove, W.M., & Meehl, P. (1996). Comparative efficiency of informal (subjective, impressionistic) and formal (mechanical, algorithmic) prediction procedures: The clinical-statistical controversy. *Psychology, Public Policy, and Law, 2,* 293–323.

Grove, W.M., Zald, D.H., Lebow, B.S., Snitz, B.E., & Nelson, C.E. (2000). Clinical vs. mechanical prediction: A meta-analysis. *Psychological Assessment, 12,* 19–30.

Grow, R., McVaugh, W., & Eno, T.D. (1980). Faking and the MMPI. *Journal of Clinical Psychology, 36,* 910–911.

Gudjonsson, G.H. (1990). One hundred alleged false confession cases: Some normative data. *British Journal of Clinical Psychology, 29,* 249–250.

Gudjonsson, G.H., Petursson, H., Skulason, S., & Siguroardottir, H. (1989). Psychiatric evidence: A study of psychological issues. *Acta Psychiatrica Scandinavica, 80*, 165–169.

Gutheil, T.G. (1992). Approaches to forensic assessment of false claims of sexual misconduct by therapists. *Bulletin of the American Academy of Psychiatry and Law, 20*, 289–296.

Gutheil, T.G., Bursztajn, H., & Brodsky, A. (1986). The multidimensional assessment of dangerousness: Competence assessment in patient care and liability prevention. *Bulletin of the American Academy of Psychiatry and the Law, 14*, 123–129.

Gutheil, T.G., & Simon, R. (1997). Clinically based risk management principles for recovered memory cases. *Psychiatric Services, 48*, 1403–1407.

Halleck, S.L. (1980). *Law in the practice of psychiatry: A handbook for clinicians.* New York: Plenum Press.

Haney, C. (1980). Psychology and legal change: On the limits of a factual jurisprudence. *Law and Human Behavior, 4*, 147–199.

Hare, R. (1991). *The Hare Psychopathy Checklist-Revised.* Toronto, Canada: Multi-Health Systems.

Hare, R.D., Harpur, T.J., Hakstian, A.R., Forth, A.E., Hart, S., & Newman, J. (1990). The revised Psychopathy Checklist: Reliability and factor structure. *Psychological Assessment: A Journal of Consulting and Clinical Psychology, 2*, 338–341.

Haroun, A., & Morris, G. (1999). Weaving a tangled web: The deceptions of psychiatrists. *Journal of Contemporary Legal Issues, 10*, 227–246.

Harris, G., Rice, M., & Quinsey, V. (1993). Violent recidivism of mentally disordered offenders: The development of a standard prediction instrument. *Criminal Justice and Behavior, 20*, 315–335.

Hart, S.D., & Hare, R.D. (1989). Discriminant validity of the Psychopathy Checklist in a forensic psychiatric population. *Psychological Assessment: A Journal of Consulting and Clinical Psychology, 1*, 211–218.

Hart, S.D., & Hare, R.D. (1992). Predicting fitness to stand trial: The relative power of demographic, criminal, and clinical variables. *Forensic Reports, 5*, 53–65.

Hawk, G.L., & Cornell, D.G. (1989). MMPI profiles of malingerers diagnosed in pretrial forensic evaluations. *Journal of Clinical Psychology, 45*, 673–678.

Heaton, R.K., Smith, H.H., Lehman, R.W., & Vogt, A.T. (1978). Prospects for faking believable deficits on neuropsychological testing. *Journal of Consulting and Clinical Psychology, 46*, 892–900.

Heilbrun, A.B. (1990). The measurement of criminal dangerousness as a personality construct: Further validation of a research index. *Journal of Personality Assessment, 54*, 141–148.

Heilbrun, K. (1987). The assessment of competency for execution: An overview. *Behavioral Sciences and the Law, 5*, 383–396.

Heilbrun, K. (1988, March). *Third party information in forensic assessment: Much needed, sometimes collected, poorly guided.* Presented at the American Psychology–Law Society/Division 41 Mid-Year Conference, Miami, FL.

Heilbrun, K. (1990). Response style, situation, third party information, and competency to stand trial: Scientific issues in practice. *Law and Human Behavior, 14*, 193–196.

Heilbrun, K. (1992). The role of psychological testing in forensic assessment. *Law and Human Behavior, 16*, 257–272.

Heilbrun, K. (1995). Child custody evaluation: Critically assessing mental health experts and psychological tests. *Family Law Quarterly, 29*, 63–78.

Heilbrun, K. (1996, March). *Daubert and forensic mental health assessment: Use and implications.* Presented at the Biennial Conference of the American Psychology–Law Society/Division 41, Hilton Head, SC.

Heilbrun, K. (1997). Prediction vs. management models relevant to risk assessment: The importance of legal context. *Law and Human Behavior, 21*, 347–359.

Heilbrun, K., & Annis, L.V. (1988). Research and training in forensic psychology: National survey of forensic facilities. *Professional Psychology: Research and Practice, 19*, 211–215.

Heilbrun, K., Bennett, W.S., White, A.J., & Kelly, J. (1990). An MMPI-based model of malingering and deception. *Behavioral Sciences and the Law, 8*, 45–53.

Heilbrun, K., & Collins, S. (1995). Evaluations of trial competency and mental state at the time of the offense: Report characteristics. *Professional Psychology: Research and Practice, 26*, 61–67.

Heilbrun, K., Hart, S., Hare, R., Gustafson, D., Nunez, C., & White, A. (1998). Mentally disordered offenders and inpatient aggression: The role of psychopathy. *Journal of Interpersonal Violence, 13*, 514–527.

Heilbrun, K., Leheny, C., Thomas, L., & Huneycutt, D. (1997). A national survey of U.S. statutes on juvenile transfer: Implications for policy and practice. *Behavioral Sciences and the Law, 15*, 125–149.

Heilbrun, K., & McClaren, H. (1988). Assessment of competency for execution? A guide for mental health professionals. *Bulletin of the American Academy of Psychiatry and Law, 16*, 205–215.

Heilbrun, K., Rosenfeld, B., Warren, J., & Collins, S. (1994). The use of third party information in forensic assessments: A two-state comparison. *Bulletin of the American Academy of Psychiatry and the Law, 22*, 399–406.

Heim, N. (1987). Psychiatric expert testimony on aggressive offenders in juvenile court proceedings. *Forensic Sciences International, 34*, 29–38.

Hellerstein, D., Frosch, W., & Koenigsberg, H. (1987). The clinical significance of command hallucinations. *American Journal of Psychiatry, 144*, 219–221.

Herman, S.P. (1990). Special issues in child custody evaluations. *Journal of the American Academy of Child and Adolescent Psychiatry, 29*, 969–974.

Hess, A. (1998). Accepting forensic case referrals: Ethical and professional considerations. *Professional Psychology: Research and Practice, 29*, 109–114.

Hiscock, M., & Hiscock, C.K. (1989). Refining the forced-choice method for the detection of malingering. *Journal of Clinical and Experimental Neuropsychology, 11*, 967–974.

Hofer, P., & Green, B. (1985). The challenge of competence and creativity in computerized psychological testing. *Journal of Consulting and Clinical Psychology, 53*, 826–838.

Hoge, R., & Andrews, D. (1994). *The Youth Level of Service/Case Management Inventory and manual.* Ottawa, Ontario: Department of Psychology, Carleton University.

Hoge, S.K., Bonnie, R.J., Poythress, N., & Monahan, J. (1992). Attorney-client decision-making in criminal cases: Client competence and participation as perceived by their attorneys. *Behavioral Sciences and the Law, 10*, 385–394.

Hoge, S.K., Bonnie, R., Poythress, N., Monahan, J., Eisenberg, M., & Feucht-Haviar, T. (1997). The MacArthur adjudicative competence study: Development and validation of a research instrument. *Law and Human Behavior, 21*, 141–182.

Hoge, S.K., & Grisso, T. (1992). Accuracy and expert testimony. *Bulletin of the American Academy of Psychiatry and Law, 20*, 67–76.

Hoge, S.K., Poythress, N.G., Bonnie, R., Monahan, J., Eisenberg, M., & Feucht-Haviar, T. (1997). The MacArthur adjudicative competence study: Diagnosis, psychopathology, and competence-related abilities. *Behavioral Sciences and the Law, 15*, 329–345.

Homant, R.J., & Kennedy, D.B. (1986). Judgment of legal insanity as a function of attitude toward the insanity defense. *International Journal of Law and Psychiatry, 8*, 67–81.

Horowitz, I., Willging, T., & Bordens, K. (1998). *Psychology of law: Integrations and applications* (2nd ed.). New York: Longman.

Howard, R.C. (1990). Psychopathy Checklist scores in mentally abnormal offenders: A re-examination. *Personality and Individual Differences, 11,* 1087–1091.

Howard, R.C., Bailey, R., & Newman, A. (1984). A preliminary study of Hare's "Research Scale for the Assessment of Psychopathy" in mentally-abnormal offenders. *Personality and Individual Differences, 5,* 389–396.

Hyler, S.E., Williams, J.B.W., & Spitzer, R.L. (1982). Reliability in the DSM-III field trials: Interview vs. case summary. *Archives of General Psychiatry, 39,* 1275–1278.

Institute of Law, Psychiatry, and Public Policy. (1995). *Basic forensic evaluation training.* Charlottesville: University of Virginia.

Jackson, M.W. (1986). Psychiatric decision-making for the courts: Judges, psychiatrists, lay people? *International Journal of Law and Psychiatry, 9,* 451–468.

Johnson, W., & Mullet, N. (1987). Georgia Court Competency Test-R. In M. Hersen & A. Bellack (Eds.), *Dictionary of behavioral assessment techniques.* New York: Pergamon Press.

Johnson, W.G., Nicholson, R.A., & Service, N.M. (1990). The relationship of competency to stand trial and criminal responsibility. *Criminal Justice and Behavior, 17,* 169–185.

Junginger, J. (1990). Predicting compliance with command hallucinations. *American Journal of Psychiatry, 147,* 245–247.

Kane, R.L., Parsons, O.A., Goldstein, G., & Moses, J.A. (1987). Diagnostic accuracy of the Halstead–Reitan and Luria–Nebraska neuropsychological batteries: Performance of clinical raters. *Journal of Consulting and Clinical Psychology, 55,* 783–784.

Kapp, M., & Mossman, D. (1996). Measuring decisional capacity: Cautions on the construction of a "capacimeter." *Psychology, Public Policy, and Law, 2,* 73–95.

Karson, S., & O'Dell, J. (1976). *A guide to the clinical use of the 16 PF.* Champaign, IL: Institute for Personality and Ability Testing.

Keilin, W., & Bloom, L. (1986). Child custody evaluation practices: A survey of experienced professionals. *Professional Psychology: Research and Practice, 17,* 338–346.

Keilitz, I., & Holmstrug, M.E. (1981). Perspectives on mental health screening and evaluation. *State Court Journal, 5,* 13–18.

Kelley, T. (1943). Cumulative significance of a number of independent experiments: Reply to A.E. Teaxler and R.N. Hilbert. *School and Society, 57,* 482–484.

Kennedy, D.B., Kelley, T.M., & Homant, R.J. (1985). A test of the "hired gun" hypothesis in psychiatric testimony. *Psychological Reports, 57,* 117–118.

Kennedy, W. (1986). The psychologist as expert witness. In W. Curran, A.L. McGarry, & S. Shah (Eds.), *Forensic psychiatry and psychology* (pp. 487–511). Philadelphia: Davis.

Kinports, K. (1988). Defending battered women's self-defense claims. *Oregon Law Review, 67,* 393–465.

Kleinmuntz, B. (1984). The scientific study of clinical judgment in psychology and medicine. *Clinical Psychology Review, 4,* 111–126.

Kleinmuntz, B. (1990). Why we still use our heads instead of formulas: Toward an integrative approach. *Psychological Bulletin, 107,* 296–310.

Kuehnle, K. (1998). Child sexual abuse evaluations: The scientist-practitioner model. *Behavioral Sciences and the Law, 16,* 5–20.

Laboratory of Community Psychiatry, Harvard Medical School. (1973). *Competency to stand trial and mental illness.* Rockville, MD: National Institute of Mental Health.

Lamb, D., Berry, D., Wetter, M., & Baer, R. (1994). Effects of two types of information on malingering of closed head injury on the MMPI-2: An analog investigation. *Psychological Assessment, 6,* 8–13.

Lambert, L.E., & Wertheimer, M. (1988). Is diagnostic ability related to relevant training and experience? *Professional Psychology, 19,* 50–52.

Lambert, M.J., Christensen, E.D., & DeJulio, S.S. (Eds.). (1983). *Assessment of psychotherapy outcome.* New York: Wiley.

Lande, R.G. (1990a). Disposition of insanity acquittees in the United States Military. *Bulletin of the American Academy of Psychiatry and Law, 18,* 303–309.

Lande, R.G. (1990b). The perils of prediction. *Military Medicine, 155,* 456–459.

Lanyon, R.I. (1986). Psychological assessment procedures in court-related settings. *Professional Psychology: Research and Practice, 17,* 260–268.

Lanyon, R.I. (1997). Detecting deception: Current models and directions. *Clinical Psychology: Science and Practice, 4,* 377–387.

Lanyon, R.I., Dannenbaum, S.E., Wolf, L.L., & Brown, A. (1989). Dimensions of deceptive responding in criminal offenders. *Psychological Assessment: A Journal of Consulting and Clinical Psychology, 1,* 300–304.

Lanyon, R.I., & Lutz, R.W. (1984). MMPI discrimination of defensive and nondefensive felony sex offenders. *Journal of Consulting and Clinical Psychology, 52,* 841–843.

Larkin, E.P., & Collins, P.J. (1989). Fitness to plead and psychiatric reports. *Medical Science and Law, 29,* 26–32.

Leary, M.R., & Miller, R.S. (1986). *Social psychology and dysfunctional behavior: Origins, diagnosis, and treatment.* New York: Springer-Verlag.

Lee, C., Beauregard, C., & Hunsley, J. (1998). Lawyers' opinions regarding child custody mediation and assessment services: Implications for psychological practice. *Professional Psychology: Research and Practice, 29,* 115–120.

Lees-Haley, P. (1992). Psychodiagnostic test usage by forensic psychologists. *American Journal of Forensic Psychology, 10,* 25–30.

Lempert, R.O., & Saltzburg, S.A. (1984). *A modern approach to evidence* (2nd ed.). St. Paul, MN: West.

Levine, M. (1980). Investigative reporting as a research method: An analysis of Bernstein and Woodward's *All the President's Men. American Psychologist, 35,* 626–638.

Lezak, M. (1995). *Neuropsychological assessment* (3rd ed.). London: Oxford University Press.

Lidz, C.W., Mulvey, E.P., & Gardner, W. (1993). The accuracy of predictions of violence to others. *Journal of the American Medical Association, 269,* 1007–1011.

Lipsitt, P., Lelos, D., & McGarry, A. (1971). Competency for trial: A screening instrument. *American Journal of Psychiatry, 128,* 137–141.

Lowery, C. (1981). Child custody decisions in divorce proceedings: A survey of judges. *Professional Psychology, 12,* 492–498.

Lunde, D.T., & Sigal, H.A. (1987). Psychiatric testimony in "cult" litigation. *Bulletin of the American Academy of Psychiatry and the Law, 15,* 205–210.

Mackie, D., & Worth, L. (1989). Cognitive deficits and mediation of positive attitude change. *Journal of Personality and Social Psychology, 57,* 27–40.

Mann, T. (1994). Informed consent for psychological research: Do subjects comprehend consent forms and understand their legal rights? *Psychological Science, 5,* 140–143.

Marlowe, D. (1995). A hybrid decision framework for evaluating psychometric evidence. *Behavioral Sciences and the Law, 13,* 207–228.

Marra, H.A., Konzelman, G.E., & Giles, P.G. (1987). A clinical strategy to the assessment of dangerousness. *International Journal of Offender Therapy and Comparative Criminology, 31,* 291–299.

Martell, D.A. (1992). Forensic neuropsychology and the criminal law. *Law and Human Behavior, 16,* 313–336.

Martell, D.A., & Sanders, S. (1991). *Mentally disordered offenders who cannot be restored to competency: A study of 20 cases converted to civil status pursuant to Jackson v. Indiana.* Unpublished manuscript, NYU/Bellevue Medical Center and Kirby Forensic Psychiatric Center, New York, NY.

Masling, M.S. (1982). *Crime seriousness and attitudes toward the accused.* Unpublished doctoral dissertation, Stanford University.

Matarazzo, J.D. (1983). The reliability of psychiatric and psychological diagnosis. *Clinical Psychology Review, 3,* 103–145.

Matarazzo, J.D. (1990). Psychological assessment versus psychological testing: Validation from Binet to the school, clinic, and courtroom. *American Psychologist, 45,* 999–1017.

McCaffrey, R.J., & Bellamy-Campbell, R. (1989). Psychometric detection of fabricated symptoms of combat-related posttraumatic stress disorder: A systematic replication. *Journal of Clinical Psychology, 45,* 76–79.

McCann, J. (1996). Standards for expert testimony in New York death penalty cases. *New York State Bar Journal, 60,* 30–33.

McCann, J. (1998). *Malingering and deception in adolescents.* Washington, DC: American Psychological Association.

McCann, J., & Dyer, F. (1996). *Forensic assessment with the Millon inventories.* New York: Plenum Press.

McGarry, A.L. (1965). Competency for trial and due process via the state hospital. *American Journal of Psychiatry, 122,* 623–631.

McGarry, A.L., et al. (1973). *Competency to stand trial and mental illness.* (DHEW Publication No. HSM 73-9105). National Institute of Mental Health.

McReynolds, P. (1989). Diagnosis and clinical assessment: Current status and major issues. *Annual Review of Psychology, 40,* 83–108.

Meehl, P.E. (1954). *Clinical versus statistical prediction: A theoretical analysis and a review of the evidence.* Minneapolis: University of Minnesota Press.

Meehl, P.E. (1989). Law and the fireside inductions (with postscript): Some reflections of a clinical psychologist. *Behavioral Sciences and the Law, 7,* 521–550.

Megargee, E. (1972). *The California Psychological Inventory handbook.* San Francisco: Jossey–Bass.

Megargee, E.I. (1982). Psychological determinants and correlates of criminal violence. In M.E. Wolfgang & N.A. Weiner (Eds.), *Criminal violence* (pp. 81–170). Beverly Hills: Sage.

Megargee, E.I., & Bohn, M.J. (1979). *Classifying criminal offenders: A new system based on the MMPI.* Beverly Hills: Sage.

Meier, S. (1994). *The chronic crisis in psychological measurement and assessment: A historical survey.* San Diego: Academic Press.

Mellsop, G., Varghese, F., Joshua, S., & Hicks, A. (1982). The reliability of Axis II of DSM-III. *American Journal of Psychiatry, 139,* 1360–1361.

Melton, G., Petrila, J., Poythress, N., & Slobogin, C. (1997). *Psychological evaluations for the courts: A handbook for mental health professionals and lawyers* (2nd ed.). New York: Guilford Press.

Melton, G., Weithorn, L., & Slobogin, C. (1986). *Community mental health centers and the courts: An evaluation of community-based forensic services.* Lincoln, NE: University of Nebraska Press.

Miller, G.H. (1986). Prohibiting psychiatric diagnosis in insanity trials. With special reference to John W. Hinckley, Jr. *Psychiatry, 49,* 131–143.

Miller, R.D. (1990). Prearraignment forensic evaluation: The odyssey moves east of the Pecos. *Bulletin of the American Academy of Psychiatry and Law, 18,* 311–321.

Miller, R.D., & Germaine, E.J. (1986). The specificity of evaluations of competency to proceed. *Journal of Psychiatry and Law, 14,* 333–347.

Miller, R., & Germain, E. (1988). The retrospective evaluation of competency to stand trial. *International Journal of Law and Psychiatry, 11,* 113–125.

Miller, R., & Germain, E. (1989). Should forensic patients be informed of evaluators' opinions prior to trial? *Bulletin of the American Academy of Psychiatry and the Law, 17,* 53–59.

Millon, T. (1993). *The Millon Adolescent Clinical Inventory manual.* Minneapolis, MN: National Computer Systems.

Millon, T. (1994). *Millon Clinical Multiaxial Inventory-III manual*. Minneapolis, MN: Interpretive Scoring Systems.

Mills, J., Kroner, D., & Forth, A. (1998). Novaco Anger Scale: Reliability and validity within an adult criminal sample. *Assessment, 5*, 237–248.

Modlin, H.C. (1989). Forensic pitfalls. *Bulletin of the American Academy of Psychiatry and the Law, 17*, 415–419.

Monahan, J. (Ed.). (1980). *Who is the client? The ethics of psychological intervention in the criminal justice system*. Washington, DC: American Psychological Association.

Monahan, J. (1981). *Predicting violent behavior: An assessment of clinical techniques*. Beverly Hills: Sage.

Monahan, J. (1984). The prediction of violent behavior: Toward a second generation of theory and policy. *American Journal of Psychiatry, 141*, 10–15.

Monahan, J. (1988). Risk assessment of violence among the mentally disordered: Generating useful knowledge. *International Journal of Law and Psychiatry, 11*, 249–257.

Monahan, J., & Steadman, H. (Eds.). (1983). *Mentally disordered offenders: Perspectives from law and social science*. New York: Plenum Press.

Monahan, J., & Steadman, H. (Eds.). (1994). *Violence and mental disorder: Developments in risk assessment*. Chicago: University of Chicago Press.

Morey, L. (1991). *Personality Assessment Inventory professional manual*. Odessa, FL: Psychological Assessment Resources.

Morse, S. (1978a). Crazy behavior, morals, and science: An analysis of mental health law. *Southern California Law Review, 51*, 527–654.

Morse, S. (1978b). Law and mental health professionals: The limits of expertise. *Professional Psychology, 9*, 389–399.

Morse, S. (1982a). Failed explanations and criminal responsibility: Experts and the unconscious. *Virginia Law Review, 68*, 971–1084.

Morse, S. (1982b). Reforming expert testimony: An open response from the tower (and the trenches). *Law and Human Behavior, 6*, 45–47.

Morse, S. (1990). The misbegotten marriage of soft psychology and bad law: Psychological self-defense as a justification for homicide. *Law and Human Behavior, 14*, 595–618.

Mossman, D. (1994). Assessing predictions of violence: Being accurate about accuracy. *Journal of Consulting and Clinical Psychology, 62*, 783–792.

Mulvey, E. (1992, March). *The advantages and challenges of using collateral reports of patient violence*. Presented at the Biennial Conference of the American Psychology–Law Society, Williamsburg, VA.

Mulvey, E., & Lidz, C. (1993). Measuring patient violence in dangerousness research. *Law and Human Behavior, 17*, 277–288.

Mulvey, E., & Lidz, C. (1995). Conditional prediction: A model for research on dangerousness to others in a new era. *International Journal of Law and Psychiatry, 18*, 129–143.

Needell, J.E. (1980). Psychiatric expert witnesses: Proposals for change. *American Journal of Law and Medicine, 6*, 425–429.

Nicholi, A. (Ed.). (1978). *The Harvard guide to modern psychiatry*. Cambridge, MA: Harvard University Press.

Nicholson, R.A. (1988). Validation of a brief form of the Competency Screening Test. *Journal of Clinical Psychology, 44*, 87–90.

Nicholson, R.A., Briggs, S.R., & Robertson, H.C. (1988). Instruments for assessing competency to stand trial: How do they work? *Professional Psychology: Research and Practice, 19*, 383–394.

Nicholson, R.A., & Johnson, W.G. (1991). Prediction of competency to stand trial: Contribution of demographics, type of offense, clinical characteristics, and psycholegal ability. *International Journal of Law and Psychiatry, 14*, 287–297.

Nicholson, R.A., & Kugler, K.E. (1991). Competent and incompetent criminal defendants: A quantitative review of comparative research. *Psychological Bulletin, 109,* 355–370.

Nicholson, R., & McNulty, J. (1992). Outcomes of hospitalization for defendants found incompetent to stand trial. *Behavioral Sciences and the Law, 10,* 371–383.

Nicholson, R.A., Robertson, H.C., Johnson, W.G., & Jensen, G. (1988). A comparison of instruments for assessing competency to stand trial. *Law and Human Behavior, 12,* 313–321.

Novaco, R. (1994). Anger as a risk factor for violence among the mentally disordered. In J. Monahan & H. Steadman (Eds.), *Violence and mental disorder: Developments in risk assessment* (pp. 21–59). Chicago: University of Chicago Press.

Nurcombe, B., & Gallagher, R. (1986). *The clinical process in psychiatry.* London: Cambridge University Press.

Office of Juvenile Justice and Delinquency Prevention. (1995). *Guide for implementing the comprehensive strategy for serious, violent, and chronic juvenile offenders.* Washington, DC: Department of Justice.

Ogloff, J. (1990). The admissibility of expert testimony regarding malingering and deception. *Behavioral Sciences and the Law, 8,* 27–43.

Ogloff, J., Roberts, C., & Roesch, R. (1993). The insanity defense: Legal standards and clinical assessment. *Applied & Preventive Psychology, 2,* 163–178.

Otto, R.K. (1989). Bias and expert testimony of mental health professionals in adversarial proceedings: A preliminary investigation. *Behavioral Sciences and the Law, 7,* 267–273.

Otto, R.K. (1992). Prediction of dangerous behavior: A review and analysis of "second-generation" research. *Forensic Reports, 5,* 103–133.

Otto, R.K. (1994). On the ability of mental health professionals to "predict dangerousness": A commentary on interpretations of the "dangerousness" literature. *Law and Psychology Review, 18,* 43–68.

Otto, R.K., & Borum, R. (1997). *Assessing and managing violence risk: A workshop for clinicians.* Tampa: University of South Florida.

Otto, R.K., Heilbrun, K., & Grisso, T. (1990). Training and credentialing in forensic psychology. *Behavioral Sciences and the Law, 8,* 217–231.

Otto, R.K., Poythress, N.G., Nicholson, R., Edens, J., Monahan, J., Bonnie, R., Hoge, S., & Eisenberg, M. (1998). Psychometric properties of the MacArthur Competence Assessment Tool–Criminal Adjudication (MacCAT-CA). *Psychological Assessment: A Journal of Consulting and Clinical Psychology, 10,* 435–443.

Otto, R.K., Poythress, N., Starr, L., & Darkes, J. (1993). An empirical study of the reports of APA's peer review panel in the congressional review of the U.S.S. Iowa incident. *Journal of Personality Assessment, 61,* 425–442.

Pankratz, L., & Binder, L. (1997). Malingering on intellectual and neuropsychological measures. In R. Rogers (Ed.), *Clinical assessment of malingering and deception* (2nd ed., pp. 223–236). New York: Guilford Press.

Paul, G. (Ed.). (1986). *Assessment in residential treatment settings.* Champaign, IL: Research Press.

Paul, G., & Lentz, R. (1977). *Psychosocial treatment of chronic mental patients: Milieu versus social learning programs.* Cambridge, MA: Harvard University Press.

Pepper-Smith, R., Harvey, W., Silberfeld, M., Stein, E., et al. (1992). Consent to a competency assessment. *International Journal of Law and Psychiatry, 15,* 13–23.

Perlin, M. (1991). Power imbalances in therapeutic and forensic relationships. *Behavioral Sciences and the Law, 9,* 111–128.

Perlin, M. (1996). "Dignity was the first to leave": *Godinez v. Moran,* Colin Ferguson, and the trial of mentally disabled criminal defendants. *Behavioral Sciences and the Law, 14,* 61–81.

Perlin, M., & Dvoskin, J. (1990). AIDS-related dementia and competency to stand trial: A potential abuse of the forensic mental health system? *Bulletin of the American Academy of Psychiatry and the Law, 18*, 349–357.

Petrella, R.C., & Poythress, N.G. (1983). The quality of forensic evaluations: An interdisciplinary study. *Journal of Consulting and Clinical Psychology, 51*, 76–85.

Petty, R., & Cacioppo, J. (1986). *Communication and persuasion: Central and peripheral routes to attitude change.* Berlin: Springer-Verlag.

Philipson, J. (1998). *Perceptions of forensic ward staff regarding patient response style.* Currently unpublished document, Allegheny University of the Health Sciences.

Pierrel, A. (1986). Competency to stand trial and the mentally retarded defendant. *Dissertation Abstracts International, 47-B*, 1282.

Pincus, H., Lieberman, J., & Ferris, S. (Eds.). (1998). *Ethics in psychiatric research: A resource manual for human subjects protection.* Washington, DC: American Psychiatric Association.

Podboy, J., & Kastl, A. (1993). The intentional misuse of standard psychological tests in complex trials. *American Journal of Forensic Psychology, 11*, 47–54.

Pope, K., Butcher, J., & Seelen, J. (1993). *The MMPI, MMPI-2, and MMMPI-A in court: A practical guide for expert witnesses and attorneys.* Washington, DC: American Psychological Association.

Popper, K. (1968). *The logic of scientific discovery.* New York: Harper & Row.

Posthuma, A., & Harper, J. (1998). Comparison of MMPI-2 responses of child custody and personal injury litigants. *Professional Psychology: Research and Practice, 29*, 437–443.

Poythress, N.G. (1981). *Conflicting postures for mental health expert witnesses: Prevailing attitudes of trial court judges.* Unpublished manuscript, Center for Forensic Psychiatry, Ann Arbor, MI.

Poythress, N.G. (1982). Concerning reform in expert testimony: An open letter from a practicing psychologist. *Law and Human Behavior, 6*, 39–43.

Poythress, N.G. (1987). Avoiding negligent release: A risk-management strategy. *Hospital and Community Psychiatry, 38*, 1051–1052.

Poythress, N.G. (1990). Avoiding negligent release: Contemporary clinical and risk management strategies. *American Journal of Psychiatry, 147*, 994–997.

Poythress, N.G. (1992). Expert testimony on violence and dangerousness: Roles for mental health professionals. *Forensic Reports, 5*, 135–150.

Poythress, N.G., Hoge, S.K., Bonnie, R., Monahan, J., Eisenberg, M., & Feucht-Haviar, T. (1988). *Journal of the American Academy of Psychiatry and the Law, 26*, 215–222.

Poythress, N., Monahan, J., Bonnie, R., & Hoge, S.K. (1999). *MacArthur Competence Assessment Tool–Criminal Adjudication.* Odessa, FL: Psychological Assessment Resources.

Poythress, N., G., Nicholson, R., Otto, R.K., Edens, J.F., Bonnie, R.J., Monahan, J., & Hoge, S.K. (1999). *Professional manual for the MacArthur Competence Assessment Tool–Criminal Adjudication.* Odessa, FL: Psychological Assessment Resources.

Poythress, N.G., Otto, R.K., Darkes, J., & Starr, L. (1993). APA's expert panel in the Congressional review of the USS Iowa incident. *American Psychologist, 48*, 8–15.

Prifitera, A., & Saklofske, D. (Eds.). (1998). *WISC III: Clinical use and interpretation.* San Diego: Academic Press.

Quay, H.C. (1986). A critical analysis of DSM-III as a taxonomy of psychopathology in childhood and adolescence. In T. Millon & G. Klerman (Eds.), *Contemporary directions in psychopathology* (pp. 151–165). New York: Guilford Press.

Rachlin, S. (1988). From impartial expert to adversary in the wake of Ake. *Bulletin of the American Academy of Psychiatry and the Law, 16*, 25–33.

Ratneshwar, S., & Chaiken, S. (1991). Comprehension's role in persuasion: The case of its moderating effects on the persuasive impact of source cues. *Journal of Consumer Research, 18*, 52–62.

Reich, J., & Tookey, L. (1986). Disagreements between court and psychiatrist on competency to stand trial. *Journal of Clinical Psychiatry, 47*, 29–30.

Reichlin, S., Bloom, J.D., & Williams, M. (1993). Excluding personality disorders from the insanity defense: A follow-up study. *Bulletin of the American Academy of Psychiatry and the Law, 21*, 91–100.

Reisner, R., Slobogin, C., & Rai, A. (1999). *Law and the mental health system: Civil and criminal aspects* (3rd ed.). St. Paul, MN: West.

Report of the Task Force on the Role of Psychology in the Criminal Justice System (1978). *American Psychologist, 12*, 1099–1113.

Resnick, P. (1995). *Malingering. Mental and emotional injuries in employment litigation.* Washington, DC: Bureau of National Affairs.

Resnick, P. (1997). Malingered psychosis. In R. Rogers (Ed.), *Clinical assessment of malingering and deception* (2nd ed., pp. 47–67). New York: Guilford Press.

Rice, M., & Harris, G. (1995). Violent recidivism: Assessing predictive validity. *Journal of Consulting and Clinical Psychology, 63*, 737–748.

Robbins, E., Waters, J., & Herbert, P. (1997). Competency to stand trial evaluations: A study of actual practice in two states. *Journal of the American Academy of Psychiatry and the Law, 25*, 469–483,

Roberts, C.F., & Golding, S.L. (1991). The social construction of criminal responsibility and insanity. *Law and Human Behavior, 15*, 349–376.

Robey, A. (1965). Criteria for competency to stand trial: A checklist for psychiatrists. *American Journal of Psychiatry, 122*, 616–622.

Robins, L., Cottler, L., & Keating, S. (1989). *The NIMH Diagnostic Interview Schedule* (Version III Revised). St. Louis, MO: Washington University.

Robins, L.N., & Helzer, J.E. (1986). Diagnosis and clinical assessment: The current state of psychiatric diagnosis. *Annual Review of Psychology, 37*, 409–432.

Rodenhauser, R., & Khamis, H. (1988). Predictors of improvement in maximum security hospital patients. *Behavioral Sciences and the Law, 6*, 531–542.

Roesch, R. (1978). A brief, immediate screening interview to determine competency to stand trial: A feasibility study. *Criminal Justice and Behavior, 5*, 241–248.

Roesch, R. (1979). Determining competency to stand trial: An examination of evaluation procedures in an institutional setting. *Journal of Consulting and Clinical Psychology, 47*, 542–550.

Roesch, R., & Golding, S.L. (1980). *Competency to stand trial.* Champaign–Urbana: University of Illinois Press.

Roesch, R., Hart, S., & Zapf, P. (1996). Conceptualizing and assessing competency to stand trial: Implications and applications of the MacArthur Treatment Competence Model. *Psychology, Public Policy, and Law, 2*, 96–113.

Roesch, R., Hart, S., & Ogloff, J. (Eds.). (1999). *Psychology and law: The state of the discipline.* New York: Plenum Press.

Rogers, R. (1984). Towards an empirical model of malingering and deception. *Behavioral Sciences and the Law, 2*, 93–112.

Rogers, R. (1986). *Conducting insanity evaluations.* New York: Van Nostrand–Reinhold.

Rogers, R. (1988). Structured interviews and dissimulation. In R. Rogers (Ed.), *Clinical assessment of malingering and deception* (pp. 250–268). New York: Guilford Press.

Rogers, R. (1990). Development of a new classificatory model of malingering. *Bulletin of the American Academy of Psychiatry and Law, 18*, 323–333.

Rogers, R. (1992). *Structured Interview of Reported Symptoms.* Odessa, FL: Psychological Assessment Resources.

Rogers, R. (1995). *Diagnostic and structured interviewing: A handbook for psychologists*. Odessa, FL: Psychological Assessment Resources.

Rogers, R. (1997a). Structured interviews and dissimulation. In R. Rogers (Ed.), *Clinical assessment of malingering and deception* (2nd ed., pp. 301–327). New York: Guilford Press.

Rogers, R. (Ed.). (1997b). *Clinical assessment of malingering and deception* (2nd ed.). New York: Guilford Press.

Rogers, R., & Bagby, R.M. (1992). Diversion of mentally disordered offenders: A legitimate role for clinicians? *Behavioral Sciences and the Law, 10,* 407–418.

Rogers, R., Bagby, R., & Chakraborty, D. (1993). Feigning schizophrenic disorders on the MMPI-2: Detection of coached simulators. *Journal of Personality Assessment, 60,* 215–226.

Rogers, R., Bagby, R.M., & Chow, M. (1992). Psychiatrists and the parameters of expert testimony. *International Journal of Law and Psychiatry, 15,* 387–396.

Rogers, R., Bagby, R.M., Crouch, M., & Cutler, B. (1990). Effects of ultimate opinions on juror perceptions of insanity. *International Journal of Law and Psychiatry, 13,* 225–232.

Rogers, R., Bagby, R.M., & Dickens, S. (1992). *Structured Interview of Reported Symptoms (SIRS) and professional manual*. Odessa, FL: Psychological Assessment Resources.

Rogers, R., Dolmetsch, R., & Cavanaugh, J. (1981). An empirical approach to insanity evaluations. *Journal of Clinical Psychology, 37,* 683–687.

Rogers, R., Dolmetsch, R., & Cavanaugh, J.L. (1983). Identification of random responders on MMPI protocols. *Journal of Personality Assessment, 47,* 364–368.

Rogers, R., & Ewing, C.P. (1989). Ultimate opinion proscriptions: A cosmetic fix and a plea for empiricism. *Law and Human Behavior, 13,* 357–374.

Rogers, R., Gillis, J., Dickens, S., & Bagby, R.M. (1991). Standardized assessment of malingering: Validation of the Structured Interview of Reported Symptoms. *Psychological Assessment: A Journal of Consulting and Clinical Psychology, 3,* 89–96.

Rogers, R., Gillis, J., McMain, S., & Dickens, S. (1988). Fitness evaluations: A retrospective study of clinical, criminal, and sociodemographic characteristics. *Canadian Journal of Behavioral Sciences, 20,* 192–200.

Rogers, R., Gillis, J.R., Turner, R.E., & Frise-Smith, T. (1990). The clinical presentation of command hallucinations in a forensic population. *American Journal of Psychiatry, 147,* 1304–1307.

Rogers, R., Harrell, E., & Liff, C. (1993). Feigning neuropsychological impairment: A critical review of methodological and clinical considerations. *Clinical Psychology Review, 13,* 255–274.

Rogers, R., & Lynette, E. (1991). The role of Canadian psychiatry in dangerous offender testimony. *Canadian Journal of Psychiatry, 36,* 79–84.

Rogers, R., Seman, W., & Wasyliw, O.E. (1983). The RCRAS and legal insanity: A cross-validation study. *Journal of Clinical Psychology, 39,* 554–559.

Rogers, R., Sewell, K., Morey, L., & Ustad, K. (1990). Detection of feigned mental disorders on the Personality Assessment Inventory: A discriminant analysis. *Journal of Personality Assessment, 67,* 629–639.

Rogers, R., & Shuman, D. (2000). *Conducting insanity evaluations* (2nd ed.). New York: Guilford Press.

Rogers, R., Wasyliw, O.E., & Cavanaugh, J.L. (1984). Evaluating insanity: A study of construct validity. *Law and Human Behavior, 8,* 293–303.

Rohde, P., Lewinsohn, P., & Seeley, J. (1997). Comparability of telephone and face-to-face interviews in assessing Axis I and II disorders. *American Journal of Psychiatry, 154,* 1593–1598.

Rosenfeld, B., & Wall, A. (1998). Psychopathology and competence to stand trial. *Criminal Justice and Behavior, 25,* 443–462.

Rosenhan, D.L. (1973). On being sane in insane places. *Science, 179,* 250–258.

Rosenhan, D.L. (1982). Psychological abnormality and law. In C.J. Scheirer & B.L. Hammonds (Eds.), *Psychology and the law* (Vol. 2, pp. 93–118). Washington, DC: American Psychological Association.

Rosenthal, P. (1983). Nature of jury response to the expert witness. *Journal of Forensic Science, 28,* 128–131.

Rotgers, F., & Barrett, D. (1996). *Daubert v. Merrell Dow* and expert testimony by clinical psychologists: Implications and recommendations for practice. *Professional Psychology: Research and Practice, 27,* 467–474.

Sacks, E. (1952). Intelligence scores as a function of experimentally established social relationships between the child and examiner. *Journal of Abnormal and Social Psychology, 47,* 354–358.

Saks, M. (1990). Expert witnesses, nonexpert witnesses, and nonwitness experts. *Law and Human Behavior, 14,* 291–313.

Sawyer, J. (1966). Measurement and prediction, clinical and statistical. *Psychological Bulletin, 66,* 178–200.

Schacter, D. (1986). Amnesia and crime: How much do we really know? *American Psychologist, 41,* 287–295.

Schneidman, E. (1981). The psychological autopsy. *Suicide and Life Threatening Behavior, 11,* 325–340.

Schretlen, D. (1988). The use of psychological tests to identify malingered symptoms of mental disorder. *Clinical Psychology Review, 8,* 451–476.

Schretlen, D. (1997). Dissimulation on the Rorschach and other projective measures. In R. Rogers (Ed.), *Clinical assessment of malingering and deception* (2nd ed.) (pp. 208–222). New York: Guilford Press.

Schretlen, D., & Arkowitz, H. (1990). A psychological test battery to detect prison inmates who fake insanity or mental retardation. *Behavioral Sciences and the Law, 8,* 75–84.

Schuller, R.A., & Vidmar, N. (1992). Battered woman syndrome evidence in the courtroom: A review of the literature. *Law and Human Behavior, 16,* 273–291.

Segal, S.P., Watson, M.A., & Nelson, S. (1986). Consistency in the application of civil commitment standards in psychiatric emergency rooms. *Journal of Psychiatry and Law, 14,* 125–148.

Sewell, K., & Rogers, R. (1994). Response consistency and the MMPI-2: Development of a simplified screening scale. *Assessment, 1,* 293–299.

Shapiro, D. (1984). *Psychological evaluation and expert testimony.* New York: Van Nostrand–Reinhold.

Shapiro, D. (1991). *Forensic psychological assessment: An integrative approach.* Boston: Allyn & Bacon.

Shea, M.T., Glass, D.R., Pilkonis, P.A., Watkins, J., & Docherty, J.P. (1987). Frequency and implications of personality disorders in a sample of depressed outpatients. *Journal of Personality Disorders, 1,* 27–42.

Shuman, D. (1986). *Psychiatric and psychological evidence.* New York: McGraw–Hill.

Shuman, D. (1997). What should we permit mental health professionals to say about "the best interests of the child"?: An essay on common sense, *Daubert,* and the rules of evidence. *Family Law Quarterly, 31,* 551–569.

Shuman, D., Champagne, A., & Whitaker, E. (1994). An empirical examination of the use of expert witnesses in the courts—Part II: A three-city study. *Jurimetrics Journal of Law, Science and Technology, 34,* 193–208.

Shuman, D., Champagne, A., & Whitaker, E. (1996). Juror assessments of the believability of expert witnesses: A literature review. *Jurimetrics Journal of Law, Science and Technology, 36,* 371–382.

Shuman, D., Greenberg, S., Heilbrun, K., & Foote, W. (1998). An immodest proposal: Should treating mental health professionals be barred from testifying about their patients? *Behavioral Sciences and the Law, 16*, 509–523.

Siegel, A., & Elwork, A. (1990). Treating incompetence to stand trial. *Law and Human Behavior, 14*, 57–65.

Silva, M., & Sorrell, J. (1988). Enhancing comprehension of information for informed consent: A review of empirical research. *IRB: A Review of Human Subjects Research, 10*, 1–5.

Simon, M.J. (1987). Use of the Proverbs Test in the assessment of competency to stand trial. *Psychological Reports, 60*, 1166.

Sivec, H., Lynn, S., & Garske, J. (1994). The effect of somatoform disorder and paranoid psychotic disorder role-related dissimulations as a response set on the MMPI-2. *Assessment, 1*, 69–81.

Skeem, J., Golding, S., Cohn, N., & Berge, G. (1998). Logic and reliability of evaluations of competence to stand trial. *Law and Human Behavior, 22*, 519–547.

Slobogin, C. (1982). *Estelle v. Smith*: The constitutional contours of the forensic evaluation. *Emory Law Journal, 31*, 71–138.

Slobogin, C. (1984). Dangerousness and expertise. *University of Pennsylvania Law Review, 133*, 97–174.

Slobogin, C. (1989). The ultimate issue issue. *Behavioral Sciences and the Law, 7*, 259–268.

Slovenko, R. (1987). The lawyer and the forensic expert: Boundaries of ethical practice. *Behavioral Sciences and the Law, 5*, 119–147.

Slovenko, R. (1991). Psychiatric expert testimony: Are the criticisms justified? *Medicine and Law, 10*, 1–29.

Smith, R.L., & Graham, J.R. (1989). Clinicians' experience and the determination of criminal responsibility. *Criminal Justice and Behavior, 16*, 473–485.

Spitzer, R.L., & Endicott, J. (1978). *Schedule of Affective Disorders and Schizophrenia.* New York: Biometric Research.

Spitzer, R.L., Forman, J., & Nee, J. (1979). DSM-III field trials: Initial interrater diagnostic reliability. *American Journal of Psychiatry, 136*, 815–817.

Spitzer, R.L., & Williams, J.B.W. (1983). *Structured Clinical Interview for DSM-III.* New York: Biometrics Research Department, New York State Psychiatric Institute.

Steadman, H.J. (1982). A situational approach to violence. *International Journal of Law and Psychiatry, 5*, 171–186.

Steadman, H.J., & Cocozza, J.J. (1978). Selective reporting and the public's misconceptions of the criminally insane. *Public Opinion Quarterly, 41*, 523–533.

Steadman, H.J., McGreevy, M., Morrissey, J., Callahan, L., Robbins, P.C., & Cirincione, C. (1993). *Before and after Hinckley: Evaluating insanity defense reform.* New York: Guilford Press.

Steadman, H.J., Mulvey, E., Monahan, J., Robbins, P., Appelbaum, P., Grisso, T., Roth, L., & Silver, E. (1998). Violence by people discharged from acute psychiatric inpatient facilities and by others in the same neighborhoods. *Archives of General Psychiatry, 55*, 1–9.

Stermac, L. (1988). Projective testing and dissimulation. In R. Rogers (Ed.), *Clinical assessment of malingering and deception* (pp. 159–168). New York: Guilford Press.

Stoller, R.J., & Geertsma, R.H. (1963). The consistency of psychiatrists' clinical judgments. *Journal of Nervous and Mental Disease, 137*, 58–66.

Stone, A. (1984). *Law, psychiatry, and morality: Essays and analysis.* Washington, DC: American Psychiatric Association.

Strasburger, L.H. (1987). "Crudely, without any finesse": The defendant hears his psychiatric evaluation. *Bulletin of the American Academy of Psychiatry and Law, 15*, 229–233.

Stricker, G. (1992). The relationship of research to clinical practice. *American Psychologist, 47*, 543–549.

Stuart, E.P., & Campbell, J.C. (1989). Assessment of patterns of dangerousness with battered women. *Issues in Mental Health Nursing, 10,* 245–260.

Thames, H. (1994). *Frye* gone, but not forgotten in the wake of *Daubert:* New standards and procedures for admissibility of scientific expert opinion. *Mississippi Law Journal, 63,* 473–505.

Thompson, J.S., Stuart, G.L., & Holden, C.E. (1992). Command hallucinations and legal insanity. *Forensic Reports, 5,* 29–43.

Traxler, A., & Hilkert, R. (1942). Effect of type of desk on results of machine-scored tests. *School and Society, 56,* 277–296.

Trueblood, W., & Binder, L. (1995, October). *Psychologists' accuracy in identifying neuropsychological test protocols of clinical malingerers.* Paper presented at the National Academy of Neuropsychology, San Francisco.

Tsudzuki, A., Hata, Y., & Kuze, T. (1957). (A study of rapport between examiner and subject). *Japanese Journal of Psychology, 27,* 22–28.

Turk, D.C., & Salovey, P. (Eds.). (1988). *Reasoning, inference, and judgment in clinical psychology.* New York: Free Press.

Tymchuk, A. (1997). Informing for consent: Concepts and methods. *Canadian Psychologist, 38,* 56–75.

Ustad, K. (1996). *Assessment of malingering on the SADS in a jail referral sample.* Unpublished doctoral dissertation, University of North Texas, Denton.

Vant Zelfde, G., & Otto, R. (1997). *Directory of practicum, internship, and fellowship training opportunities in clinical-forensic psychology.* Pittsburgh, PA: American Academy of Forensic Psychology.

Vitiello, B., Malone, R., Buschle, P.R., Delaney, M.A., & Behar, D. (1990). Reliability of DSM-III diagnoses of hospitalized children. *Hospital and Community Psychiatry, 41,* 63–67.

Walker, L. (1979). *The battered woman.* New York: Harper & Row.

Walker, L. (1984). *The battered woman syndrome.* Berlin: Springer.

Walker, L. (1990). Psychological assessment of sexually abused children for legal evaluation and expert witness testimony. *Professional Psychology: Research and Practice, 21,* 344–353.

Walker, L., & Monahan, J. (1996). *Daubert* and the Reference Manual: An essay on the future of science in law. *University of Virginia Law Review, 82,* 837–857.

Walker, L., Thyfault, R.K., & Browne, A. (1982). Beyond the juror's ken: Battered women. *Vermont Law Review, 7,* 1–14.

Walters, G.D. (1988). Assessing dissimulation and denial on the MMPI in a sample of maximum security, male inmates. *Journal of Personality Assessment, 52,* 465–474.

Walters, G.D., White, T.W., & Greene, R.L. (1988). Use of the MMPI to identify malingering and exaggeration of psychiatric symptomatology in male prison inmates. *Journal of Consulting and Clinical Psychology, 33,* 143–150.

Warren, J., & Fitch, W.L. (1993). *Virginia Forensic Information Management System annual report.* Charlottesville: University of Virginia, Institute of Law, Psychiatry, and Public Policy.

Warren, J., Fitch, W.L., Dietz, P., & Rosenfeld, B. (1991). Criminal offense, psychiatric diagnosis, and psycholegal opinion: An analysis of 894 pretrial referrals. *Bulletin of the American Academy of Psychiatry and the Law, 19,* 63–69.

Wasyliw, O.E., Cavanaugh, J.L., & Rogers, R. (1985). Beyond the scientific limits of expert testimony. *Bulletin of the American Academy of Psychiatry and the Law, 13,* 147–158.

Wasyliw, O.E., Grossman, L.S., Haywood, T.W., & Cavanaugh, J.L. (1988). The detection of malingering in criminal forensic groups: MMPI validity scales. *Journal of Personality Assessment, 52,* 321–333.

Webster, C., & Cox, D. (1997). Integration of nomothetic and ideographic positions in risk assessment: Implications for practice and the education of psychologists and other mental health professionals. *American Psychologist, 52,* 1245–1246.

Webster, C., Douglas, K., Eaves, D., & Hart, S. (1997). *HCR-20: Assessing risk for violence* (version 2). Vancouver: Simon Fraser University.

Webster, C., Eaves, D., Douglas, K., & Wintrup, A. (1995). *The HCR-20 Scheme: The assessment of dangerousness and risk*. Vancouver: Simon Fraser University and Forensic Psychiatric Services Commission of British Columbia.

Webster, C., Harris, G., Rice, M., Cormier, C., & Quinsey, V. (1994). *The Violence Prediction Scheme: Assessing dangerousness in high risk men*. Toronto, Canada: University of Toronto, Centre of Criminology.

Wechsler, D. (1981). *Manual for the Wechsler Adult Intelligence Scale—Revised*. San Antonio, TX: The Psychological Corporation.

Wechsler, D. (1992). *Wechsler Individual Achievement Test: Manual*. San Antonio, TX: The Psychological Corporation.

Weiner, I., & Hess, A. (Eds.). (1987). *Handbook of forensic psychology*. New York: Wiley.

Weinstock, R., Leong, G.G., & Silva, J.A. (1991). Opinions by AAPL forensic psychiatrists on controversial ethical guidelines: A survey. *Bulletin of the American Academy of Psychiatry and Law, 19,* 237–248.

Weissman, H. (1991). Child custody evaluations: Fair and unfair professional practices. *Behavioral Sciences and the Law, 9,* 469–476.

Wetter, M., Baer, R., Berry, D., & Reynolds, S. (1994). The effect of symptom information on faking on the MMPI-2. *Assessment, 1,* 199–207.

Wetter, M., Baer, R., Berry, D., Robinson, L., & Sumpter, J. (1993). MMPI-2 profiles of motivated fakers given specific symptom information: A comparison to matched patients. *Psychological Assessment, 5,* 317–323.

Wiener, D.N. (1948). Subtle and obvious keys for the MMPI. *Journal of Consulting Psychology, 12,* 164–170.

Wildman, R., Batchelor, E., Thompson, L., Nelson, F., Moore, J., Patterson, M., & de Laosa, M. (1980). *The Georgia Court Competency Test: An attempt to develop a rapid, quantitative measure for fitness for trial*. Unpublished manuscript, Forensic Services Division, Central State Hospital, Milledgeville, GA.

Wildman, R.W., White, P.A., & Brandenburg, C.E. (1990). The Georgia Court Competency Test: The base-rate problem. *Perceptual and Motor Skills, 70,* 1055–1058.

Winick, B. (1984). Incompetency and insanity. From *Supplement to Florida criminal rules and practice*. Tallahassee: Florida Bar Association.

Winick, B.J. (1992). Competency to be executed: A therapeutic jurisprudence perspective. *Behavioral Sciences and the Law, 10,* 317–337.

Wirshing, D., Wirshing, W., Marder, S., Liberman, R., & Mintz, J. (1998). Informed consent: Assessment of comprehension. *American Journal of Psychiatry, 155,* 1508–1511.

Wyda, J., & Black, B. (1989). Psychiatric predictions and the death penalty: An unconstitutional sword for the prosecution but a constitutional shield for the defense. *Behavioral Sciences and the Law, 7,* 505–519.

Yates, K. (1994). Therapeutic issues associated with confidentiality and informed consent in forensic evaluations. *New England Journal on Criminal and Civil Confinement, 20,* 345–368.

Ziskin, J. (1981). *Coping with psychiatric and psychological testimony* (Vols. 1–3, 3rd ed.). Marina Del Rey, CA: Law and Psychology Press.

Ziskin, J., & Faust, D. (1988). *Coping with psychiatric and psychological testimony* (Vols. 1–3, 4th ed.). Marina Del Rey, CA: Law and Psychology Press.

Zonana, H. (1994). *Daubert v. Merrell Dow Pharmaceuticals*: A new standard for scientific evidence in the courts? *Bulletin of the American Academy of Psychiatry and the Law, 22,* 309–325.

Zonana, H., Crane, L.E., & Getz, M.A. (1990). Training and credentialing in forensic psychiatry. *Behavioral Sciences and the Law, 8,* 217–231.

CASES

Ake v. Oklahoma, 105 S.Ct. 1087 (1985).
Arizona State Board of Medical Examiners v. Clark, 97 Arizona 205, 398 P.2d 908 (1965).
Barefoot v. Estelle, 463 U.S. 880 (1983).
Berry v. City of Detroit, 25 F.3d 1342 (6th Cir. 1994).
Brandt v. Medical Defense Association, 856 S.W.2d 667 (1993).
Buchanan v. Kentucky, 483 U.S. 402 (1987).
Burkhart v. Washington Metro. Area Transit Auth., 112 F.3d 1207 (D.C. Cir. 1997).
Canterbury v. Spence, 464 F.2d 787 (D.C. Cir 1972).
Carmichael v. Samyang Tire, Inc., 131 F.3d 1433 (1997).
Chambers v. Mississippi, 410 U.S. 284 (1973).
Chester v. State, 473 S.E.2d 759 (Ga. 1996).
Connecticut v. Villano, 634 A.2d 907 (Conn. App. Ct. 1993).
Daubert v. Merrell Dow Pharmaceuticals, Inc., 113 S.Ct. 2786 (1993).
Dinco v. Dylex, Ltd., 111 F.3d 964 (1st Cir. 1997).
Dusky v. United States, 362 U.S. 402 (1960).
Estelle v. Smith, 451 U.S. 454 (1981).
Frohne v. State, 928 S.W. 2d 570 (Tex. Ct. App. 1996), petition for cert. filed, 65 U.S.L.W. 3799
    (U.S. May 20, 1997) (No. 96-1864).
Frye v. United States, 293 F. 1013 (D.C. Cir 1923).
Funk v. Commonwealth, 8 VA App 91 (1989).
Gier v. Educational Service Unit No. 16, 845 F. Supp. 1342 (D. Neb. 1994).
Godinez v. Moran, 509 U.S. 389 (1993).
Hiser v. Randolph, 126 Ariz. 608, 617 P.2d 774 (1980).
Hoult v. Hoult, 57 F.3d 1 (1st Cir. 1995).
Idaho v. Snow, 815 P.2d 475 (Idaho Ct. App. 1991).
In re Fleshman, 82 B.R. 994 (Bankr. W.D. Mo., 1987).
In re Payment of Court-Appointed Expert Witness, 59 Comp. Gen. 313 (1980).
In re TMI Litigation Consolidated Proceedings, 927 F. Supp. 834 (M.D. Pa. 1996).
Isely v. Capuchin Province, 877 F. Supp 1055 (E.D. Mich 1995).
Jackson v. Indiana, 406 U.S. 715 (1972).
Jenson v. Eveleth Taconite Co., 130 F.3d 1287 (1997).
Jones v. United States, 103 S.Ct. 3043 (1983).
Karabian v. Columbia University, 930 F. Supp. 134 (S.D. N.Y. 1996).
Kumho Tire Company, Ltd. v. Carmichael, 526 U.S. 137 (1999).
Levine v. Torvik, 986 F.2d 1506 (6th Cir. 1993).
Marx & Co. v. Diners' Club, Inc., 550 F.2d 505 (2d Cir. 1977).
Mayer v. Baiser, 497 N.E.2d 827 (1986).
McKendall v. Crown Control Corp., 122 F.3d 803 (1997).
McKinney v. Anderson, 924 F.2d 1500 (9th Cir. 1991), *vacated on other grounds sub nom.*
Miranda v. Arizona, 384 U.S. 436 (1966).
Moore v. Ashland Chemical, Inc., 126 F.3d 679 (1997).
Nash v. Wennar, 645 F. Supp. 238 (1986).
Nathanson v. Kline, 350 P.2d 1093 (Kan. 1960).
Noble v. Sartori, 1989 Ky. App. LEXIS 67 (1989).
Pennington v. State, 913 P.2d 1356 (Okla. Crim. App. 1995), cert. denied, 177 S.Ct. 121 (1996).
Rock v. Arkansas, 107 S.Ct. 2704 (1987).
Rodriguez Cirilo v. Garcia, 908 F. Supp. 85 (D.P.R. 1995).

Rosen v. Ciba-Geigy Corporation, 892 F. Supp. 208 (N.D. Ill. 1995).
Rutigliano v. Valley Business Forms, 929 F. Supp. 779 (D. N.J. 1996).
Shahzade v. Gregory, 923 F. Supp. 286 (D. Mass. 1996).
Sieling v. Eyman, 478 F.2d 211 (9th Cir. 1973).
Soutear v. United States, 646 F. Supp. 524 (E.D. Mich. 1986).
Specht v. Jensen, 853 F.2d 805 (10th Cir. 1988).
State v. Alberico, 861 P.2d 192 (N.M. 1993).
State v. Cavaliere, 663 A.2d 96 (N.H. 1995).
State v. Foret, 628 So.2d 1116 (La. 1993)
State v. Jarbath, 555 A.2d 559 (N.J. Sup. Ct. 1989).
State v. Maelega, 907 P.2d 758 (Haw. 1995).
State v. Martens, 629 N.E.2d 462 (Ohio App. 3 Dist. 1993).
State v. Parkinson, 909 P.2d 647 (Idaho Ct. App. 1996).
State v. Picklesimer, No. 96CA2, 1996 WL 599425 (Ohio Ct. App. Oct. 15, 1996).
State v. Spencer, 459 S.E.2d 812 (N.C. App. 1995).
Steward v. State, 652 N.E.2d 490 (Ind. 1995).
S.V. v. R.V., 933 S.W.2d 1 (Tex. 1996).
Thompson v. Sun City Community Hospital, Inc., 141 Ariz. 597, 688 P.2d 605 (1984).
Tungate v. Commonwealth, Ky. 901 S.W.2d 41 (1995).
Unique Concepts, Inc. v. Brown, 659 F. Supp. 1008 (S.Dist. N.Y. 1987).
United States v. Alvarez, 519 F.2d 1036 (3rd Cir. 1975).
United States v. Alzanki, 54 F.3d 994 (1st Cir. 1995), cert. denied, 116 S.Ct. 909 (1996).
United States v. Bighead, 128 F.3d 1329 (1997).
United States v. Brewer, 783 F.2d 841 (9th Cir. 1986).
United States v. Brown, 891 F. Supp. 1501 (D. Kan. 1995).
United States v. Coleman, 762 F. Supp. 1513 (D. D.C. 1991).
United States v. Downing, 753 F.2d 1224 (3rd Cir. 1985).
United States v. Evanoff, 10 F.3d 559 (8th Cir. 1993).
United States v. Gallo, 20 F.3d 7 (1st Cir. 1994).
United States v. Green, 548 F.2d 1261 (6th Cir. 1977).
United States v. Jones, 107 F.3d 1147, cert. denied, 117 S.Ct. 2527 (1997).
United States v. Mason, 1996 U.S. Dist. LEXIS 10524 (1996).
United States v. McMurray, 833 F. Supp. 1454 (D. Neb. 1993).
United States v. Michigan, 680 F. Supp. 928 (W.D. Mich. 1987).
United States v. Newman, 49 F.3d 1 (1st Cir. 1995).
United States v. Poff, 926 F.2d 588 (7th Cir. 1991).
United States v. Powers, 59 F.3d 1460 (4th Cir. 1995).
United States v. Reynolds, 77 F.3d 253 (8th Cir. 1996).
United States v. Rouse, 111 F.3d 561 (8th Cir. 1997).
United States v. Ruklick, 919 F.2d 95 (8th Cir. 1991).
United States v. Smith, 736 F.2d 1103 (6th Cir. 1984).
United States v. Speight, 726 F. Supp. 861 (D. D.C. 1989).
United States v. Studley, 907 F.2d 254 (1st Cir. 1990).
Waldorf v. Shuta, 916 F. Supp. 423 (1996).
Washington v. McNallie, 870 P.2d 295 (Wash. Sup. Ct. 1994).
Washington v. Pryor, 799 P.2d 244 (Wash. Sup. Ct. 1990).
Watkins v. Telsmith, Inc., 121 F.3d 984 (1997).
Wood v. Upjohn Company, No. 6093-I-II (Sept 4, 1984) (LEXIS, States library, Wash. file).
Woods v. Lecureux, 110 F.3d 1215 (1997).

Author Index

Ackerman, M., 6, 106, 113
Allen, A., 85
American Academy of Psychiatry and the
  Law, 6, 17, 27, 28, 33, 38, 47, 53, 59, 68,
  75, 90, 101, 109, 116, 124, 131, 133, 144,
  154,167, 177,192, 229, 236 , 243, 247,
  250, 259, 269
American Bar Association, 17, 30, 61, 71,
  79, 91,116, 124, 131, 146, 158, 220, 271
American Psychiatric Association, 17, 27,
  38, 47, 52, 59, 68, 75, 101, 109, 116, 124,
  131, 144, 154, 167, 177, 192, 215, 229,
  243, 247, 250, 259, 264, 269
American Psychological Association, 17,
  26,28, 33, 34, 37, 46, 52, 58, 66, 72, 73,
  84, 87, 90, 100, 105,109, 115, 122, 124,
  130, 136, 137, 138, 141, 142, 147, 152, 154,
  158, 167, 177, 191, 197, 207, 214, 215,
  222, 223, 228, 233, 235, 242, 246, 249,
  252, 258, 268
Anastasi, A., 138
Andrews, D., 118
Appelbaum, K., 119
Appelbaum, P.S., 3, 6, 62, 88, 108,113, 117,
  153, 155, 156, 157, 158, 172, 219

Baer, R., 180, 181
Bagby, R.M.,113, 181, 185, 218
Bartol, A.., 4
Bartol, C., 4
Barrett, D., 199
Bazelon, D.L., 36
Beauregard, C., 69
Bell, F., 137
Bem, D., 85

Bennett, E., 271
Bennett, W.S., 179
Berge, G., 133
Berry, D.T., 180, 181
Bersoff, D., 17, 28, 33, 34, 200
Binder, L., 183, 186
Bishop, T., 69
Black, B., 113
Black, H.C., 6
Blau, T., 56, 57, 70, 105, 205
Bonnie, R.J., 25, 84, 85, 87, 112, 132, 203,
  213, 223
Bordens, K., 6
Borum, R., 25, 102, 118, 125, 140, 171, 194,
  209, 218, 219, 220, 232, 288
Brehm, S., 270
Bricklin, B., 106
Brigham, J., 4, 5
Brodsky, S.L., 6, 37, 169, 194, 205, 211, 234,
  226, 227, 248, 261, 267, 274, 280
Brodzinsky, D.M., 105
Buis, T., 185
Butcher, J., 180

Cacioppo, J., 270
Campbell, D., 104, 105, 107
Carlin, A., 180
Cavanaugh, J.L., 73, 78
Cecil, J., 53
Chaiken, S., 270
Chakraborty, D., 181
Champagne, A., 270, 271
Chow, M., 218
Cocozza, J., 54
Coggins, M., 193, 194

335

Cohn, N., 133
Colbach, E.M., 43
Collins, S.,102, 125, 170, 218, 219, 221
Committee on Ethical Guidelines for
    Forensic Psychologists, 4, 17, 23, 27,
    34, 38, 41, 47, 52, 59, 60, 66, 74, 90, 100,
    109, 115, 123, 131, 136, 143, 154, 167, 177,
    191, 198, 206, 214, 228, 235, 242, 246,
    250, 259, 269
Committee on Government Policy, Group
    for the Advancement of Psychiatry,
    117
Conte, J., 203
Coons, P., 173
Cooper, D., 204, 270, 271, 272, 273
Cormier, C., 113
Cox, D., 127
Crouch, M., 218
Crowder, J., 194
Cruise, K., 203
Curran, W., 133
Cutler, B., 218

Dahlstrom, W. G., 180
Dammeyer, M., 202
Darkes, J., 100
Dawes, R., 108, 126
Dennis, D., 117
Dickens, S., 113
Dietz, P., 194
Dodds, L., 200
Douglas, K., 118, 127
Duncan, J., 182
Dvoskin, J., 193, 194

Eaves, D., 118, 127
Eckl, L., 200
Eisenberg, M., 112, 132
Ekman, P., 117, 166, 167
Elwork, A., 105
Emery, R.E., 50, 70
Endicott, J., 182
Ewing, C.P., 213, 214, 217, 221

Farber, S., 69
Faust, D., 36, 44, 104, 105, 108, 114, 170, 183,
    266
Federal Judicial Center, 53
Federal Rules of Evidence for United
    States Courts and Magistrates, 53

Fein, R., 62, 194
Fein, S., 270
Felner, R., 69
Ferris, S., 158
Feucht-Haviar, T., 112, 132
Fisher, D., 110
Fisher, W., 54
Fiske, D., 104, 105, 107
Fitch, W.L., 44
Fletcher, K., 108
Florida Mental Health Institute, 25, 62
Flynn, J., 158
Foote, W., 70, 173
Frazen, M., 170
Frederick, R., 184
Freedman, A., 139
Funder, D., 85

Gallagher, R., 138
Gardner, W., 103
Garske, J., 181
Giannelli, P., 30
Gillis, J.R., 181
Glass, D. R., 200
Glassman, J., 69
Goldberg, J., 181
Golding, S., 6, 25, 29, 62, 108, 111, 112, 128,
    132, 133
Gothard, S., 180
Gough, H.G., 180
Graham, J., 180
Green, B., 137
Greenberg, S., 6, 37, 41, 42, 70, 169, 194,
    205, 211, 234, 248
Greene, R.L., 180, 186
Greer, A, 54
Grisso, T., 3, 6, 8, 15, 25, 26, 36, 54, 62, 84,
    88, 93, 102, 104, 105, 108, 110, 113, 120,
    125, 127, 128, 130, 132, 133, 153, 155-158,
    166, 171, 173, 190, 194, 195, 204, 205,
    209, 213, 218-220, 223, 224, 232, 248,
    251, 278, 288, 290
Grove, W.M., 126
Guilmette, T., 183
Gutheil, T.G., 3, 107

Halleck, S.L., 50, 56, 71, 79
Haney, C., 189
Hare, R., 118, 167
Haroun, A., 273

Harper, J., 180
Harrel, E., 177
Harris, G., 113, 118, 127, 132
Harris, M.J, 180
Hart, K., 183
Hart, S.D., 6, 127, 145
Hata, Y., 138
Heaton, R.K., 183
Heilbrun, K., 21, 30, 32, 41, 42, 70, 101, 102, 106, 110, 113, 114, 119, 125, 127, 128, 169, 170, 173, 175, 179, 185, 189, 193, 194, 200, 204, 209, 218, 219, 221
Herbert, P., 171
Hess, A., 6, 25, 79, 80, 133
Hewitt, P., 180
Hilkert, R., 137
Hill-Fotouhi, C., 113
Hiscock, C.K., 183
Hiscock, M., 183
Hoff, A., 137
Hofer, P., 137
Hoge, R., 118
Hoge, S.K., 25, 112, 132, 203
Homant, R.J., 42
Horowitz, I., 6
Hoyt, K., 137
Huneycutt, D., 21, 189, 193
Hunsley, J., 69

Institute of Law, Psychiatry, and Public Policy, 25, 62
Imwinkelried, E., 30

Johnson, W. G., 203

Kaemmer, B., 180
Kane, A., 6, 106
Kaplan, H., 139
Kapp, M., 108
Karson, S., 180
Kassin, S., 270
Kastl, A., 105
Kelley, T., 137
Kelley, T.M., 42
Kelly, J., 179
Kelly, M., 183
Kennedy, W., 248
Kennedy, D.B., 42
Kuehnle, K., 202
Kuze, T., 138

Laboratory of Community Psychiatry, Harvard Medical School, 111
Lamb, D., 181
Lanyon, R.I., 166
Lebow, B.S., 126
Leheny, C., 21, 189, 193
Lee, C., 69
Lees-Haley, P., 125
Lehman, R.W., 183
Lelos D., 203
Levine, M., 172, 292
Lewinsohn, P., 171
Lezak, M., 158
Liberman, R., 157
Lidz, C.W., 103
Lieberman, J., 158
Liff, C., 177
Lipsitt P., 203
Lowery, C., 24
Lynn, S., 181

Mann, T., 157
Marder, S., 157
Marlowe, D., 114, 185
Martell, D., 194
Matarazzo, J.D., 107
Matthews, D., 194
McCann, J., 6, 114, 170, 185
McClaren, H., 118
McGarry, A. L., 24, 128, 133, 203
Meehl, P., 105, 108, 126, 210
Megargee, E., 118, 180
Meier, S., 104
Melton, G., 3, 6, 16, 25, 36, 60-62, 93,107, 118, 119, 128, 133, 145, 147, 150, 151, 155, 166, 169, 173, 177, 179, 187, 194, 195, 199, 201, 205, 209, 213, 215, 217, 219, 224, 243, 247, 248, 250, 251, 255, 256, 261, 270, 274, 278, 280, 299
Millon, T., 180, 185
Mintz, J., 157
Monahan, J., 6, 10, 25, 62, 92, 103, 112, 117, 118, 132, 278
Morey, L., 180, 181
Morris, G., 273
Morse, S., 15, 84, 91, 93,122, 127, 213, 214, 223, 265
Mossman, D., 108
Mullet, N., 203
Mulvey, E.P., 103, 108

Nelson, C.E., 126
Neuhaus, I., 270, 271, 272, 273
Nicholi, A., 139
Nicholson, R., 185
Nurcombe, B., 138

O'Dell, J., 180
Office of Juvenile Justice and Delinquency
  Prevention, 118, 128
Ogloff, J., 6, 178, 187
Otto, RK., 28, 36, 100, 103, 112, 132, 140, 173,
  195
O'Sullivan, M., 117, 166, 167

Pankratz, L., 183, 186
Parry, C., 194
Pepper-Smith, R, 157
Perlin, M., 86
Peters, L., 200
Petrella, R.C., 94, 125, 221, 247
Petrila, J., 3, 6, 16, 25, 36, 60-62, 93,107, 118,
  119, 128, 133, 145, 147, 150, 151, 155, 166,
  169, 173, 177, 179, 187, 194, 195, 199, 201,
  205, 209, 213, 215, 217, 219, 224, 243,
  247, 248, 250, 251, 255, 256, 261, 270,
  274, 278, 280, 299
Petty, R., 270
Philipson, J., 176
Pincus, H., 158
Podboy, J., 105
Popper, K., 207
Posthuma, A., 180
Poythress, N.G., 3, 6, 16, 24, 25, 36, 60-62,
  93, 94, 100, 107, 112, 118, 128, 133, 145,
  147, 150, 151, 155, 166, 169, 173, 177, 179,
  187, 194, 195, 199, 125, 132, 187, 201,
  205, 209, 213-215, 217, 219, 221, 224,
  243, 247, 250, 251, 255, 256, 261, 262,
  270, 274, 278, 280, 299
Prifitera, A., 158
Primavera, J., 69
Pynchon, M.R., 193, 194

Quinsey, V., 113, 118

Rachlin, S., 78, 79
Rai, A., 155
Rector, N., 185
Reisner, R., 155
Resnick, P., 173, 187

Reyonlds, S., 181
Rice, M., 113, 118
Robbins, E., 171
Robey, A., 111
Robinson, L., 181
Roesch, R., 6, 25, 62, 108, 111, 145
Rogers, R., 6, 11, 25, 50, 70, 73, 78, 103, 113,
  126, 132, 165, 166, 170, 176, 180-186, 203,
  213, 214, 217, 218, 221, 251, 278
Rohde, P., 171
Rosa, J., 203
Rosenfeld, B, 102
Rosenthal, P., 271
Rotgers, F., 199
Rowlison, R., 69

Sacks, E., 137, 233
Sadock, B., 139
Saklofske, D., 158
Saks, M., 268
Sawyer, J., 37, 105, 126
Schacter, D., 167, 173, 187
Schneidman, E., 100
Schoendorf, K., 113
Schreiber, J., 112
Schretlen, D., 181
Seeley, J., 171
Seeman, M., 185
Sewell, K., 180, 181
Shapiro, D., 3, 6, 25, 57, 62, 83, 107, 133,
  173, 194
Shah, S., 133
Shuman, D., 41, 42, 70, 193, 201, 251, 270
Silva, M., 158
Sivec, H., 181
Skeem, J., 133
Slobogin, C., 3, 6, 16, 25, 36, 60-62, 93,107,
  113, 118, 119, 128, 133, 145, 147, 150, 151,
  155, 166, 169, 173, 177, 179, 187, 194, 195,
  199, 201, 205, 209, 213, 215, 217, 219,
  222, 223, 224, 243, 247, 248, 250, 251,
  255, 256, 261, 270, 274, 278, 280, 299
Smith, H., 183
Snitz, B.E., 126
Sorrell, J., 158
Spitzer, R.L., 182
Starr, L., 100
Steadman, H.J., 6, 25, 54, 85, 103, 118, 172, 278
Stermac, L.,181
Stewart, T., 194

Stone, A., 223
Sukel, H., 271
Sumpter, J., 181
Swanson, J., 118
Swartz, M., 118

Tellegen, A., 180
Thames, H., 110
Thomas, L., 21, 189, 193
Toner, B., 181
Traxler, A., 137
Trueblood, W., 183
Tsudzuki, A., 138
Tymchuk, A., 158

Ustad, K., 181, 182

Van Dayne, C., 194
Vant Zelfde, G., 28, 36
Vogt, A.T., 183
Vossekuil, B., 194

Walker, L., 92
Warren, J., 44, 102, 173, 175, 194
Wasyliw, O.E., 73, 78
Waters, J., 171
Webster, C., 113, 118, 127, 132
Wechsler, D., 158
Weiner, I., 6, 25, 133
Wetter, M., 181
Whitaker, E., 270
White, A.J., 179
Wildman, R.W., 179
Willging, T., 6, 53
Willis, S., 183
Wintrup, A., 118
Wirshing, D., 157
Wirshing, W., 157
Wyda, J., 113

Yates, K., 146

Zaitchik, M., 117, 119
Zald, D.H., 126
Zapf, P., 145
Ziskin, J., 36, 44, 114, 266
Zonana, H., 199

Cases
    Ake v. Oklahoma, 48, 55, 60, 76

Cases (cont.)
    Arizona State Board of Medical Examiners
        v. Clark, 17
    Barefoot v. Estelle, 201
    Berry v. City of Detroit, 201, 215
    Brandt v. Medical Defense Association, 17
    Buchanan v. Kentucky, 60
    Burkhart v. Washington Metro. Area Transit
        Auth., 215, 216
    Canterbury v. Spence, 155
    Carmichael v. Samyang Tire, Inc., 201
    Chester v. State, 200
    Chambers v. Mississippi, 113
    Connecticut v. Villano, : 117
    Daubert vs. Merrell Dow Pharmaceuticals,
        Inc., 15, 29, 101, 108, 109,110, 169, 178,
        192, 209, 212, 231, 236, 260
    Dinco v. Dylex, Ltd., 216
    Dusky v. United States, 23, 111, 223
    Estelle v. Smith, 48, 60, 145, 153
    Frohne v. State, 200
    Frye v. United States, 91, 101, 178, 199, 212,
        231, 236, 260
    Funk vs. Commonwealth, 76
    Gier v. Educational Service Unit No. 16,
        110, 200
    Godinez v. Moran, 86, 89, 92
    Helling v. McKinney, 53
    Hiser v. Randolph, 17
    Hoult v. Hoult, 200
    Idaho v. Snow, 117
    In re Fleshman, 53
    In re Payment of Court-Appointed Expert
        Witness, 53
    In re TMI Litigation Consolidated
        Proceedings, 231
    Isely v. Capuchin Province, 29, 110, 200
    Jenson v. Eveleth Taconite Co., 231
    Jackson v. Indiana, 204
    Jones v. United States, 116
    Karabian v. Columbia University, 200
    Kumho Tire Company, Ltd. v. Carmichael,
        201, 260
    Levine v. Torvik, 132
    McKinney v. Anderson, 53
    Marx & Co. v. Diners' Club, Inc., 215
    Mayer v. Baiser, 169, 260
    McKendall v. Crown Control Corp., 231
    Moore v. Ashland Chemical, Inc., 231
    Nash v. Wennar, 17

Cases (cont.)
  Nathanson v. Klein, 155
  Newkirk v. Commonwealth, 200
  Noble v. Sartori, 17
  Pennington v. State, 200
  Rosen v. Ciba-Geigy Corporation, 231
  Rock v. Arkansas, 113
  Rodriguez Cirilo v. Garcia, 200
  Rutigliano v. Valley Business Forms, 231
  Shahzade v. Gregory, 200
  Sieling v. Eyman, 93
  Soutear v. United States, 132
  Specht v. Jensen, 215
  State v. Alberico, 110, 200
  State v. Cavaliere, 110, 200
  State v. Foret, 110, 200
  State v. Jarbath, 116
  State v. Maelega, 200
  State v. Martens, 110, 200
  State v. Parkinson, 200
  State v. Picklesimer, 200
  State v. Spencer, 110
  Steward v. State, 110
  S.V. v. R.V., 200
  Thompson v. Sun City Community
    Hospital, Inc., 17
  Tungate v. Commonwealth, Ky.,110, 200
  Unique Concepts, Inc. v. Brown, 53
  United States v. Alzanki, 200
  United States v. Alvarez, 146
  United States v. Bighead, 231
  United States v. Brewer, 23
  United States v. Brown, 110, 200
  United States v. Coleman, 116
  United States v. Downing, 23, 192
  United States v. Evanoff, 200
  United States v. Garcia, 23
  United States v. Gallo, 117

Cases (cont.)
  United States v. Green, 23
  United States v. Mason, 24
  United States v. McMurray, 833 F.Supp
    1454 (D. Neb. 1993). Chapter V: 116
  United States v. Michigan, 680 F.Supp. 928
    (W.D.Mich. 1987). Chapter II: 53
  United States v. Newman, 49 F.3d 1 (1st
    Cir.1995). Chapter IX: 215
  United States v. Poff, 926 F.2d 588 (7th
    Cir. 1991). Chapter V: 117
  United States v. Powers, 59 F.3d 1460 (4th
    Cir. 1995). Chapter V: 110
  United States v. Reynolds, 77 F.3d 253 (8th
    Cir. 1996). Chapter VIII: 200
  United States v. Rouse, 111 F.3d 561 (8th
    Cir. 1997). Chapter VIII: 200
  United States v. Ruklick, 919 F.2d 95 (8th
    Cir. 1991). Chapter V: 116
  United States v. Smith, 736 F.2d 1103 (6th
    Cir. 1984). Chapter II: 23
  United States v. Speight, 726 F.Supp. 861
    (D.D.C. 1989). Chapter V: 116
  United States v. Studley, 907 F.2d 254 (1st
    Cir. 1990). Chapter V: 117
  Waldorf v. Shuta, 916 F.Supp 423 (1996).
    Chapter V: 102
  Washington v. McNallie, 870 P.2d 295
    (Wash.Sup.Ct. 1994). Chapter V: 117
  Washington v. Pryor, 799 P.2d 244
    (Wash.Sup.Ct. 1990). Chapter V: 117
  Watkins v. Telsmith, Inc., 121 F.3d 984
    (1997). Chapter IX: 231
  Wood v. Upjohn Company, No. 6093-I-II
    (Sept 4, 1984) (LEXIS, States library,
    Wash. file). Chapter I: 17
  Woods v. Lecureux, 110 F.3d 1215 (1997).
    Chapter IX: 216

Subject Index

Accuracy of information, problems with
  bias, 174–175
  expertise, 174–175
  memory loss, 174–175
  suggestibility, 174–175
Ackerman-Shoendorf Patient Evaluation of
  Custody Tests, 113
Administration of psychological tests
  conditions generally, 136–138, 304
  empirical evidence, 137–138
  privacy, 135
  setting, 135
  security, 136, 139
American Psychological Association, 5
American Psychology Law Society, 3
Assessment measures, nature of
  objective versus subjective, 122
  clinical versus actuarial, 122, 129
Attribution, 242–246
Authorization, 58

Brodsky's maxims for expert witnesses
  (generally), 261–266

Child custody evaluation, 87, 173
Child sexual abuse, 202–203
Civil forensic mental health evaluations
  competencies, 88
  generally, 234–235
Clinical versus statistical prediction, 108,
  126
Collateral sources of information
  accuracy, problems of, 173–175
  empirical evidence, 170–172, 292–293
  generally, 10, 83

Collateral sources of information (*cont.*)
  hearsay problem, 169
  standard of practice, 172
Competence consent to treatment
  assent to evaluation, 157–158
  evaluation, 156
Competence to stand trial
  assessment of, 203–204
  generally, 23, 92–93, 111–113
  notification of purpose, 150
  waiver of constitutional rights, 93
Competence to Stand Trial Assessment
  Instrument, 111, 203
Competency Assessment Instrument, 128
Competency Screening Test, 128, 203
Confidentiality
  evaluation setting, 137
  limits of, 142, 144
Contrary quotient, 43
Court appointed experts, 53–54
Credibility, elements of, 270–273
Criminal Justice Mental Health Standards,
  71, 79, 91, 124, 131, 146, 158, 220

Deliberate indifference, 216–217
Diagnostic and Statistical Manual of Mental
  Disorders, 11
Dual roles
  child custody evaluations, 69
  empirical data, 68–69
  examiner-examinee relationship, 37–39,
  294, 302
  possible exception, 75
  problems associated with, 69–72
  standard of practice, 78

Dual roles (*cont.*)
  tests of impartiality, 42–45

Error rate, 108
Ethical issues
  competence, 27–28
  confidentiality, 137, 142, 144
  documentation, 242–243
  dual roles, 37–39, 66–68, 73
  expertise, 27
  fees, 52
  forensic activities, 100, 191–192, 259, 268–269
  informed consent, 23, 142–145
  interpretation of tests, 168, 208, 228
  maintain documentation, 90
  misuse of assessment techniques, 207
  notification, 141–142
  personal contacts, 208
  psychological test construction, 109, 177
  relevance, 109
  role clarification, 47
  scientific or professional judgment, 90
  substantiation of findings, 100, 229
  testing special populations, 109, 208
Ethics, sources of
  Ethical Guidelines for the Practice of Forensic Psychiatry, 6, 17, 27–28, 38, 53, 58–59, 66, 68, 75, 109, 116, 137, 144, 154, 168, 177, 192, 197, 209, 215, 229–230, 243, 247, 250, 259, 269
  Ethical Principles of Psychologists and Code of Conduct, 17, 26, 28, 37, 46, 52, 66, 73–74, 90, 100, 109, 115, 122, 130, 136, 141–142, 154, 167, 177, 190–191, 197–198, 205, 207–208, 214, 228, 235, 242, 246, 249, 258–259, 268–269, 281
  Guidelines for Child Custody Evaluations in Divorce Proceedings, 72, 87, 105, 147, 222, 233, 252
  Specialty Guidelines for Forensic Psychologists, 17, 27–28, 38, 47, 52, 59, 66, 74, 90, 100, 109, 115, 122, 131, 136, 143, 154, 168, 177, 191, 197, 205, 208–209, 214, 228–229, 235, 246–247, 250, 259, 269
  Standards for Educational and Psychological Testing, 137–138, 152

The Principles of Medical Ethics with Annotations Especially Applicable to Psychiatry, 17, 26, 28, 38, 47, 52, 59, 68, 75, 90, 100, 109, 116, 122, 131, 137, 142, 154, 168, 177, 192, 197, 209, 215, 229, 243, 247, 250, 259, 269
Evidentiary standards of admissibility, 91–92
Expert
  assessing expertise, 32–35
  credibility, elements of, 270–273
  defined, 29
  expert versus fact witness, 41
  impression management, 273–274, 305
  maxims for, generally, 261–266, 274–281
  mental health expertise, 29
  professional appearance, 270–273, 274
  substantive expertise, 32
Expert testimony
  admissibility of, generally, 23, 91, 260
  admissibility of, psychological techniques, 110–111, 178
  cross-examination of, 120
  evidentiary standards, 91–92, 199–202, 230–231
  generally, 15, 305
  inadmissibility, examples of, 110
  malingering, 178
  multiple sources of information, 105
  reasonable clinician test, 155
  relevance, 192–193
  standards of practice, 234–236

Federal Rules of Civil Procedure, 179
Federal Rules of Evidence
  court appointed experts, 53–54
  exclusion of evidence, 178
  expert testimony, 29, 41, 108–110, 200, 209
  opinion testimony, 192
  opinion testimony of experts, basis of, 169, 209, 260
  relevant evidence defined, 23, 25–28, 121, 178
  ultimate issue, 215–216
Financial arrangements
  generally, 51–53, 297
  funding, sources of, 54–55
Forced-choice testing defined, 183

Forensic issues
    civil evaluations, 234–235
    defined, 21
    distinguished, 21
    empirical research on, 24
    relevance, 114
Forensic mental health assessment
        principles
    criticisms of, 8
    defined, 3
    derivation, 16–18
    established vs. emerging, 8
    organization of, 14–16
    policy, 8
    principles defined, 6–7
    research on, 7
    role of, 299–300
    training model, 7
    value of, 7
Forensic psychology
    defined, 4
    specialization in, 289–300
Forensic psychiatry defined, 6
Forensic versus therapeutic assessment
    comparison of, 9–14
    data sources, 11
    examiner-examinee relationship, 10
    limits of knowledge, 12
    notification of purpose, 10
    report writing, 12–13
    response style, 11
    standard, 11
    testimony, role of, 13

Georgia Court Competency Test, 179, 203
Georgia Court Competency Test—
        Mississippi Version Revised, 203

HCR-20, 118
Historical information, 115, 118
Hypothesis testing, 92, 105–106, 119–120,
        129, 194–196, 206, 211

Idiographic information, 189–190, 194–196
Impartiality
    defined, 36
    empirical evidence, 41–44
    in court, 40
    role of forensic clinician, 39–41, 294–295

Impression management, 273–274
Inference, levels of, 209–210
Informed consent, 23, 142-145, 293–294, 304
Instruments for Assessing Understanding
        and Appreciation of Miranda
        Rights, 113
Interdisciplinary Fitness Interview
        Revised, 25, 111, 132
Investigative journalism, 303

Juvenile decertification,
    assent, request for, 148
    example, 149
    generally, 128

Law and psychology
    debate, 4–5
    distinguished, 189
    generally, 4
    training, 34, 285, 289–300
Legal competencies, 84, 88, 130

MacArthur Competence Assessment Tool-
        Criminal Adjudication, 25, 112, 132
MacArthur Competence Assessment Tool-
        Treatment, 113, 132
MacArthur Research Network, 103, 112, 156
MacArthur Structured Assessment of
        Competencies of Criminal
        Defendants, 112, 132, 203
MacArthur Treatment Competence
        Research Instruments, 156
Malingering
    admissibility of, evidence about, 178–179,
        187
    assessment of, 180–184
    confrontation, 187
    defined, 165
    empirical evidence, 179–184
    forced-choice testing defined, 183
    neuropsychological impairment, 186
Mental disease or defect, 124, 127
Millon Clinical Multiaxial Inventory, 181,
        184–185
Minnesota Mulitphasic Personality
        Inventory-Adolescents, 185
Minnesota Multiphasic Personality
        Inventory-2, 102, 126, 179, 181, 184–
        186

Models, use of in forensic mental health assessment
generally, 83, 295–296
child custody evaluations, use of in, 87
Grisso's model, 84
Morse's model, 84
advantages of, 85
criticisms, 85
Multi-trait multi-method matrix, 105
Multiple sources of information
empirical evidence, 102–104
generally, 99
validity of, 104–106

Nomothetic information, 196–197
Notification, 141–153, 304

Personality Assessment Inventory, 180–181, 184
Principles of forensic mental health assessment: see Forensic mental health assessment principles
Psychological tests
generally, 105
selection of sources, 107–108, 204–206
Psychopathy Checklist-Revised, 118
Punishment
philosophy of, 116–117

Reasonable clinician test, 155
Reliability, 108–109, 267
Report writing
attribution, 241–246
clinical functioning section, 128
empirical evidence about, 132–133
organization of, 249–252
organization of, insanity evaluations, 251–252
psychiatric jargon, 94, 246–249
Research, future implications for, 286–289
Response style
collateral information,167
empirical evidence, 179–184
face validity, 120, 166
multiple sources of information, 103
testing of, 176
styles of, 165
Role clarification, 46–47, 294

Scientist-practitioner model, 202
Selection of psychological tests, 107–108, 204–206
Setting for testing: see Testing setting
Slippage, 155, 160
Special populations, testing of, 109, 208
Standards of practice
generally, 93–95
rating forensic evaluation reports, 94
Structured Instrument of Reported Symptoms, 113, 182–183

Testimony: see also Expert testimony
basis of, 257–258
effectiveness, 256–257, 267–268, 281–282
maxims for, 261–266
Testing setting, 304

Ultimate legal question
communication of, 213, 219–220
debate, 213, 220–226, 298, 304–305
empirical evidence, 217–219
generally, 6, 21, 298
report writing, 94–95
testimony, 215–217
United States Supreme Court
competence restoration, 204
criminal competencies, 89
expert testimony, 30, 201, 2090
informed consent, 145–146
sanity at the time of the offense, 76

Validity
convergent, 252
generally, 108
Validity Indicator Profile, 184
Violence Prediction Scheme, 113, 118
Violence Risk Appraisal Guide, 113, 118, 127
Violence risk assessment, 118, 128

Wechsler Adult Intelligence Scale-Third Edition, 102, 126

Youth Level of Service/Case Management Inventory, 118